Clinical Handbook of
Feline Behavior
Medicine

Clinical Handbook of Feline Behavior Medicine

Edited by

Elizabeth Stelow
University of California
Davis, CA, USA

WILEY Blackwell

Registered Office
John Wiley & Sons, Inc., 111 River Street, Hoboken, NJ 07030, USA

Editorial Office
111 River Street, Hoboken, NJ 07030, USA

For details of our global editorial offices, customer services, and more information about Wiley products visit us at www.wiley.com.

Wiley also publishes its books in a variety of electronic formats and by print-on-demand. Some content that appears in standard print versions of this book may not be available in other formats.

Library of Congress Cataloging-in-Publication Data
Names: Stelow, Elizabeth Ann, 1959- editor.
Title: Clinical handbook of feline behavior medicine / edited by Elizabeth Stelow,
    University of California Davis, California, USA.
Description: Hoboken, NJ : John Wiley & Sons, 2023. | Includes bibliographical references and index.
Identifiers: LCCN 2022026720 (print) | LCCN 2022026721 (ebook) | ISBN 9781119653219 (paperback) |
    ISBN 9781119652816 (pdf) | ISBN 9781119653042 (epub) | ISBN 9781119653271 (ebook)
Subjects: LCSH: Cats--Behavior. | Cats--Behavior therapy.
Classification: LCC SF446.5 .C59 2023 (print) | LCC SF446.5 (ebook) | DDC 636.8--dc23/eng/20220822
LC record available at https://lccn.loc.gov/2022026720
LC ebook record available at https://lccn.loc.gov/2022026721

Cover image: © Elizabeth Stelow
Cover design by Wiley

Set in 9.5/12.5pt STIXTwoText by Integra Software Services Pvt. Ltd, Pondicherry, India

SKY10037975_110422

While this volume has been a labor of love, it has also been a bit of a distraction from my other commitments. I would not have had the time, emotional fortitude, and humor to see this commitment through without the unending support of my husband, Joe DiNunzio. I would have been equally stymied without the benign neglect of our teenage twins, Ainsley and Rowan. Had they not been happily out there living their own best lives, I would never have found the time to complete this volume. To all three of you, I am forever grateful and dedicate this book to you.

Contents

Contributors

Melissa Bain, DVM, MS, DACVB, DACAW
Professor of Clinical Animal Behavior
Department of Medicine and Epidemiology
UC Davis School of Veterinary Medicine
Davis, CA, USA

Jeannine Berger, DVM, DACVB, DACAW, CAWA
Senior Vice President, Rescue and Welfare
San Francisco Society for the Prevention of
Cruelty to Animals
San Francisco, CA, USA

C. A. Tony Buffington, DVM, MS, PhD, DACVN
Clinical Professor
Department of Medicine and Epidemiology
UC Davis School of Veterinary Medicine
Davis, CA, USA

Sharon Crowell-Davis, DVM, PhD, DACVB
Department of Anatomy and Physiology
College of Veterinary Medicine
University of Georgia
Athens, GA, USA

Gina Davis, DVM
Resident
Clinical Animal Behavior Service
UC Davis School of Veterinary Medicine
Davis, CA, USA

Mikel Delgado, PhD
Feline Minds
Cat Behavior Consulting
Berkeley, CA, USA

Emma Grigg, MA, PhD, CAAB
Lecturer, Dept. of Population Health and
Reproduction
UC Davis School of Veterinary Medicine
Davis, CA, USA

Ilana Halperin, DVM, DABVP (Canine and Feline Practice)
Health Sciences Assistant Clinical Professor in
Community Practice
UC Davis School of Veterinary Medicine
Davis, CA, USA

Kathryn Houpt, VMD, PhD, DACVB
James Law Professor Emeritus, Section of
Behavior Medicine
Department of Clinical Sciences
Cornell University College of Veterinary Medicine
Ithaca, NY, USA

Sun-A Kim, DVM, MS
Clinical Professor of Clinical Animal Behavior
Veterinary Medical Teaching Hospital,
Chungbuk National University,
Cheongju, Korea

Rachel Malamed, DVM, DACVB, CABC
Dr. Rachel Malamed Behavior Consulting
Los Angeles, CA, USA

Amanda Rigterink, DVM, DACVB
Veterinarian/Owner
Veterinary Behavior of Indiana
Carmel, IN, USA

Margie Scherk, DVM, DABVP (Feline Practice)
catsINK Feline Consultant
Vancouver, BC, Canada

Judi Stella, PhD
Head of Standards & Research
Good Dog, Inc.
Columbus, OH, USA

Karen Sueda, DVM, DACVB
Veterinary Specialist, Behavior
VCA West Los Angeles Animal Hospital
Los Angeles, CA, USA

Wailani Sung, MS, PhD, DVM, DACVB
Director of Behavior and Welfare Programs
San Francisco Society for the Prevention of
Cruelty to Animals
San Francisco, CA, USA

Kristyn Vitale, PhD
Assistant Professor
Animal Health & Behavior
Unity College
New Gloucester, ME, USA

Preface

When the publishers proposed a book on feline behavior, I knew I wanted to develop something that the veterinary general practitioner, veterinary technician, and veterinary student would find clinically useful. My initial research included a meeting with a friend and general practice veterinarian, Dr. Aine Coil. I asked – and she told me – what challenges she faces with feline behavior and what resources would be most helpful.

Based on that conversation, the framework of the book was born: A book that serves both as a quick reference during a patient appointment and a "deep dive" resource for when the clinician, technician, or student has time to read and prepare for a case ahead of time.

There are a number of "background" chapters that can inform clinical cases but are not quick-reference oriented. These include normal social behavior, preventing problem behaviors, play, cat relationships in the home, and cats in the clinic.

Most of the clinical chapters have a section on what's normal and what's not, formatted in a way that can be easily consumed during a patient appointment. Some have flow charts for quick decision making. Others have forms for the clients to complete to further discussions.

Ultimately, the volume serves to aid the veterinary practitioner as they guide their medicine and their clients toward better welfare for their feline patients.

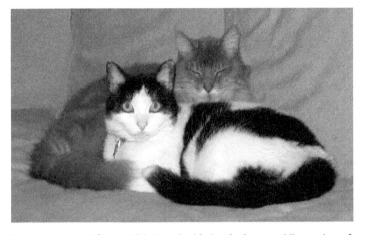

Dublin (gray) and Chantal (black and white) enjoying a cuddle on the sofa.

Acknowledgments

This volume would not have come to be without the faith of the publishers, my colleagues, and a cadre of gifted and insightful contributing authors.

I thank all of this book's editors at Wiley. They have been enthusiastic, supportive, and extremely patient. I don't recommend trying to pull together a book during a global pandemic and a breast cancer diagnosis. But, if you must do so, you want this Wiley team on your side.

I thank my friend and colleague, Dr. Aine Coil, for sharing what the general practitioner needs to know about feline behavior.

I thank my colleagues and friends at the UC Davis Behavior Service for their key role in shaping the skeleton of the book and reviewing the proposal. Without Dr. Sun Kim and our technician Michelle Borchardt, there is no telling the structure the book would have taken. Drs. Bain, Buffington, Delgado, Grigg, and van Haaften were extremely supportive and insightful.

I cannot even begin to express sufficient gratitude to the contributing authors for this book. Throughout the stops and starts, they have been dedicated, flexible, and so very giving of their writing talents and knowledge. I thank each and every one of them for contributing. The world of feline care is considerably richer for their involvement in it.

About the Companion Website

This book is accompanied by a companion website:

www.wiley.com/go/stelow/behavior

QR Code:

This website includes patient history forms, client handouts, how-to videos, and other support materials for preventing, diagnosing, and treating behavior problems in cats.

1

Introduction to Feline Veterinary Behavior

Elizabeth Stelow

Background

There is little doubt that a veterinarian can be one of the most influential participants in the life of an owned cat. Clinicians assist with preventative, emergent, and chronic medical care and should provide the majority of counseling the owners receive regarding the prevention and treatment of problem behaviors. An owner's knowledge about the needs of their cat cannot be underestimated in its impact on the cat's overall welfare: The owner who understands cat behavior and has a stronger bond reports fewer problem behaviors, while the owner that does not understand their cat is more likely to respond to unwanted behaviors with punishment, leading to worsened welfare.[1]

It is estimated that up to 40% of owned cats in the United States have exhibited problem behaviors of some kind.[2,3]

Feline behavior problems can lead to injury of owners and other pets, erosion of the human–animal bond, and the owner's unwillingness to keep the cat.[4] In fact, behavior problem is the number two reason given for a cat being relinquished to a shelter; the number one is dropping off entire litters to be placed in homes.[5]

But, many owners don't come to veterinarians with behavior problems. In a 2002 study by Dr. Laurie Bergman, only 26% of owners with urine marking cats had presented this problem to their veterinarians. Why? It may be because owners

1) think veterinarians are interested in only medical issues
2) believe veterinarians aren't competent or trained in addressing behavior problems
3) aren't always asked about behavior proactively during a routine or "medical" visit.

Unfortunately, these owners are somewhat justified in their beliefs. In 2001, McMillan found that only 25% of veterinarians make behavior questions a standard part of their history taking.[6] And, in one study, only 2/3 of the 70 veterinarians surveyed could correctly distinguish between urine marking and toileting based on a case presented to them.[7] In yet another study, six veterinarians willingly had their vaccine consultations recorded. The viewers of those recordings noted that only 10 of the 58 behavior problems mentioned by owners to their veterinarians were addressed.[8]

In fact, veterinarians should be on the front line of preventing or addressing behavior problems; but they often aren't. There appear to be two key reasons from the standpoint of the veterinarian.

First, it is possible that veterinarians don't see the value in exploring and treating problem behaviors. One 2004 study reported that, when veterinarians in small-animal practice ranked the skills needed by new graduates from veterinary schools, "behavior" averaged 16th in importance.[9] We tend to put effort into what we value.

Second, it may be that clinicians see the value, but don't feel comfortable asking about behavior because they're not certain they can help. In one study, half of the clinicians surveyed in small-animal practice said they lacked the training in behavior to provide consultations with owners, despite behavior issues being raised by owners weekly.[10,11] In the study with the six veterinarians video recorded during their appointments, five of the six reported feeling unable to meet their clients' expectations regarding behavior problems, mainly due to inadequate training on the subject.[12]

This is not a new concern. In 1999, Gary Patronek raised the issue of the disconnect between the level of behavioral advice required by clients and the level offered by veterinarians.[13]

The challenge is that this lack of intervention on behalf of feline patients has measurable effects, as seen in the statistics about relinquishment and human–animal bond maintenance noted above. Further, the curious owner will find information in websites, books, or from friends that may not be current, appropriate, or safe; and they may not have the ability to see the potential harm.

Another hazard of lack of veterinary behavior guidance is that not all clients are aware that their behavior with kittens can prevent – or lead to – problem behaviors in the future. These behaviors can include "nuisance" behaviors like scratching items or climbing on people (See Figures 1.1, 1.2) but can also include aggression toward people or other cats. Client information can help, as long as the veterinarian knows what to tell the client and the client trusts the veterinarian to understand.[14]

Certainly, if clinicians are to be of assistance to clients in dealing with their cats' behavior problems, they will need to want to do it and be prepared to do it. One role of this book is to provide the interested clinician a resource to feel more prepared.

If we are to encourage owners to turn to us, we must be proactive in asking about their cat's behaviors and have a plan for diagnosing and treating the problems we uncover. The purpose of this introduction, then, is to provide the practitioner with useful tools for gathering behavior

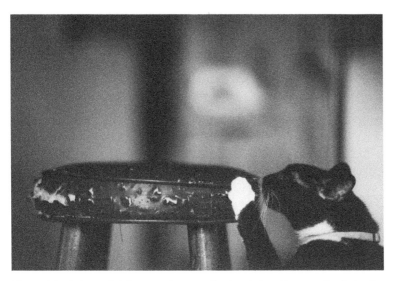

Figure 1.1   It is crucial that veterinary professionals be able to assist their clients with feline behavioral issues before the human–animal bond is irrevocably damaged. Craig Adderley/Pexels.

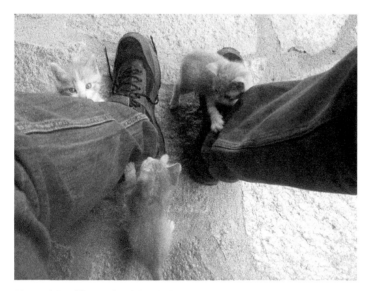

Figure 1.2   Clients should be led to prevent future behavior problems in cats through their interactions with kittens in the home. hansiline/pixabay.

information and common treatment options. Individual clinical chapters (5–12) will provide detailed information on diagnosing and treating the specific problems presented there.

When a practitioner finds that a cat is engaging in a problem behavior, it's important to approach the diagnosis and treatment in an efficient and systematic way.

Behavioral Diagnosis

A behavioral diagnosis requires the following:[15]

- A detailed history, both medical and behavioral
- Observation of the problem in person or via video
- A way to rule out medical differentials (CBC, serum biochemistry, specialized lab tests, imagery, etc.) and knowledge of key medical differentials for the specific problem behavior
- Understanding of specific diagnostic criteria for the specific problem behavior

History

A detailed history is the basis for making a tentative behavioral diagnosis. To gather the most comprehensive information, it is most useful to request that the owners complete a form that prompts them for a wide variety of background details.[16] An example of a thorough history form is provided in Appendix 3 and also on the website for this book. Follow-up questions to be asked during the actual appointment are based on the information in – and missing from – the owner-prepared form.

The types of information to be gathered include:

Table 1.1   Path to a thorough behavioral history.

Basic information	Signalment: pet's name, age, reproductive status, breed
	Acquisition: age, source, known conditions at previous home, and disposition of littermates
	Family: Names, ages, move-in dates of all household members (people and animals)
	Medical history: Include both disease/injury history and any previous behavioral assessments
Environmental information	Feeding routine: diet, how/where fed, appetite, behavior toward people when eating
	Litter box and hygiene information: number, locations, substrates, cleaning schedule, and routine
	Household enrichment: toys, interactive play time, window perches, trees/shelves, outdoor time
Owner information	Goals of this and future appointments
	Willingness and ability of owner to implement treatment elements
	If aggression, how severe does the owner perceive the aggression to be?
	Each family member's relationship with the cat, including trust in their safety
Incident information (for aggression problems)	Please see chapters on aggression for this information

Basic Information

The signalment will be the key identifiers in the cat's medical record. But it is important to gather such basic information as how and at what age the cat was acquired, what humans and other pets live in the household or frequently interact with the cat, and any past medical problems and how they were resolved.

There can be clues about the cat's current behavior in even the most basic aspects of its history. For instance, other pets in the household can be an underlying stressor or may provide a good outlet for appropriate play; but it's important to know which. People moving in or out of the home frequently can be a source of stress that owners don't always consider when they think about triggers for the aggression. And, there may be a medical problem that coincides with the onset of the aggression that the owners did not equate with a possible cause.

Environmental Information

The cat's environment can have a profound impact on its behavior; so it is important to review the layout of the house, the enrichment provided, and the litter box and other routines. Because lack of suitable outlets for play and predatory behaviors can be implicated in aggression problems,[17] it is crucial to understand what resources are provided to your feline patients.

Relationships of Owners and Cats

Aside from the cat's motivation, little has more of an impact on outcome than the cat's relationships in the home, the owners' goal, and their ability to implement an effective plan. So, this area of investigation is very important and often overlooked in the interest of time or the avoidance of difficult discussions. Here are ways to think of and explore these factors:

Owner relationships with the cat. Ask each owner to describe his/her relationship with the cat. Consider these answers as you focus on different elements of the plan. Who is most invested? Who feels most detached?

The role of owner in the outcome. The owners must be open to – and see value in implementing – all of the elements of the treatment plan. It pays to mention early in the appointment that the treatment of this problem will require some changes in the way the household runs; then ask if the owners are ready to know how. Simply asking for their permission before proceeding can influence how open they are to hearing the plan. Then, as you discuss actual plan elements, you can check in further about what can and can't be implemented easily.

Owner goals. Ask for the owners' goals directly. It's best not to assume that you understand what the owners need as an outcome – or even that all of the owners present need the same outcome. This is especially true of the person most likely to be attacked versus the others. So, look from person to person and ask directly what each one is looking for as a goal. There's no need to address whether those goals are reasonable or not – this discussion is fact finding for the practitioner.

Assess owners' ability to implement a treatment plan. As you determine how complicated a given case likely will be, begin to assess each owner's ability to implement the plan that is taking shape. Ability may be affected by an owner's limitations (physical problems, age – especially children, and available time to devote to the plan) or household limitations (schedules, physical space and home layout, and overall activity levels – chaos versus quiet). As the practitioner presents the plan, these limitations will need to be taken into consideration and may affect the outcome of the appointment itself if the plan simply cannot be implemented at all. These appointments may lead to conversations about rehoming or euthanasia.

Owner assessment of the problem. Ask each owner how severe they consider the aggression to be. This is a set up for the next conversation (if needed) about trust.

Owner risk tolerance and trust. If the presenting complaint is aggression, and the owners have assessed the aggression as severe, ask each owner how risky that owner thinks life is with the cat and how much the owner trusts the cat (and can envision trusting the cat in the future). It is best to get this information into the open, in case owners are feeling differently about the cat. The plan may be a non-starter if one owner states that he/she will never be able to trust the cat again. It's best at that point to focus on all owners seeing that rehoming/euthanasia is the only solution possible for that owner.

While objective descriptions of the behaviors are more useful than subjective assessments in supporting a diagnosis, studies have shown there is a limit to what the owners can tell you about both body language and specific triggers, because most owners lack more than a superficial awareness of behavior in their pets.[18]

Observation

Observation of the behavior can be in-person during the appointment or via video provided in advance by the owner. Depending on the type of behavior problem, the clinician will prefer either of these options. It is entirely possible that, even with both types of observation, the clinician will not see the behavior being reported by the owner; this makes the details in the history form even more important.

Medical Differentials

Each behavior problem presented in this book will contain a list of medical differentials that the clinician should try to rule out before proceeding with treatment of a behavioral cause.

Diagnostic Criteria

Likewise, each behavioral diagnosis presented in the book will also present the diagnostic criteria for that diagnosis.

Once a diagnosis has been established, the clinician will turn their attention to the treatment plan.

Treatment

While treatment for behavior issues varies depending on the diagnosis, signalment, owner lifestyle and commitment, and other factors, there are some general treatment categories that should be considered for each plan. These include management, tools, cat–owner relationship, behavior modification, and medications. Here's a sensible way to think about these areas of treatment:

Management

The goal of management is to change the circumstances around the problem behavior in such a way that the behavior is less likely to occur while the remainder of treatment is implemented. In short, management often comes down to avoidance – of the cat being in places where the behavior most often happens, of people interacting in a way that leads to the behavior, of the cat having access to target items/people/other pets. By avoiding situations, we accomplish two things: First, the harm to the targets of aggression, the soiling of carpets, and other possible damage due to the behavior is minimized. Second, the cat has a break from engaging in the behavior we hope to treat, thus making the behavior less of a habit while we try to replace it.

Examples:

- Avoid interacting with the cat when it's displaying the body language of arousal (dilated pupils, twitching tail, rippling muscles along its back), if those signs often predict aggression (see Figure 1.3)
- Separate fighting cats when they aren't being supervised

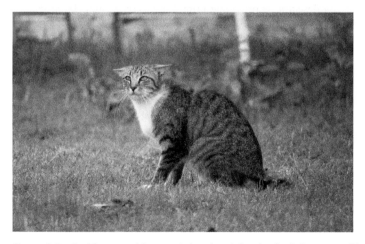

Figure 1.3   Avoid approaching a cat showing defensive body language. Photo from pxhere.

- Keep the household cat from viewing outdoor cats if he redirects aggression to his owners or urine marks when he sees them
- If visitors are a fear or aggression trigger, put the cat in a separate room with lots of resources when people visit
- Close bedroom doors at bedtime if the cat wakes people in the middle of the night for attention

Also considered a part of management, environmental enrichment is key to the happiness of indoor cats.[19] Please see Chapter 2 for more information.

Tools

Many management ideas require tools to implement. For instance, blocking visual access to outdoor cats is easiest with opaque window privacy film. Offering a variety of litter boxes may help the owner solve a toileting issue. And enrichment is often about things (toys, perches, hiding spots, etc.) being added to the living spaces. (See Figure 1.4).

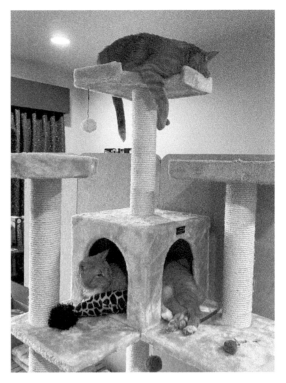

Figure 1.4   Cat trees offer extensive enrichment, including climbing, playing, and the sense of vertical space. Photo courtesy of Liz Stelow.

Cat–Owner Relationship

There are a couple of ways to enhance the relationship between a cat and its family members:

- Predictable interactions. If the cat is anxious or fearful, or if the owners have responded harshly to the cat's behavior in the past, the first step in relationship-building is to be predictable around the cat. Studies have shown that an animal's ability to predict stimuli, even those that are aversive, has an impact on the stress associated with those stimuli.[20,21] Depending on the behavioral diagnosis, "predictable" interactions may require the owner(s) to decide on the amount or style of physical restraint, play, and handling the cat will receive; on how to respond when the cat does something they do or don't like; or on whether the cat is always or never allowed in certain rooms, on furniture, or on countertops. Each case is unique in the "unpredictable" situations the cat faces.
- Training. Cats can be trained to do a number of "tricks," some of which can be helpful in redirecting the cat's attention when necessary and others that are just for fun. Training should always be done with treats or other valuable rewards, and may or may not be done using a clicker.
- Avoidance of punishment. Regardless of the way they manifest, behavior problems are most often based in fear, anxiety, frustration, or other emotional motivation. As such, they are not easily controlled by punishment. In fact, punishment can aggravate a tense situation by increasing the chance of aggression and exacerbating any underlying stress or fear.

Behavior Modification

The most common way to change how a cat feels about its triggers is systematic desensitization and counterconditioning. The principles of this technique are:

- The cat is exposed to a very small "dose" of the triggering stimulus (item, noise, person, cat)
- He is rewarded for this exposure
- He can leave any time he wants if the intensity is too much
- He always remains calm and relaxed throughout the exposure
- Over time, exposure is increased by moving closer to the item or person, or having the volume of the sound increased. All previous rules apply at this increased exposure

The final goal is to have a cat that is no longer concerned about its triggers. This may take a few sessions or many. Everything must happen at the cat's pace.

Medications

For many behavior problems that have an emotional underpinning, medications may be either helpful or necessary. Please refer to individual chapters for suggestions and Appendix 1 for greater detail on options.

References

1 Grigg EK, Kogan LR. Owners' attitudes, knowledge, and care practices: Exploring the implications for domestic cat behavior and welfare in the home. *Animals*. 2019;9(11):978.

2 Amat M, Ruiz de la Torre JL, Fatjo' J, et al. Potential risk factors associated with feline behavior problems. *Appl Anim Behav Sci*. 2009;121:134–139.

3 Martinez AG, Pernas GS, Casalta FJD, et al. Risk factors associated with behavioral problems in dogs. *J Vet Behav*. 2011;6:225–231.

4 Dawson LC, Dewey CE, Stone EA, Guerin MT, Niel L. Evaluation of a canine and feline behavioral welfare assessment tool for use in companion animal veterinary practice. *Appl Anim Behav Sci*. 2018;201:67–76.

5 Salman MD, Hutchison JM, Ruch-Gallie R, et al. Behavioral reasons for relinquishment of dogs and cats to 12 shelters. *J Appl Anim Welf Sci*. 2000;3:93–106.

6 McMillan FD, Rollin BE. The presence of mind: On reunifying the animal mind and body. *J Am Vet Med Assoc*. 2001;218(11):1723–1727.

7 Bergman L, Hart BL, Bain M, et al. Evaluation of urine marking by cats as a model for understanding veterinary diagnostic and treatment approaches and client attitudes. *J Am Vet Med Assoc*. 2002;221:1282–1286.

8 Roshier AL, McBride EA. Canine behaviour problems: Discussions between veterinarians and dog owners during annual booster consultations. *Vet Rec*. 2013;172(9):235.

9 Greenfield CL, Johnson AL, Schaeffer DJ. Frequency of use of various procedures, skills, and areas of knowledge among veterinarians in private small animal exclusive or predominant practice and proficiency expected of new veterinary school graduates. *J Am Vet Med Assoc*. 2004;224(11):1780–1787.

10 Golden O, Hanlon AJ. Towards the development of day one competences in veterinary behaviour medicine: Survey of veterinary professionals experience in companion animal practice in Ireland. *Irish Vet J*. 2018;71(12). doi:10.1186/s13620-018-0123-3.

11 Goins M, Nicholson S, Hanlon A. Veterinary professionals' understanding of common feline behavioural problems and the availability of "cat friendly" practices in Ireland. *Animals*. 2019;9(12):1112. doi:10.3390/ani9121112.

12 Roshier AL, McBride EA. Veterinarians' perceptions of behaviour support in small-animal practice. *Vet Rec*. 2013;172(10):267.

13 Patronek GJ, Dodman NH. Attitudes, procedures, and delivery of behavior services by veterinarians in small-animal practice. *J Am Vet Med Assoc*. 1999;215(11):1606–1611.

14 Gazzano A, Bianchi L, Campa S, Mariti C. The prevention of undesirable behaviors in cats: Effectiveness of veterinary behaviorists' advice given to kitten owners. *J Vet Behav*. 2015;10(6):535–542.

15 Landsberg G, Hunthausen W, Ackerman L. Behavior counseling and behavioral diagnostics. In: *Behavior problems of the dog and cat*, 3rd ed. St Louis: Elsevier; 2013:65–73.

16 Overall KL. How to use these handouts an protocols. In: Overall KL, ed. *Manual of clinical behavioral medicine for dogs and cats*. St Louis: Elsevier; 2013:535–538.

17 Amat M, Manteca X. Common feline problem behaviours: Owner-directed aggression. *J Feline Med Surg*. 2019 Mar;21(3):245–255.

18 Mariti C, Guerrini F, Vallini V, et al. The perception of cat stress by Italian owners. *J Vet Behav*. 2017;20:74–84.

19 Buffington CAT, Westropp JL, Chew DJ, et al. Clinical evaluation of multimodal environmental modification (MEMO) in the management of cats with idiopathic cystitis. *J Feline Med Surg*. 2006;8(4):261–268.

20 Beerda B, Schilder MBH, van Hooff JARAM. Behavioural, saliva cortisol and heart rate responses to different types of stimuli in dogs. *Appl Anim Behav Sci*. 1998;58:365–381.

21 Weiss JM. Influence of psychological variables on stress-induced pathology. In: Porter R, Knight J, eds. *Physiology, emotion and psychosomatic illness*. Amsterdam and New York: Associated Scientific Publishers; 1972:253–280.

2

Normal Feline Social Behavior

Kristyn Vitale

When attempting to address problem behaviors in cats, it is first important to have a solid foundation in typical feline social behaviors. This chapter will cover several topics including normal social behaviors cats engage in with other cats, cat body language cues, the structure of feline social groups, and characteristics of the human–cat relationship. Although we lack a common verbal language with cats, we can examine cat social behavior and body language as an indicator of the mental state of the cat and apply this to inform the best ways to enact our interactions with them.

Social Communication and Body Language

Normal Social Behaviors

Social behavior is any interaction between two or more individuals.[1] Social behavior may occur among members of the same species or between members of different species. Domestic cats display an array of social behaviors with one another. Even cats which do not live in social groups display social behavior, such as during mating and the rearing of kittens. Cats have behaviors which fit into several categories of social behavior; these include affiliative, agonistic, and investigatory behaviors.

Affiliative behaviors are any social behavior that strengthens group cohesion and social bonds, often reducing aggression between the individuals. Common affiliative behaviors displayed by cats include allorubbing, allogrooming, social rolling, spending time in contact or near to one another, and social play.[2,3] In an allorub, a cat presses the head or side of their body against an individual while moving, effectively rubbing up against the social partner. During allogrooming a cat uses their tongue to lick the body of another individual (Figure 2.1). In a social roll, the cat turns over onto their back and exposes their belly in the presence of a social partner (Figure 2.2). Exposing the ventral area in a social roll or sitting with the stomach exposed can be taken as a sign of trust. The belly is a location of vital organs and to expose this vulnerable location to another cat or a human can indicate the cat is not threatened. Cats also spend time near social partners. They will lay together, sit together while in physical contact, or sit in close proximity to one another, a behavior also known as huddling.

In social play, a cat interacts with a social partner in a non-harmful manner.[2,3] When two cats play with one another, the style of play can very much depend on the two individuals involved. Play can sometimes appear rough and look almost like aggression to the untrained observer.

Clinical Handbook of Feline Behavior Medicine, First Edition. Edited by Elizabeth Stelow.
© 2023 John Wiley & Sons, Inc. Published 2023 by John Wiley & Sons, Inc.
Companion Website: www.wiley.com/go/stelow/behavior

Figure 2.1 Two cats sit together after a short bout of play. One cat begins to groom the other with their tongue.

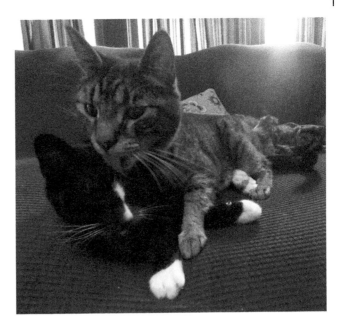

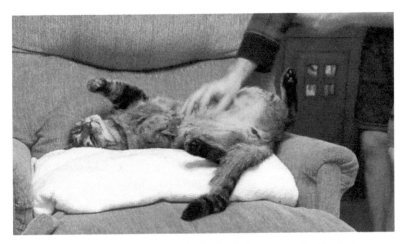

Figure 2.2 A cat engages in a social roll after being approached by their owner.

During social play, two cats may chase and wrestle with one another, bite each other's necks, smack each other with their paws (also known as cuffing), and rake their back legs against the conspecific's belly in a motion very similar to dissecting a prey animal.[2] Although this may sound like an aggressive encounter, during play, the more salient signs of aggression are missing. There is a lack of aggressive vocalizations and the behaviors the cats display are inhibited, or not produced to their full potential. A bite during play is not enough to break the skin, a play cuff does not typically involve the claws being extended, and the belly raking does not rip the conspecific's belly open. During play the interaction is mutually initiated and there will be brief pauses in which both cats take turns reinitiating the play bout. Sometimes play will end with the cats sitting together or allogrooming, as seen in Figure 2.1. So, when is it not play?

Agonistic behaviors include any behavior that occurs during competition. This includes aggressive behavior as well as behavior that serves for conflict resolution, such as submissive behaviors. Several of the play behaviors already mentioned can also be aggressive behaviors under different contexts. Common aggressive behaviors include cuffing, chasing, charging, or biting.[2] Unlike in play, these behaviors are not inhibited. Claws are extended during a cuff and teeth may actually break the skin during a bite. Cats also display behaviors that are aimed at preventing a physical altercation. One such behavior is head aversion in which cats avert their heads at right angles to avoid a direct stare.[3]

Cats also display investigatory behaviors. These behaviors aid in the discrimination of other individuals and include behaviors such as following a conspecific or sniffing the body of another cat. Investigatory behaviors are important to recognize the identity of the social partners around them and to know which cats are familiar and which may be a threat. Cats mainly do this through the use of olfactory (or scent/chemical) cues. Olfactory cues can communicate the sexual status and identity of the cat producing the cue. Free-roaming cats spend more time sniffing the urine and feces markings of unfamiliar cats compared to markings of familiar cats, of whom the scent was recognizable. Urine and feces are not the only olfactory cues cats produce. Cats also deposit chemical cues through scratching behavior and object rubbing, in which a cat rubs their head or body against an item or area in their environment.[4] Although the location and existence of scent glands on the cat's body is still debated,[5] several chemical compounds have been identified from the cat facial area (F1-F5 Pheromones), from the mammary glands of a queen during lactation (Feline Appeasing Pheromone), and from between the digits on the cat's toes (Feline Interdigital Semiochemical).[4] More remains to be learned about cat chemical communication and investigatory behaviors, but we will return to this topic shortly.

Common Vocalizations

In addition to the affiliative, aggressive, and investigatory social behaviors just described, cats also produce a number of vocalizations in a variety of different contexts. Kittens create at least 9 different vocalizations and adult cats produce at least 16 different vocalization patterns.[6] Murmur patterns of vocalizations are produced when the cat's mouth is closed and the breath passes through the nose. Murmur pattern vocalizations include the purr vocalization and the trill vocalizations, which is like a combination of a purr/meow. These vocalizations are often used in an affiliative context such as during a greeting and in kitten–mother communication to request or acknowledge receipt of something. Vowel pattern vocalizations are produced when the mouth opens and then gradually closes and the breath passes through mouth, creating "maou" or "wa-ou" vocalizations of various intensities.[6] This includes meows used when soliciting for resources, such as food or to be let outside. It also includes more intense complaint meows and anger wails. Finally, strained intensity vocalization patterns are those produced when the cat's mouth is held rigidly open and the breath forced through the mouth, creating an array of often aggressive vocalizations such as growling, snarling, and spitting. Mating cries are also produced in this way.

Preliminary research has examined the frequency of cat vocalizations produced in a variety of different contexts. Specifically, researchers looked at how the contours, or the pitch of the vocalization, changed though an utterance of the call.[7] Researchers found that the pitch of the vocalization signals a pet cat's mental state. Meows produced in affiliative contexts, such as during greeting, play, or when being picked up, were short, high pitched, and had a rising pitch to them. On the other hand, meows produced in negative situations, such as when the cat was stressed or being transported in a carrier, had a falling pitch to them. In all, vocalizations with rising frequency pitch signaled positive, or affiliative states, and vocalizations with falling contours signaled negative or stressed states. It appears that an analysis of a meow's pitch and vocal characteristics can be one accurate signal of cat mental states.

This idea is further supported by analysis of cat purr vocalizations. Scientists have shown that purrs are altered to convey meaning. Cats produce both solicitation and non-solicitation purrs. A solicitation purr is similar to a typical purr, except that there is a high-frequency voiced component overtop the purr.[8] This sounds like a high-pitched cry in addition to the low-pitched purr. Interestingly, the peak of this cry occurs at similar frequencies to that of a human infant's cry (between 300 and 600 Hz). Humans who listened to the vocalizations also deemed the solicitation purrs to sound "more urgent and less pleasant" than the typical non-solicitation purr.[8] The characteristics of these vocalizations make them difficult to ignore. Just as a baby's high-pitched cry is an indication that they need food or care, the solicitation purr may also be an indication of the cat's needs. Indeed, the solicitation purr is produced when the cat is seeking food from the owner, and this has led the researchers to propose that there may be a mammalian tendency to respond to these types of high-frequency cries with caregiving behaviors. To date, it is not known if cats produce the solicitation purr in other contexts, such as when seeking attention from their owner or whether it is isolated to food-getting behavior.

Cat Body Language

In addition to social behaviors and vocalizations, body language can also be an indicator of cat mental states. When looking at body language, a calm or confident posture is one that is open and in which muscles are relaxed. As discussed above, a relaxed cat may sit with their vulnerable belly exposed (Figure 2.2). They may sit with their eyes closed, resting, or their eyes open and the cat's pupils may be only slightly dilated. A relaxed cat's ears will face forward on the head. The tail may slowly move side to side or may be in a "tail up" position in which the tail sticks straight upright into the air. A tail up is seen as an affiliative signal that is often displayed during friendly interactions.[9] A cat with confident, relaxed body posture can be seen in Figure 2.3. Cats with this body posture may engage in other affiliative behaviors, such as allorubbing, and solicit for attention from social partners. They may also produce vocalizations such as meows, purrs, or trills.

Figure 2.3   A cat displays confident body posture despite being in a novel location. Note the forward-facing ears, the "tail up," fur flat against the body, and only slightly dilated pupils.

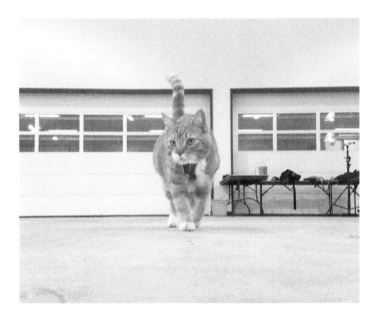

A cat that is aggressive or threatened will display very different body positioning. Instead of having an open and relaxed body posture, the cat may have a small, tense body. As seen in the cat on the right side of Figure 2.4, a threatened cat will appear hunched like a tight little ball with the tail stiffly tucked to the side of their body.[10] Alternatively, a threatened cat may also use their body to appear larger. The cat may arch their back, similar to a typical Halloween style cat, and may exhibit piloerection, that is, the fur on the body and tail standing up on its ends (Figure 2.5). In both of these postures, cats will often have ears rotated sideways or held flat against their head (Figure 2.4). The pupils will be mostly or fully dilated. Cats with this body posture may also bare their teeth and rapidly flick the tip of their tail from side to side. They may also engage in frequent swallowing or lip-licking, in which the cat quickly licks their lips or nose with their tongue.[11] They will also produce vocalizations such as growling, hissing, or caterwauling. If a cat is noted to display more than

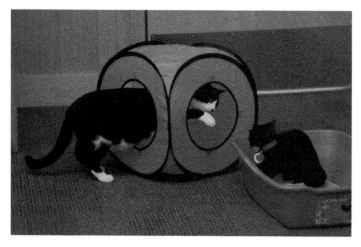

Figure 2.4   An uncertain meeting. The kitten on the right displays flattened ears, a tense and tight body posture, and holds the tail directly against its body.

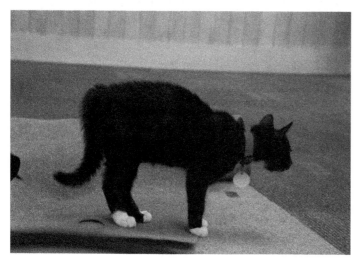

Figure 2.5   A cat begins to display an arched back and fur piloerection in response to an unfamiliar conspecific.

one of these behavioral indicators, it is best to cease social interaction and give the cat space in order to avoid potential aggression or unnecessary stress for the cat.

A final indicator to look for is the cat's facial expression. Cats have facial expressions associated with fear, frustration, and relaxation.[11] Researchers found that cat facial expressions connected with fear include eye blinking and half-blinking as well as a bias to turn the head and gaze to the left side. Expressions related to frustration include dropping of the jaw, raising of upper lip, nose wrinkling, parting of lips, mouth stretching, lip-licking, and showing of tongue. These expressions were often accompanied by a hissing vocalization. Finally, a bias to turn the head and gaze to the right side was noted during relaxed engagement. Even extremely subtle facial expression can signal a large amount of information for a careful observer.

In all, an examination of the cat's body posture, ear positioning, tail positioning, and facial expression can be an important starting point for determining a cat's comfort level in a given situation. Now that we have covered typical social behaviors and body language in cats, let's move on to typical social structure of both free-roaming and pet cats.

Feline Social Structure

Despite common stereotypes, cats display great variability and flexibility in their social behavior and do not strictly live asocial lives.[3,12,13] For a better understanding of the structure of feline social behavior, let us first explore the early social development of kittens, and then move on to characteristics of group living in domestic cats.

Social and Behavioral Development in Kittens

Kittens are born into the world altricial which means they are completely dependent on their mother for survival. Because of this, the early life of a kitten is focused on social interactions with the mother and littermates.[14] Tactile and olfactory senses are functional at birth and a series of experiments highlights the importance of thermal and olfactory cues in the behavior of young kittens. Newborn kittens primarily use temperature as a guiding tool for their behavior, seeking to be in the warmest area of the nest. However, after about 1 week of age this dependence on thermal cues shifts to a dependence on olfactory cues. Kittens now rely heavily on scent cues to orient and navigate in their surroundings.[15] Researchers found that kittens displayed distress when near to strange odors.[16] However, kittens' stress responses were reduced when near to familiar odors. This may indicate that familiar scents let a kitten know they are in a safe location and therefore exert a calming effect.[14] As we have already discussed, scent-related behaviors continue to be important aspects of investigatory behavior as kittens mature into an adult cat.

The ability to detect auditory stimuli is the next sense to develop at around 11–16 days old and the sense of sight develops slightly later at 14–21 days old. After 24 days, kittens will follow moving objects and the sensory systems begin to function holistically.[17] Now that the kitten's senses allow for slightly more coordinated movement, social play begins. A kitten's first social partners are the mother and littermates (unless the kitten has been orphaned). Kittens will begin to engage in social play with their siblings, practicing the wrestling, chasing, and cuffing behaviors we have already discussed. They will learn how hard of a bite is too hard and how rough is too rough through feedback from their littermates.

It is important that during a kitten's development they are exposed to social partners, both conspecifics and humans, within a specific time frame. Both cats and dogs have a sensitive period for socialization in which they learn that social partners are nothing to fear. For cats, this period is between 2 and 7 weeks.[18] Without proper socialization during this time a cat can become feral, or unsocialized, and can be extremely difficult to socialize as an adult. This is not to say that socialization for older kittens and adult cats does not continue to serve an important role. Although much remains to be learned about this topic, kitten socialization and training classes are becoming more popular, even for older kittens 3–8 months old,[19] and such experiences have the potential to increase the welfare of cats.

Solitary or Social?

In popular media, there is disagreement as to whether cats are really social animals. However, with millions of cats living in human homes around the world, it appears there is more to the story. Cats display a large amount of flexibility in their ability to live socially. An examination of the behavior of outdoor free-roaming cats indicates that their social behavior is greatly shaped by the distribution of important resources, namely the location and abundance of food, shelter, and mates.[12,20] Cats form social groups when these vital resources are clumped together in one location, like at a fishing port or garbage area. Cats live mainly solitary lives when these resources are dispersed out, as would be the case for typically occurring wild prey.[20] Similar to dogs,[21] cats appear to be social generalists and display plasticity in their social behavior, living solitarily or socially depending on environment and life experience.[3]

Cats are capable of forming social groups with conspecifics, known as cat colonies. As noted by Macdonald et al.,[20] free-roaming cats within these colonies were often thought to be random groupings of individuals that showed up to exploit resources rather than a group with a social structure. However, it later "became clear that the behavior of individuals in these colonies is far from socially random."[20] Within the colony exist "preferred associates" or cats that prefer to be near one another and engage in frequent affiliative behavior with one another.[3,20,22] Cats that are more familiar with one another or are relatives are more likely to spend time near one another and engage in affiliative interactions.[3] This supports the idea that cats should be adopted in sibling pairs (or groups) or in pairs of cats that are already familiar to each other.

The demographics of these cat colonies can vary. The typical demographic of many of the colonies reported in the literature are that the core is comprised of actively reproducing females (and their close kin) and male toms often live on the peripheries of the colony.[20] However, in colonies where individuals are predominately spayed and neutered, the demographics of the colony are altered. The colony I studied for my Master's thesis was comprised of 17 adult males and 10 adult females, and 83% of the colony was spayed/neutered. With more males in the colony than females (sex ratio 1.7:1) the core of this colony was predominately neutered males (see unpublished work Shreve, 2014).[23] Much more remains to be learned about factors influencing social group formation and behavior in free-roaming cats. But it appears both female and male cats have the capacity to live socially in groups and prefer to spend time near certain conspecifics over others.[3] This may be true for cats living in colonies, but what about the social nature of the pet cats living in our homes?

Just like cats living outdoors, cats in human homes live in a variety of social situations. One study examined if stress levels differed for cats living alone or in multi-cat homes. They found there was no significant difference in level of stress, as measured through fecal cortisol, for cats that lived alone compared to those living with other cats.[24] Cats that lived with other cats were not significantly more stressed than singly living cats. Instead, aligned with the flexible social nature of cats, there was much variability between cats regardless of housing situation. Some cats were more stressed while other cats were less stressed, and it did not have much to do with the number of social partners in the environment. One important note is, there was some impact of the cat's age. Younger cats, less than 2 years old, were more likely to be stressed living alone and less likely to be stressed in multi-cat homes. So, the behavioral outcomes for living socially or solitarily may also depend on age of the cat. In all, whether a cat prefers social partners or not depends on the individuality and life experience of the cat involved. Some cats may be stressed from living alone while others may be stressed from living socially.

The ability of pet cats to live in highly dense social groups is illustrated by the house cats studied by Bernstein and Strack (1996).[25] Fourteen pet cats lived in a one-story 1,340 square foot home, that's about 1 cat per 96 square foot of home! The cats chose to spend time in certain locations of the home over others. In areas where several cats preferred that location, cats were observed "time-sharing" the spot instead of directly engaging in aggressive behavior for access to the location. In all, the cats tended to engage in affiliative behaviors with one another and little aggressive behavior was described. Given that cats were willing to share access to locations with one another, does this mean that cats defend a territory or do they instead "time-share" certain locations?

Territorial or Space-Sharing?

Even for cats living mainly solitary lives, there can be considerable overlap in home ranges.[20] Much of cat behavior, such as the tendency to rub, or "mark," objects, allorubbing on humans, and urine spraying has been described as territorial behavior.[5] If cats were using these behaviors to deposit territorial markers (i.e. to indicate active defense of a location) then scent markings should serve as a warning to other cats that they should avoid the location. However, research with cats living in an outdoor enclosure did not find clear evidence for the use of scent markers in this way. Instead, Feldman states "Scent marking in this study supports the idea that cats do not defend territories, instead patrolling and reinforcing marks throughout a looser home range. The suggestion has been made that different forms of marking may serve separate signalling functions."[26] Other studies of non-enclosed outdoor cats have supported this idea, finding that home ranges of cats will often overlap with one another extensively with little evidence of active defense of these locations.[27]

Given the social plasticity of cats, it is possible that certain environmental conditions promote territorial behavior and other conditions promote more flexible behavior tolerating range overlap. It appears the majority of cats studied to date do display more tolerant space-sharing behavior and are not engaging in territorial behavior. If this is the case, then what is the purpose of these scent markings? Feldman stated that the study cats tended to scent mark along common routes and in areas where they tended to spend the most time. As mentioned, research with newborn kittens indicates they rely heavily on olfactory cues to orient and navigate their surroundings[15] and that being near to familiar odors reduces kitten distress.[16] In all, this indicates that scent can serve as a spatial reference tool and being near to familiar scents may promote stress-relief for the cat.

All of these factors are important considerations when setting up a cat's environment to promote proper social behaviors. Some owners may incorrectly assign a cat's inappropriate scent marking behavior as territorial yet, in reality the problem behavior could be occurring due to stress related to inadequacy of the captive environment or from lack of environmental enrichment, not from the cat attempting to mark off and actively defend the home area. If an owner has an issue with inappropriate scent marking in the home, then they should evaluate the layout of the cat's resources in the house. Cats should have access to objects in which they can deposit their scent (through scratching, litter box use, rubbing/rolling on cat beds) and these objects should be spread throughout the home, in areas where the cat spends time. Scent areas can be placed so cats can use them as they patrol their preferred locations within the home. Proper access and placement of scent spots can help reduce problem behaviors, such as inappropriate scratching, and help increase cat welfare.[4]

The Human–Cat Relationship

Many of the typical social behaviors observed in the human–cat relationship are not all that different from those described in the cat–cat relationship. Cats frequently engage in affiliative behavior with humans, such as rubbing against or grooming a person or engaging in a social roll (Figure 2.2). Cats also prefer human interaction to other forms of appetitive stimuli. In a preference assessment of pet and shelter cats, 50% of cats (or 19 out of 38 cats) most preferred human interaction (playing, petting, or being talked to) over other forms of appetitive stimuli.[28] The flexible social nature of cats has also been seen in a study of pet and shelter cat sociability in which a wide range of responses were noted from cats. Some cats were highly social, spending the entire session with the human, other cats were less social, spending the entire session out of reach, and other cats spent intermediate amounts of time with the person.[13] Although a variety of sociability responses were noted, a bias toward anti-social behavior was not observed. This was especially true in the shelter cats, who spent on average 47% of the session with a person when the person ignored the cat and spent 75% of the session with the person when they paid attention to the cat. There was also a significant difference between pet and shelter cat sociability, with shelter cats spending significantly more time with the inattentive person compared to the pet cats. This aligns with research conducted with pet and shelter dogs, which has demonstrated that shelter animals are more likely to seek out interaction with a human, even if the person is a stranger who is ignoring them.[29] This may be because shelter cats are more deprived of social interaction since they lack a primary caregiver and do not have consistent social interactions like pet cats. In these cases, social interaction may be a viable form of enrichment for shelter cats.[30] In all, cat sociability appears to be highly individual and depend on the individuality of the cat, the behavior of the human, and population in which that cat lives.

Cats also have the ability to form secure attachments with humans. Secure attachments are characterized by the ability to be comforted by the presence of an attachment figure and use them as a "secure base" from which to feel comforted and explore the world around them.[31] In a study of 108 cats, it was found that the majority of kittens and adult cats display a secure attachment toward their owner.[19] In this study, cats were brought to an unfamiliar location with their owner and experienced three short phases in which their owner was present (baseline phase), their owner left the room (alone phase), and the owner returned to the room (reunion phase). A cat was categorized as securely attached when, during the reunion phase, the cat ceases their separation distress and openly seeks out and greets the owner before returning to exploring the room around them, effectively being soothed by the return of the owner (Figure 2.6). Sixty-four percent of kittens aged 3–8 months were categorized as securely attached and 36% were categorized as insecurely attached. Insecurely attached individuals are those that do not display a reduction of stress upon reunion with their owner, and either excessively cling to their owner or avoid their owner. Of the adult cats, 65.8% were categorized as securely attached and 34.2% of adult cats as insecurely attached. This indicates that for the majority of cats, human owners serve as a source of comfort and stress reduction.

In another study utilizing similar secure base methods previously described, it was found that not just any characteristic of the owner reduces stress for cats.[32] When presented with a scent object belonging to the owner following the alone phase (such as a shoe or shirt with the owner's

Figure 2.6 Typical behavior of a secure cat. After greeting the owner following a brief separation, the cat returns to exploring the novel location with little signs of distress. Note the upright tail, open body posture, and forward ears.

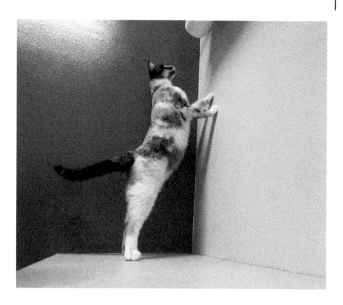

scent) cats did not display a reduction in stress and, in some instances, stress behaviors increased in response to the scent object. Only the owner's true presence was enough to reduce stress in cats. Additionally, the allorub was identified as an important reunion behavior. It was found that 83% of adult cats rub their owner following the separation. This behavior was displayed significantly more toward the owner when they returned to the room as compared to baseline, before the owner left the room. This indicates that in addition to being an affiliative greeting behavior, allorubbing may also be used to calm the cat or reduce stress.

If cats are capable of forming attachment bonds, then cats may also be capable of developing separation anxiety syndrome (SAS). Indeed, research has found that cats display many of the classic symptoms of separation anxiety when separated from their owner.[33] This includes behaviors like inappropriate urination and defecation, excessive vocalization, destructiveness, and overgrooming. Much research remains to be done in this area, but to date it appears that separation from the owner can be a source of distress for the cat that may lead to more severe behavioral problems in certain individuals. It is possible that insecure individuals, who do not display a stress reduction at the return of their owner, may be more susceptible to developing separation anxiety. However, this has yet to be explored by researchers to date.

Cats are also sensitive to several human social cues and behavior.[13,34] These include the ability to follow human pointing gestures, human gaze, and reference human emotions. However, that is not to say that all cats have these abilities. As mentioned, cats that lack critical experiences with humans early on, during their sensitive period for socialization, may have an increased fear response to humans and may not have the same capacity to respond to human social cues or form attachments to humans. One study examined if human socialization impacted usage of cat vocalizations.[35] They compared the vocalizations of feral (unsocialized) cats to house cats. They found feral cats tended to show extremely aggressive/defensive behavior and produced higher call rates. The agonistic growling and hissing vocalizations of the feral cat were higher in frequency and longer in duration than that of the house cat vocalizations. On the other hand, house cats' meow vocalizations were higher in frequency than the feral cat meows. In all, the level of socialization a cat has received can very much impact the social behaviors and vocalizations that cat produces toward humans as an adult.

Millions of cats live worldwide in homes or are free-roaming outdoors. Cats share homes with a variety of species, not only humans but other cats, dogs, birds, rodents, rabbits, reptiles, the list can go on. Given the plastic social behavior of cats, their ability to respond to human social cues, to live in a variety of environments, and their capacity to form secure attachment bonds, it is not surprising cats have become such popular companion animals. Although much remains to be learned about feline social behavior and the human–cat relationship, the existing evidence points to the fact that cats display a rich repertoire of social behaviors and can form strong ties with social partners.

References

1 Jasso del Toro C, Nekaris KA-I. Affiliative behaviors. In: Vonk J, Shackelford T, eds. *Encyclopedia of animal cognition and behavior*. Cham, NY: Springer International Publishing; 2019:1–6. ISBN 978-3-319-47829-6.

2 Stanton LA, Sullivan MS, Fazio JM. A standardized ethogram for the felidae: A tool for behavioral researchers. *Appl Anim Behav Sci*. 2015;173:3–16. doi:10.1016/j.applanim.2015.04.001.

3 Vitale KR. The social lives of free-ranging cats. *Animals*. 2022;12(1):126. doi:10.3390/ani12010126.

4 Vitale KR. Tools for managing feline problem behaviors: Pheromone therapy. *J Feline Med Surg*. 2018;20(11):1024–1032. doi:10.1177/1098612X18806759.

5 Spotte S. *Free-ranging cats behavior, ecology, management*. Wiley; 2014. http://public.eblib.com/choice/publicfullrecord.aspx?p=1742829

6 Moelk M. Vocalizing in the house-cat: A phonetic and functional study. *Am J Psychol*. 1944;57(2):184. doi:10.2307/1416947.

7 Schötz S, van de Weijer J, Eklund R. Melody matters: An acoustic study of domestic cat meows in six contexts and four mental states [Preprint]. *PeerJ Preprints*. 2019. doi:10.7287/peerj.preprints.27926v1.

8 McComb K, Taylor AM, Wilson C, Charlton BD. The cry embedded within the purr. *Curr Biol*. 2009;19(13):R507–R508. doi:10.1016/j.cub.2009.05.033.

9 Crowell-Davis SL, Curtis TM, Knowles RJ. Social organization in the cat: A modern understanding. *J Feline Med Surg*. 2004;6(1):19–28. doi:10.1016/j.jfms.2003.09.013.

10 Leyhausen P. *Cat behaviour: The predatory and social behaviour of domestic and wild cats*. (Tonkin B. A., trans.). New York, NY, USA: Garland STPM Press; 1979.

11 Bennett V, Gourkow N, Mills DS. Facial correlates of emotional behaviour in the domestic cat (Felis catus). *Behav Process*. 2017;141:342–350. doi:10.1016/j.beproc.2017.03.011.

12 Izawa M, Doi T. Flexibility of the social system of the feral cat, Felis catus. *Physiol Ecol Jpn*. 1993;29:237–247.

13 Vitale KR, Udell MAR. The quality of being sociable: The influence of human attentional state, population, and human familiarity on domestic cat sociability. *Behav Process*. 2019;158:11–17. doi:10.1016/j.beproc.2018.10.026.

14 Vitale Shreve KR, Udell MAR. Stress, security, and scent: The influence of chemical signals on the social lives of domestic cats and implications for applied settings. *Appl Anim Behav Sci*. 2017;187:69–76. doi:10.1016/j.applanim.2016.11.011.

15 Freeman N, Rosenblatt J. Specificity of litter odors in the control of home orientation among kittens. *Dev Psychobiol*. 1978a;11(5):459–468. doi:10.1002/dev.420110509.

16 Freeman NCG, Rosenblatt JS. The interrelationship between thermal and olfactory stimulation in the development of home orientation in newborn kittens. *Dev Psychobiol*. 1978b;11(5):437–457. doi:10.1002/dev.420110508.

17 Bradshaw JWS, Casey RA, Brown SL. *The behaviour of the domestic cat*, 2nd ed. Oxfordshire, OX, UK: CABI; 2012.

18 Karsh EB, Turner DC. The human–cat relationship. In: Turner DC, Bateson PPG, eds. *The domestic cat: The biology of its behaviour*, 1st ed. Cambridge, UK: Cambridge University Press; 1988;157–177.

19 Vitale KR, Behnke AC, Udell MAR. Attachment bonds between domestic cats and humans. *Curr Biol*. 2019;29(18):R864–R865. doi:10.1016/j.cub.2019.08.036.

20 Macdonald DW, Yamaguchi N, Kerby G. Group-living in the domestic cats: Its sociobiology and epidemiology. In: Turner DC, Bateson PPG, eds. *The domestic cat: The biology of its behaviour*, 2nd ed. Cambridge, UK: Cambridge University Press; 2000;95–115.

21 Udell MAR, Brubaker L. Are dogs social generalists? Canine social cognition, attachment, and the dog-human bond. *Curr Dir Psychol Sci*. 2016;25(5):327–333. doi:10.1177/0963721416662647.

22 Curtis TM, Knowles RJ, Crowell-Davis SL. Influence of familiarity and relatedness on proximity and allogrooming in domestic cats (Felis catus). *Am J Vet Res*. 2003;64(9):1151–1154. doi:10.2460/ajvr.2003.64.1151.

23 Shreve (Vitale) KR. *The influence of food distribution and relatedness on the social behaviours and proximities of free-roaming cats (Felis silvestris catus)*. Miami University; 2014. http://rave.ohiolink.edu/etdc/view?acc_num=miami1414773468 (accessed March 10, 2022).

24 Ramos D, Reche-Junior A, Fragoso PL, Palme R, Yanasse NK, Gouvêa VR, Beck A, Mills DS. Are cats (Felis catus) from multi-cat households more stressed? Evidence from assessment of fecal glucocorticoid metabolite analysis. *Physiol Behav*. 2013;122:72–75. doi:10.1016/j.physbeh.2013.08.028.

25 Bernstein PL, Strack M. A game of cat and house: Spatial patterns and behavior of 14 domestic cats (Felis catus) in the home. *Anthrozoos*. 1996;9(1):25–39.

26 Feldman HN. Methods of scent marking in the domestic cat. *Can J Zool*. 1994;72(6):1093–1099.

27 Liberg O, Sandell M, Pontier D, Natoli E. Density, space organisation and reproductive tactics in the domestic cat and other felids. In: Turner DC, Bateson PPG, eds. *The domestic cat: The biology of its behaviour*, 2nd ed. Cambridge, UK: Cambridge University Press; 2000;119–147.

28 Vitale Shreve KR, Mehrkam LR, Udell MAR. Social interaction, food, scent or toys? A formal assessment of domestic pet and shelter cat (Felis silvestris catus) preferences. *Behav Process*. 2017;141(3): 322-328. doi:10.1016/j.beproc.2017.03.016.

29 Barrera G, Jakovcevic A, Elgier AM, Mustaca A, and Bentosela M. Responses of shelter and pet dogs to an unknown human. *J Vet Behav*. 2010;5(6): 339–344. https://doi.org/10.1016/j.jveb.2010.08.012.

30 Houser B, Vitale K. Increasing shelter cat welfare through enrichment: A review. *Appl Anim Behav Sci*. 2022;248:105585.

31 Bowlby J. *Attachment and loss: Attachment*, 2nd ed., Vol. 1. New York, NY, USA: Basic Books; 1982.

32 Behnke AC, Vitale KR, Udell MAR. The effect of owner presence and scent on stress resilience in cats. *Appl Anim Behav Sci*. 2021;234:105444. doi:10.1016/j.applanim.2021.105444.

33 Schwartz S. Separation anxiety syndrome in cats: 136 cases (1991–2000). *J Am Vet Med Assoc*. 2002;220(7):1028–1033.

34 Vitale Shreve KR, Udell MAR. What's inside your cat's head? A review of cat (Felis silvestris catus) cognition research past, present and future. *Anim Cogn*. 2015;18(6):1195–1206. doi:10.1007/s10071-015-0897-6.

35 Yeon SC, Kim YK, Park SJ, Lee SS, Lee SY, Suh EH, Houpt KA, Chang HH, Lee HC, Yang BG, Lee HJ. Differences between vocalization evoked by social stimuli in feral cats and house cats. *Behav Process*. 2011;87(2):183–189. doi:10.1016/j.beproc.2011.03.003.

3

Preventing Behavior Problems in Domestic Cats

Emma K. Grigg

Introduction

Domestic cats are very popular companion animals in many parts of the world. For example, the American Pet Products Association estimates that 92.4 million cats live as pets in homes in the United States, and over a third of all Americans currently own a cat.[1] Although ownership of pets has been linked to health benefits for humans,[2,3] the relationship does not always work out for all concerned. Living with a pet with behavior problems can be stressful and can have negative impacts on the lives of human owners,[4–6] and behavior problems are a primary reason for relinquishment of pets to shelters, and euthanasia.[7]

In many cases, behavior problems in domestic cats can be avoided through conscientious environmental management and enrichment tailored for the needs of this species.[8,9] The relationships between environmental stressors and domestic cat welfare, health and behavior problems have been well-documented in shelters and cat colonies,[10–13] and for pet cats living in private homes.[14,15] Although more research is needed on the lives of pet cats living in private homes, available information suggests that many of these cats are not provided with the resources they need for optimal behavioral health and welfare.[13,16–19] Insufficient provision of resources in the home can be a significant source of stress for pet cats.[17,20] Lower levels of owner knowledge of normal cat behavior and environmental requirements have been linked to higher reported behavior problems in pet cats,[19] and studies have reported that many cat owners lack even basic knowledge about cat behavior and appropriate cat care.[21–24] For multi-cat homes, current recommendations state that the initial introduction of new cats needs to be done carefully and gradually, working at the comfort level of the cats involved, in order to minimize or avoid future social conflict between the cats.[25,26]

One framework that is frequently put forth for helping owners ensure that their pets' physical and mental needs are met is the Five Freedoms,[27] or the similar frameworks known as the Five Pillars[28] or the five Pet Welfare Needs[18] (Box 3.1). Familiarity with these frameworks and provision of these resources to pet cats can help prevent behavior problems, a common negative "side effect" of suboptimal welfare.[15,28–30]

The goal of this chapter is to provide an overview of recommendations for new and existing cat owners for avoiding the development of behavior problems, although many of these suggestions can also be a useful part of treating existing behavior problems, as other chapters in this volume will show. As the saying goes, however, an ounce of prevention is worth a pound of cure, and behavior problems are generally much easier to prevent than to treat once established. Many feline behavior

---

The Five Freedoms[27]

The Five Freedoms concept was published following an enquiry into the (suboptimal) welfare of farm animals in the UK in the 1960s and is designed to capture the minimum requirements for animals to have good welfare. This concept has since been adopted by a number of organizations dedicated to animal welfare, including many focused on the welfare of companion animals. Attention to each of these Five Freedoms will help ensure owners and caretakers are meeting the basic needs of the animals in their care.

1) *Freedom from hunger and thirst*: by ready access to fresh water and a diet to maintain full health and vigor.
2) *Freedom from discomfort*: by providing an appropriate environment including shelter and a comfortable resting area.
3) *Freedom from pain, injury or disease*: by prevention through rapid diagnosis and treatment.
4) *Freedom to express normal behavior*: by providing sufficient space, proper facilities and company of the animal's own kind.
5) *Freedom from fear and distress*: by ensuring conditions and treatment which avoid mental suffering.

The Five Pillars of a Healthy Feline Environment[8]

A number of organizations have modified the Five Freedoms to be more specific to a particular species; for example, the American Association of Feline Practitioners (AAFP) and the International Society of Feline Medicine (ISFM) developed the Five Pillars for owners and caretakers of domestic cats, to highlight the most important aspects of the cats' environment. Familiarity with and provision of these resources to pet cats can improve welfare and help prevent behavior problems.

Pillar 1: Provide a safe place
Pillar 2: Provide multiple and separated key environmental resources, such as food, water, scratching areas, litterboxes, resting/sleeping areas
Pillar 3: Provide opportunities for play and exercising natural behaviors (such as predatory behaviors)
Pillar 4: Provide positive, consistent, and predictable human–cat interactions
Pillar 5: Provide an environment that respects the cat's sense of smell

---

problems can be avoided through (for example) careful introductions, excellent litterbox management, provision of plentiful resources important to cats, and management/mitigation of stressors.

Best Practices for Preventing Problems

Realistic Expectations and Understanding of Natural Cat Behavior, and Individual Variation in Cat "Personality"

Harmonious relationships with pet cats can be aided by an understanding of the origins of the domestic cat, and the changes that likely occurred (and, didn't occur) during the domestication process. This sets the stage for realistic expectations, awareness of popular misconceptions about cats, and promotes understanding of otherwise mystifying cat behaviors. Box 3.2 provides a brief

---

Box 3.2   The natural history of the domestic cat – setting the stage for understanding and realistic expectations

---

One important resource for avoiding behavior problems in pet cats is to understand the normal behavior (and corresponding environmental needs) of this species. Modern day domestic cats are descended from the African wildcat, *Felis silvestris lybica*, which has DNA almost identical to that of today's domestic cat.[34] *F.s. lybica* still exists today as a solitary and highly territorial species, a nocturnal hunter that preys primarily on small mammals, reptiles and insects, and that physically resembles a slightly large tabby domestic shorthair.[35]

The domestication of the cat most likely began about 10,000 years ago, in the Fertile Crescent region of the Middle East.[36] (36 Driscoll et al. 2007). Once humans began to settle in a place and cultivate crops, grain and other types of food needed to be stored. This abundance of food stored in one central location attracted rodents (and other pests), which could do significant damage to human food reserves; cats, in turn, began to use this high density of rodent prey as a food resource, coming to the grain storage areas at night to hunt. In order to take advantage of this resource, however, individual cats needed to be somewhat tolerant of not just human proximity,[37] but also the proximity of other cats attracted to the abundant food resource. Over the course of their domestication, therefore, cats became more tolerant and less wary of humans, and more tolerant of the proximity of other members of their species.[38] So, while the ancestor of the domestic cat was a solitary and territorial predator, modern domestic cats have a much more fluid social life, and can often live peacefully with another familiar cat or cats. Nonetheless, cats are not, as a rule, highly and indiscriminately gregarious by nature (in the way that many domestic dogs can be). An abundance of resources was required to enable cats to adapt to a more social way of life. This is important to bear in mind, particularly in when introducing a new cat to the home, and/or in multi-cat homes.

Cats today are both a predator and a prey species; they are drawn to high places and perches (a good vantage point for scouting out the nearby environment, locate prey, and avoid other animals), and small, dark hiding places (good for avoiding predators, or waiting to ambush an unwary prey animal). Their small prey often hide in small holes and crevices, driving cats to investigate such places in the environment, or even to squeeze themselves into these locations. Cats are primarily nocturnal, and so may be more comfortable in dim, quiet areas, away from harsh lighting and loud noises, particularly when feeling anxious or threatened.

These aspects of their natural history can inform our care of domestic cats today, and their wellbeing is dependent on the ability to express natural behaviors to some degree; the sufficient availability of resources; and some ability to control their own environment.

---

overview of aspects of the natural history of cats most relevant to living with a pet cat today; a brief, entertaining video on the origins of many natural cat behaviors can be found at https://youtu.be/sI8NsYIyQ2A.[31] For more detail on normal cat social behavior, see Chapter 2 in this volume.

For example, the concept of cats as "low maintenance" (or low cost) pets is largely inaccurate. Cats display individual variation in behavior and personality,[32,33] so while some cats may be more aloof and independent, many cats require considerable human attention (Figure 3.1). All pets, including cats, require commitment for the life of the pet (which, for cats, may be well over 15 years). Regardless of the cat's apparent independence, providing an enriched environment (which may include toys, interactive play, positive human attention) is important for the cat's quality of

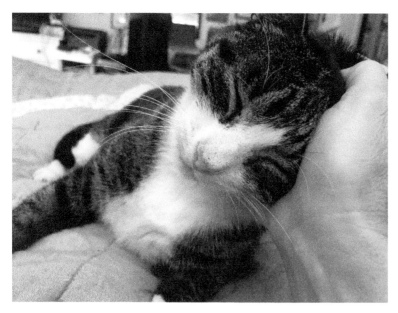

Figure 3.1   Cats' social needs vary, but many companion cats seek out and value attention from and physical contact with their human companions (photo: E. Grigg).

life, particularly for indoor-only cats. Although physically smaller than many dog breeds, cats do require sufficient space to explore, including vertical space, and space for resting locations to choose from, and multiple, separated resources such as food, water, and litterboxes. Boredom and stress caused by a sterile, unchanging environment can cause or exacerbate behavior problems, and ignoring the cat may be inhumane. All pet cats incur costs associated with, at minimum, food, toileting needs, parasite control, and veterinary care.

As noted in Box 3.2, the modern domestic cat has a more flexible sociality than its ancestor the African wildcat. Nonetheless, cats do tend to be very selective of their feline companions (much more so than most domestic dogs, for example), and some thought and planning should be put into the introduction of unfamiliar cats within the home in order to avoid conflict and stress-related behaviors (Figure 3.2). More on this issue is covered in the "Selecting a new cat or kitten" and "Introductions" sections that follow.

Selection of a New Kitten or Cat

For households without a resident cat, the experience of bringing a new kitten or cat into the home and getting to know the new feline family member can be wonderful. A new kitten can be highly entertaining, full of energy, curiosity, and charm. On the other hand, bringing a boisterous, energetic kitten home also entails a significant amount of adjustment and work (for example, kitten-proofing the household, socializing the new kitten, and training a few basic life skills like tolerance of the carrier, nail trims, and even "come when called" – see the following sections for strategies). Animal shelters and rescue organizations are full of wonderful adult and senior cats looking for homes, and many households may prefer adopting an older cat, who will likely be calmer and more self-sufficient. In addition, an adult cat may be perfect for a new cat owner or an elderly person looking for companionship. If the household has a resident dog, it may be helpful to select

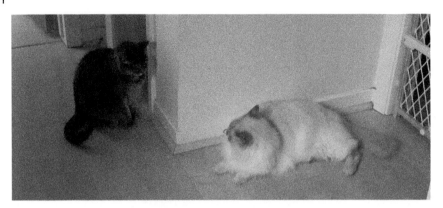

Figure 3.2 Without careful and patient introductions between new and resident cats, social conflict can occur, leading to stress-related behavior and medical issues down the line. Based on body language, these two cats are not best friends (photo: E. Grigg).

a cat who has lived with a friendly dog in the past, as such cats are likely to be less fearful of dogs and adjust more easily to the presence of the dog in their new home.

There is little research-based information as to differences in temperament, etc., between pedigree cat breeds, although one study reported Persian cats were presented more frequently for elimination problems than other breeds.[15] Nonetheless, a client looking to purchase a pedigree should research the breed and be aware of any special requirements such as grooming, and any breed-specific disease risks (International Cat Care provides a list of inherited disorders in purebred cats; available at https://icatcare.org/advice/inherited-disorders-in-cats). Many beautiful and good-tempered mixed breed cats are available for adoption in local shelters or rescue organizations.

For households that already have a resident cat (or cats), prospective adopters should be aware that there is a significant possibility that their resident cat may be more stressed than benefitted by the addition of another cat. Consideration should be given to the age and temperament of the resident cat when choosing the new addition. For example, adult cats may be more tolerant of the addition of a kitten than another adult cat; but geriatric cats may be less tolerant of an overly rambunctious kitten, and it may be preferable to select a cat of similar age and temperament. If neutered, sex of the cat may not play much role in the chances that the two cats will form a bond, although anecdotally, neutered male cats are often said to be more tolerant than females.[35] Given the importance of resource availability to domestic cat behavior, owners considering adding another cat to their household should be made aware of the need for a corresponding increase in the provision of resources (such as number of litterboxes, food and water stations, and beds) necessary to avoid conflicts between cats.[19,39]

For people hoping to have more than one pet cat in their home, the best-case scenario may be to simultaneously adopt littermates, a bonded pair of adult cats, or two unrelated but compatible kittens of same age (Figure 3.3). Cats appear to place high value on the security of their territory,[33] and introducing new cats simultaneously may minimize the conflicts and stress that can occur when adding a new, unfamiliar cat to the home of a resident cat.

Understanding Cat Body Language

One important tool for preventing the development or exacerbation of behavior problems in cats is an understanding of feline body language, particularly signs of stress in cats. Although many

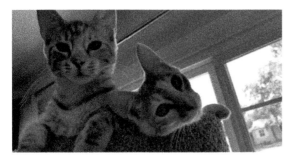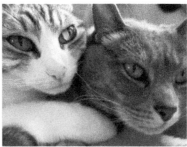

Figure 3.3   For people hoping to have more than one pet cat in their home, one way to increase the chances that the cats will get along well appears to be to simultaneously adopt littermates, a bonded pair of adult cats, or two unrelated but compatible kittens of same age (Photos: M. Delgado).

owners can recognize prominent signs of stress in cats (such as excessive vocalization, posture with ears back, and house soiling), they often miss the more subtle signs of stress in cats.[24] Cats Protection (UK) has a helpful video for cat owners on how to interpret body language in cats (available at https://youtu.be/bvsfB7sf4QU), and owners can download a free illustrated handout on "Cat Language" at https://www.doggiedrawings.net/freeposters.[40] A more comprehensive (text-based) seven-level cat stress scale ranging from 1 (fully relaxed) to 7 (terrorized) is available in Kessler and Turner.[41]

Introductions (Between Cats, between Cats and Dogs, between Cats and Children)

As noted earlier, domestic cats can form close bonds with other members of their species, but when introducing unfamiliar cats (such as when bringing a new cat or kitten into the household), considerable care must be taken to maximize the chances that the resident cat will accept the new addition. Social stress is common between cats,[38] and often contributes to behavior problems such as inappropriate elimination and aggression.[8,29] For these reasons, it is worth taking the time and effort to introduce cats gradually and systematically.

Recommendations for introductions between cats are as follows. (e.g., Overall et al.[42]; Horwitz and Neilson[43]; Atkinson 2018).[35] This process can be divided into three phases: olfactory habituation, visual habituation, and finally, direct contact habituation:[15]

1) Start by establishing a private, safe space for the new cat to live in while resident cat(s) gets used to their presence (and, vice versa). This space should ideally be a room with a door that securely closes, and should be equipped with all the resources needed by the cat: food, water, scratching post, litterbox, a soft place to sleep, a perch or two, and a few toys. The new cat should be brought, in the carrier, to this room upon first arriving home. Pheromone diffusers (such as Feliway™) placed around the home may be helpful in supporting calm during this process, although research findings are mixed regarding the efficacy of these products (e.g., Griffith et al.[44]; Prior and Mills[45]; but see also Frank et al.[46]).
2) While in the safe room, the new cat should be allowed to explore and adjust to the new space at his/her own pace. Interacting with the new cat in a friendly way (feeding, providing treats and playtime) is highly recommended, but if the cat hides (under furniture etc.), do not attempt to physically remove the cat from their hiding place in order to interact with them. Attempts to force social interactions with cats are rarely helpful.[8]

3) Place food bowls and/or favorite treats near both sides of the closed door, to encourage cats to spend time in close proximity. Identify a favorite food treat for both the new and resident cats, to use during introductions.

4) Given the importance of scent to cats' perception of their world, a "scent exchange" should be done before the cats are allowed visual or physical access to each other. As a first step, take bedding used by the resident cat, and place it in the new cat's safe room; similarly, take bedding used by the new cat, and place it near a location frequented by the resident cat. In addition, if the cats enjoy such handling, a clean towel or cloth can be wiped gently over the new cat (concentrating on the sides of the head) and then wiped on furniture within the resident cat's space, and vice versa, to facilitate scent exchange between the two areas. The goal is to allow each cat plenty of time to familiarize themselves with their new roommate's scent, so that once they meet "in person," they are more likely to accept the other as a member of their social group or colony.

5) When both cats appear to be relaxed about their situation, you can begin to allow brief (3–5 minutes) visual access between the cats. Potential ways to do this include: using a mesh or screen door; a baby gate (or >1 baby gate stacked one above the other in a doorway); or latching a door open just enough to allow visual access, but not wide enough to allow cats to fit through the door (Figure 3.4). Containing one or both cats in a crate (such as a dog crate) is generally not recommended, as it may be very stressful for the contained cat(s), as they cannot escape at will. Some experts make an exception for introducing very young kittens, who might be comfortable contained in a large crate in the corner of a room during initial introductions, provided that the kitten has access to a hiding box within the crate should they wish to retreat there. Cats who are harness-trained could be on harness during these interactions.

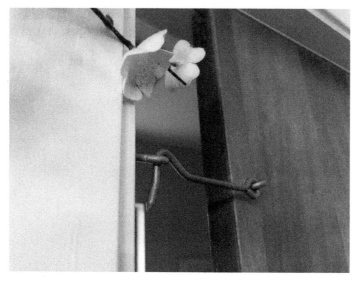

Figure 3.4   One way to allow visual access without physical access is to install a gate latch or similar to a door frame, allowing the door to remain open just enough for cats to see each other, but not fit through the gap. This technique can also be used, with a larger latch/wider gap, to provide cats with a dog (or child) free room in the house, complete with litterbox, etc. (Photo: E. Grigg).

Allow the resident cat(s) to investigate the new arrival without direct physical contact, starting with short exposure periods to avoid either cat becoming overly fearful or excited. Do this a few times a day for at least a few days, providing favorite treats to both cats during each exposure to help make the experience positive. If any overt aggression or extreme fearfulness is seen (hissing, swatting, etc.), cats should be immediately redirected using a toy or treat; do not punish the cats if this happens, as that will only add to the aversive nature of the exchange. In these cases, return to full separation in the safe room for a few days and then try again.

6) Once both cats appear relaxed in the (partial) presence of the other cat, you can begin allowing supervised direct interactions. Continue to provide positive experiences (such as treats or play with a favorite toy) during these initial face-to-face meetings. During such meetings, it is important to ensure that there are "escape routes" for both cats, such as by ensuring accessible perches, or room under furniture to which either cat can retreat.

7) If things are going well and the cats appear tolerant of each other, you can gradually increase the duration of time the cats are allowed access to each other, and relax your supervision. It is a good idea to leave the new cat's safe room in place, perhaps using a baby-gate or screen to separate the room from other cats (and dogs, small children, etc.) until the new cat is fully comfortable in their new home.

Note that these steps can be followed if conflict develops between two cats living together in a home; separation and gradual reintroductions may help restore harmony, as part of an overall plan to assess and treat the cause of the conflict (see Ch. 11 of this volume or Pachel[47] for guidelines for addressing inter-cat aggression).

When introducing cats and dogs, the primary consideration should be safety of the cat; cats can be injured or killed by dogs, who may see them as prey. Anecdotally, a dog who has grown up with cats is much more likely to easily accept a new cat into their home (Figure 3.5), but many dogs still need gradual introduction to new (vs. familiar) cats. Similarly, a cat who has lived with friendly dogs in the past will likely be much quicker to adjust to the presence of the dog in their new home. The process described above for introducing cats can be followed for introducing a new cat to a home with dogs, who also rely heavily on sense of smell in evaluating social interactions. During

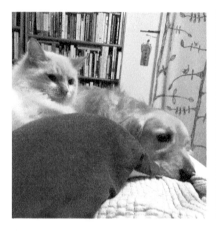 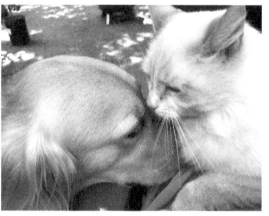

Figure 3.5 Many cats and dogs, introduced later in life, can coexist quite peacefully together. This is generally easier if the individuals involved were exposed to calm, friendly members of the other species when young, and introductions between dogs and cats should always be done with attention to the safety of both parties (see text for detailed information) (Photos: E. Grigg).

step 5, above, it is best to contain the dog on leash, rather than having the cat in a crate and allowing the dog to approach unrestrained, as this can be very threatening to a cat.[35] (35 Atkinson 2018.) The dog's behavior during step 5 can help determine how quickly the process can proceed to direct interactions; ideally the dog will be interested in the new cat, but not obsessively so, without growling or barking, and be easily distracted away from the cat with treats or trained cues. Direct supervision, and multiple "escape routes" for the cat, are essential until both dog and cat are comfortable with each other; maintaining a "dog free zone" (such as the safe room described in step 1, above, with a baby gate or cat door preventing access by the dog) is a good way to minimize stress for the household cat(s). There is some evidence that use of canine calming pheromone diffusers (Adaptil™) may be helpful when integrating cat and dog households.[45]

When introducing cats and children, again the initial focus should be on safety, for both parties. Prior to introducing a new cat, teach children to approach and handle cats gently (Figure 3.6), to recognize body language of stress in cats such as tail twitching and lowered ears, and to respect any attempts by the cat to retreat or hide. Supervise initial interactions closely to avoid stressing the cat (or overstimulating the child, for whom a new pet can be a very exciting experience). Continue supervising interactions until you are confident that both parties are comfortable with their new roommate, and ensure that the cat has a "safe room" to get away from the child when desired.

Declawing

Declawing (onychectomy, i.e., amputation of the third phalanx) is ethically controversial; as an elective procedure, declawing is strongly opposed by the AAFP, discouraged by the American Veterinary Medical Association,[48] and illegal in some countries, including the UK. Scratching surfaces and sharpening their claws is a natural behavior for cats, and thus declawing prevents cats from engaging in certain species-typical behaviors. There is some evidence that declawing

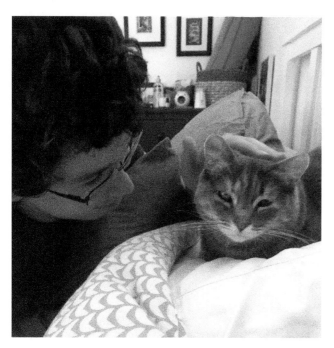

Figure 3.6 Children and pets can be a wonderful combination, with potential benefits for both. Children do need to be taught how to interact appropriately with any pet, for the safety and welfare of both parties. (Photo: E. Grigg).

increases the risk of behavior problems,[19,49] and thus if the goal is to prevent behavior problems, declawing is strongly discouraged. Instead, cats should be provided with suitable scratching surfaces, and redirected to these if they scratch other surfaces (such as furniture). More information on appropriate scratching surfaces can be found in the "Preparation of the environment" section, below, and additional tips for owners to prevent inappropriate scratching can be found in the AAFP's Position Statement on declawing (available at https://catvets.com/guidelines/position-statements).[50]

Maintain Regular Veterinary Care

Medical issues (such as external parasites and associated allergies, endocrine disorders, gastrointestinal/urinary problems, skin irritations, injuries) left undiagnosed and/or untreated can often contribute to, or exacerbate, behavior problems (e.g., Carney et al.[29]; Horwitz and Rodan[30]). Owners should be aware of the common warning signs of illness in cats (aka sickness behaviors), such as vomiting; housesoiling; fearful, aggressive or avoidance behavior (including hiding); changes in food intake; and self-scratching or overgrooming.[51] Regular veterinary visits and prompt attention to medical concerns is an essential part of preventing behavior problems.

Preparation of the Environment

Perhaps the most important piece of advice for current and perspective cat owners is to ensure that the cat's environmental needs are met. Competition (real or perceived) for resources between cats, or inability to easily access important resources can result in increased stress.[8] An "environment of plenty" is key, particularly for indoor-only cats! Resources important to cats are listed below, provision of which will help meet the Five Pillars of a healthy feline environment (Box 3.1; Ellis et al.[8]). An individual cat may frequently utilize all these resources, or may use only some, but it is important to ensure that cats have access to these resources to ensure quality of life and reduce risk of development of behavior problems. To prevent behavior problems, owners should attend to the cat's environmental needs from the time the cat enters the home, rather than waiting until problems develop. [See also client handout: Resources Important to Domestic Cats]

- Litterboxes: Good litterbox maintenance is essential to avoiding undesirable housesoiling behavior. An abundance of research exists on cat preferences for litter style, box shape, cleanliness, etc. (see Carney et al.[29] or Atkinson[35] for more detail). In general, recommendations are as follows:
  - *Number*: The number of litterboxes available to cats in homes should be equal to the number of resident cats plus one. Litterboxes should be in separate locations that are easily accessible to the cats (e.g., at least one on each floor, in multilevel homes), but away from high traffic locations and food/water stations. The goal is to maximize the probability that there will be a clean litterbox (unguarded by another cat, in multi-cat homes) available to the cat when needed.
  - *Size*: Litterboxes should be large enough for the cat to turn around easily (e.g., 1.5 times the length of the cat from nose to base of tail), to investigate and dig in different areas of the box when selecting a toileting location, and easy for the cat to enter and exit. Many feline behavior experts recommend using plastic storage containers, with smooth bottoms for ease of scooping, as these tend to be larger than many commercially available litterboxes. A low entry can be cut into one side of the storage box to facilitate access (particularly for small or senior cats).

– *Style*: The use of a covered vs. uncovered litterbox appears to be a matter of individual preference, with some cats preferring one sort or the other, and other cats using both equally.[52] It may be helpful to offer both styles to the cat, and allow him/her to indicate their preference. One note of caution regarding covered litterboxes is that this style makes it more difficult to see the conditions within, and may result in less frequent cleanings (and consequent avoidance of the box by the cat) if the owner is not vigilant about regular cleaning.

– *Litter type*: The most commonly recommended type of litter is fine-grained, unscented, clumping clay litter, maintained at a depth of 1.5–2 in. Low dust formulas may reduce the amount of dust inhaled by the cat and in the box vicinity. Highly scented litters or litter deodorizers may be off-putting to cats, and litterbox liners may get caught in cat claws when digging in the substrate. Here again it may be helpful to offer a choice of litters to the cat, allowing them to select a preferred type. One commercially available litter brand contains an herb designed to attract cats to the box (Cat Attract™), and may be helpful in encouraging cats to (or, back to) the box.

– *Cleaning*: Cleanliness of the box is essential.[53] All boxes should be scooped at least once per day, with the goal being to keep the box free of physical/visual evidence of previous use by other cats.[28] Periodic complete replacement of the litter and cleaning of the box itself is recommended, to minimize odor.

- Food/water stations: Multiple food and clean water bowls should be available, in separate locations (even in single cat homes), away from litterboxes; some cats prefer running water, so provision of a cat fountain (Figure 3.7) may be beneficial.[35]

- Places for rest and retreat: A selection of comfortable places to sleep, and quiet, safe, comfortable, and perhaps dark hiding places, should be available in the cat's living space (Figure 3.8). The addition of a box for hiding in was found to reduce stress in shelter cats, compared to cats

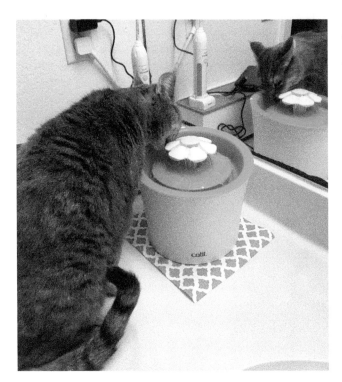

Figure 3.7 Cat drinking from a cat water fountain (Catit Flower Fountain; Rolf C. Hagen, Inc.; Quebec, CA). Cat fountains can be a great way to provide running water options for cats, but must be cleaned, and new filters installed, regularly (Photo: E. Grigg).

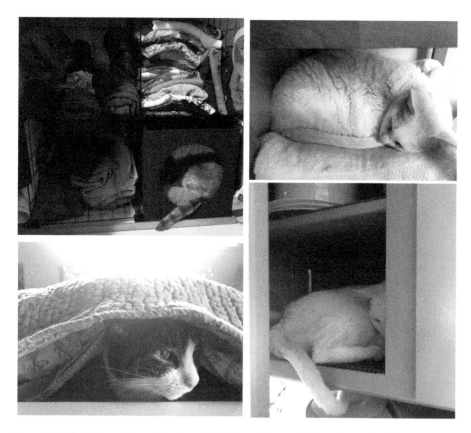

Figure 3.8 Provision of a variety of comfortable resting and hiding places is an important aspect of companion cat care; if these are not provided (or sometimes, even when they are), many cats will seek out their own favorite locations. (Photos: E. Grigg).

not provided boxes.[54] Most cats like to have an escape route available when they feel stressed, and to be able to social distance on occasion (away from other household cats, dogs, small children, or unfamiliar human visitors). Provide a way for the cat to retreat to his safe space when he needs a break.

- Scratching options: As noted above, cats need to scratch their claws regularly; this serves to sharpen and condition their claws, and as visual and chemical communication. At least two options should be offered, and perhaps more in multi-cat homes if space permits, in different and prominent locations; failure to provide at least one appropriate scratching surface makes inappropriate scratching (on furniture, rugs, etc.) almost inevitable. A variety of substrates are available for both commercial products and homemade scratching posts, such as jute rope, cardboard, and carpet. One recent study found that cats preferred vertical, standing scratchers over horizontal ones, and jute and cardboard surfaces over sofa fabric or carpet,[55] although cats will display individual preferences in surface type and location. Sprinkling the surface with catnip or silver vine may help stimulate use of the scratching post.
- Vertical space (perches, cat trees): Access to vertical space increases the overall space available to the cat, enables the cat to survey his/her surroundings, and allows for social distancing between cats in multi-cat homes. Vertical space can consist of commercially available "cat trees," or purpose-built ramps, ledges, or shelving (Figure 3.9).

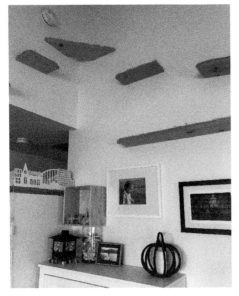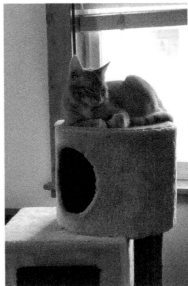

Figure 3.9 Places to climb and perch are high value 'real estate' for cats, and are an important resource to provide (especially for indoor-only cats, and in multicat homes). (Photos: E. Grigg).

- Positive and consistent interactions with, and attention from, familiar humans: Despite the popular misconception that cats as pets are aloof and independent, many cats seek affection and social interactions with their human companions, and positive human–animal interactions (including interactive play) can be an essential part of maintaining cat welfare.[13,16] Cats appear to prefer to be the initiators of social interactions with their humans, and interactions initiated by the cat tend to last longer.[56-58] Owners who interact often and regularly with their cats on a daily basis report fewer problematic behaviors.[59]

- Enrichment (human, visual, toys): Ellis et al.[28] define environmental enrichment as "any addition to the environment of an animal resulting in a presumed increase in the environment's quality, and a subsequent presumed improvement to the animal's welfare". Hal Markowitz, the father of environmental enrichment, noted that enrichment "should be a synonym for 'more like nature,'" [60] i.e., meeting an animal's needs as closely as possible to how they would have been met in nature, "in order to empower them to engage in species-typical behaviors in healthy and appropriate ways."[61] Cats evolved to live an outdoor lifestyle, and indoor cats in particular may show increased stress from the presence of (incompatible) conspecifics, competition for resources, insufficient mental stimulation, and lack of physical exercise.[62] Providing enrichment is one important route to decreasing stress, and correspondingly decreasing the risks for development of stress-related behavior problems.[14,54] Suggestions for providing enrichment for cats usually fall into three areas: hiding opportunities, elevated perching opportunities, and toys,[28] much of which is covered above. Some additional ideas include:
  - Interactive toys (e.g., toys which require participation of a human, and allow the cat to practice natural predatory behaviors, such as wand toys); small toys that resemble catchable prey (such as self-propelled or stuffed mice; Hall et al.[63]) (Figure 3.10); and/or food puzzle toys that can stimulate cats' natural foraging behavior; (Dantas et al.[64] http://foodpuzzlesforcats.com). Toys should be rotated regularly to maintain interest, and chosen with safety in mind (for

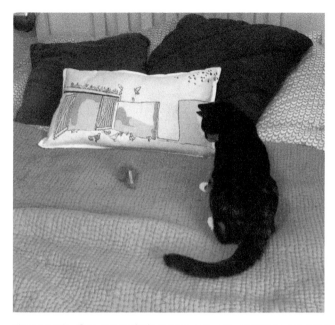

Figure 3.10 Cats, particularly indoor-only cats, should be provided with both toys and interactive play. Toys for independent play are usually preferred if they resemble small prey (like the toy mouse in this photo), or are filled with (or 'marinated in') catnip or silvervine; food puzzle toys are popular with some cats. Toys for independent play should be regularly rotated, to maintain the cat's interest, and removed if damaged. Interactive play involving cat wands or 'fishing pole' style toys that mimic hunting behavior and require the participation of the human in the game are often particularly valuable to the cat. (Photo: E. Grigg).

example, to minimize risk of ingestion of toy parts by the cat). Encouraging play and biting behaviors directed towards fingers and feet is discouraged, however, as this may teach the cat that it is rewarding to stalk, pounce on, and bite the owner.[65] See also Chapter 4 on Play behaviors, this volume.

- Resting place or perch allowing view of wildlife and activity outdoors[66] (Figure 3.11). Note that while many cats appear to enjoy surveying the outside world, some cats may be stressed if there are other, unfamiliar cats in view; if the latter, reduce visibility of intruder cats using temporary opaque window film, or plantings in front of the window.[35] Some authors suggest daily spraying of a pheromone product (such as Feliway™) around the "viewing area"; or discouraging unfamiliar cats from frequenting areas near house using humane methods (e.g., don't leave food outside near the home, use mild, motion-activated deterrents).
- Many additional resources for enrichment ideas exist; see "Sources of Additional Information" at the end of this chapter.

● Safety (cat-proofing): It is the responsibility of anyone bringing a cat into a home to ensure that obvious hazards to pets are removed. For example, many common houseplants are toxic to cats; for a sample list, see https://www.aspca.org/pet-care/animal-poison-control/toxic-and-non-toxic-plants. Some cats like to chew electric cables and cords; these should be secured and covered (e.g., using cable sleeves or covers) in such a way as to avoid electric shock. Similarly, linear objects like string and elastic bands can be attractive to many cats, and consuming these objects can lead to dangerous foreign body obstructions; these items should be removed from the cat's environment and kept out of reach. Additional information on household products, etc., toxic to cats can be found at the ASPCA's Poison Control page, https://www.aspca.org/pet-care/animal-poison-control.

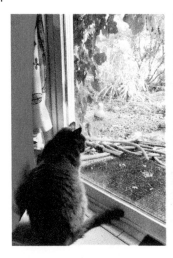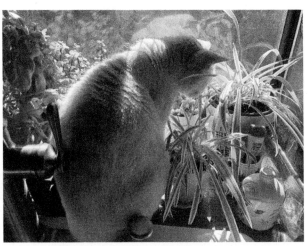

Figure 3.11   Perches or resting spots that allow the cat to view the world outside are an excellent way to provide dynamic enrichment for many cats. If, conversely, the cat becomes fearful (for example, by viewing other neighborhood cats outside), cling window film is one way to block visual access while still allowing in natural light (see the text for more ideas) (Photos: E.Grigg).

Indoor vs. Outdoor?

Do cats need outdoor access to be happy? Not necessarily. Access to the outdoors undeniably provides cats with ample opportunities to perform natural behaviors such as exploring their environment, hunting, and climbing. However, it also poses increased risks of injury, disease, predation, ingestion of toxins, and even death.[67] Due to these risks, along with risks to birds, small mammals, and other wildlife caused by cat predation, the AVMA recommends counseling cat owners about the risks and suggesting alternate ways to meet the cat's environmental needs without allowing unrestrained outdoor access.[47] Careful attention to the environmental and behavioral needs can provide an excellent quality of life for indoor-only cats. Alternately, supervised outdoor access (on harness, or in purpose-built cat enclosures; Figure 3.12) can allow cats time outdoors while ensuring their safety and the safety of local wildlife. If allowed outside, a cat flap should be installed (and the cat trained to use the flap), to allow the cat to retreat indoors when desired; if unfamiliar cats use the cat flap, an electronic version (activated by a collar on the resident cat) can limit access. Electronic containment systems (such as "invisible fence" systems) are not recommended.

Socialization and Handling of Kittens and Young Cats

One of the Five Pillars of an optimal environment for domestic cats (Box 3.1) is the provision of positive, consistent, and predictable human–cat social interaction.[8] This should be done ideally from an early age, so that the kitten grows into a cat who is comfortable and friendly with humans. As noted earlier, cats' social preferences vary by the individual, and are influenced by genetics, early life experiences, and learning throughout their lifetime.[68] Nonetheless, gentle handling by humans during the socialization period (between approximately 2 and 7 weeks of age) predisposes the cat to more resilience and a better ability to bond with humans.[69] Care should be taken during socialization to avoid overwhelming or stressing the cat (see "Understanding cat body language", above). Lack of exposure to and positive experiences with humans, or worse, negative experiences during this period, may result in lifelong fearfulness or avoidance of humans.[68,70]

Figure 3.12   Supervised access to the outdoors, such as in a purpose-built enclosure or "catio", can provide a safe way for the cat(s) to benefit from the many natural enrichment opportunities (visual, scent, sound) provided by the outside world (Photo: M. Delgado).

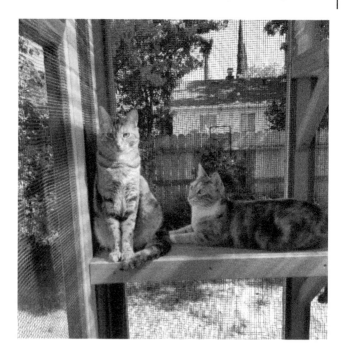

Owners of kittens or young cats should be gradually and gently acclimated to the kinds of handling that the cat will encounter later in life (nail trims, grooming, etc.), using favorite food treats or toys to make the experience a pleasant one and to build positive associations.[71] Similarly, young cats should be introduced to a variety of aspects of the life of a companion animal, such as children, dogs, other cats, the cat carrier, and the veterinary clinic, again using careful supervision and classical conditioning (see Box 3.3) to build calm acceptance and minimize the development of fearfulness. Given the struggles many cat owners have getting their cats into a cat carrier for veterinary visits, crate training the cat should be part of this socialization process. A client handout on crate training cats can be found in Yin,[72] and a short video demonstrating crate training cats can be found at https://youtu.be/b1wDsJ5snFk (Fundamentally Feline 2013).

Spaying/Neutering and Risk of Behavior Problems

The primary reason for neutering cats is to prevent unwanted litters, and the majority (87%) of pet cats in the US are neutered.[73] In addition, cats who remain intact (i.e., who are not spayed or neutered) may display markedly higher rates of certain reproduction-related behaviors generally considered very undesirable by cat owners, such as spraying (territorial and social marking), roaming, vocalizing, and inter-cat aggression (particularly in males).[74,75] Intact females will go into estrus multiple times per year (starting as young as 4 months of age; and during this time they will "call" loudly and frequently, may roam, and will often spray.[76] They may also attract intact males to the property, who in turn will spray, vocalize, and potentially antagonize resident male cats. Owners considering delaying or declining elective neutering should be aware of the realities of living with an intact cat. As the experience is likely to be stressful for cats, some experts recommend scheduling neutering so that it does not coincide with other stressful events, such as vaccination or rehoming.[35]

Box 3.3   How Cats Learn – Three forms of learning are highly relevant to life with companion animals

---

Habituation: Considered one of the simplest forms of learning, habituation refers to a decrease in the animal's response to an (inconsequential) stimulus following repeated exposure to that stimulus. The opposite of habituation is *sensitization*, in which an animal becomes increasingly reactive to a repeated stimulus; sensitization often occurs when the stimulus is very loud, frightening and/or unpredictable.

> *Real-world example*: A new kitten in the household may initially be startled by the sounds of a household appliances like the dishwasher or computer printer, but over repeated exposures (without any other negative experiences associated with these sounds), most cats will learn to ignore (i.e., will habituate to) these sounds.

Classical Conditioning: This is the process of building an association in the animal's mind between two things that would not necessarily have been associated previously; this is accomplished (deliberately or accidentally) by the two events or other stimuli repeatedly occurring simultaneously or in close proximity. A classically conditioned response requires no decision-making on the part of the animal, but rather is a reflex-like, emotional one.

> *Real-world example*: The sound of a cat-food can being opened, followed immediately (and repeatedly) by the arrival of tasty canned food, can result in the sound causing an immediate anticipatory emotion (i.e., of dinner) in the cat.

Operant Conditioning: In operant conditioning, the animal's behavior determines the outcome, and thus whether the behavior continues and/or will be repeated in the future; this is "learning based on consequences." A behavior followed by a reward (reinforcement) is likely to be repeated; a behavior followed by an unpleasant outcome (punishment) is less likely to be repeated.

> *Real-world examples*: A cat who jumps onto a kitchen counter and discovers an uncovered butter dish (resulting in a tasty snack for the cat) will likely repeat the behavior in the future, particularly if food is regularly left unattended on the countertop.

Cats can be easily "target trained" to touch a target stick (or hand, marked location, etc.) – the target is presented near the cat's nose or paw, so that the cat will likely move toward the target to sniff or investigate it. The moment the cat touches the target, a food treat is presented. This process is repeated until the cat learns that touching the target results in a reward.

Training and Learning

Fortunately, the old misconception that cats cannot be trained has lost ground among cat owners in recent years,[19] although it is still often repeated in popular culture. The recommendation that cats can (and should) be trained as a way to reduce the likelihood of behavior problems, increase welfare, and strengthen the bond with their owner is a newer one,[77] despite the widespread acceptance of the parallel concepts for domestic dogs. Cats learn throughout their lives, in the same ways as dogs, humans, and other animals, and as described in learning theory: operant conditioning, classical conditioning, habituation, and so on (Box 3.3). Karen Pryor's book *Getting Started: Clicker Training for Cats* (2003) and the online "Cat School" (https://www.catschool.co) are two great starting points for owners and caretakers wishing to train their cats; see "Sources of Additional Information" at the end of this chapter for more information. Training can also be useful for preparing the cat for veterinary visits, travel, and boarding (see "Socialization and handling," above); it is particularly effective to start this type of training when the cat is still a kitten.

Training can be a very useful part of ensuring appropriate behavior, and redirecting undesirable behavior – instead of focusing on how to stop the cat performing an unwanted behavior, it is generally more effective (and less frustrating) to focus on what we want the cat to do, and rewarding this desirable behavior (with training for that behavior if necessary).

All cat owners (regardless of whether or not they plan to train their cat) should be aware of cats as lifelong learners, and their own human role in shaping their cat's behavior. A behavior by the cat that is rewarded will be repeated; a behavior that is not rewarded, or that results in unpleasant or painful consequences for the cat, is much less likely to be repeated. So, for example, a cat who wakes her owner up before dawn by jumping on the bed and crying for food will continue to do this if the behavior is promptly rewarded by the owner with breakfast. A cat who scratches at a closed door to be let through will eventually stop this behavior if the door is not ever opened in response to this behavior. Importantly, owners should also be aware of the risks of responding to "misbehavior" with positive punishment (i.e., by adding something unpleasant, scary or painful in response to the cat's behavior). Positive punishment is difficult to use effectively, can increase fear and the likelihood of defensive aggression, and damage the human–animal bond.[20,78]

Stress Reduction

Given the established and negative relationship between stress and the welfare and behavior of domestic cats (e.g., Amat et al.),[15] cat owners should be aware of common stressors for cats (e.g., changing or unpredictable environments, competition for resources, loud noises, strong odors, conflict with other cats, and inability to perform natural behaviors;[11,12,42] and should attempt to minimize stress to their pet cats whenever possible. Provision of the environmental needs listed earlier in this chapter (see "Preparation of the environment", above) is an important step in stress reduction for domestic cats. The best way to recognize feline stress is through their body language and vocalization (see "Understanding cat body language" above). Additional guidelines for recognizing and minimizing stress in pet cats can be found in Overall et al.[42] The "Five Freedoms" and "Five Pillars" (Box 3.1) can be used as a guideline to help owners assess the quality of their cat's environment, and perhaps highlight areas where improvements would be beneficial to the cat's behavior and welfare.

In some cases, cats may be particularly sensitive to stress, and environmental management alone may be insufficient for avoiding behavior problems. These cats may benefit from further interventions to reduce stress, which (depending on the individual cat, and preferences of the owner) may range from special diets, to nutraceuticals, to psychoactive medication. Consult chapters in this text focusing on stress-related behavior problems for more detail on diagnosis and treatments for these cats.

Recommendations for veterinary clinic staff for minimizing stress in feline patients (and thus avoiding the development of fearful or aggressive behaviors in the clinic) can be found in Hammerle et al.[79] and Yin,[72] and through the Low Stress Handling® University (https://lowstresshandling.com) or Fear Free® veterinary certification programs (https://fearfreepets.com).

Role of Owner

Ensuring best welfare (optimal physical and mental health) is one of the best ways to prevent behavior problems in the cat. The owner's role is to provide the necessary resources initially, and throughout the life of the cat, using an "adaptive management" strategy to discover what works best for the individual cat or cats in the household. For example, some cats may rely heavily on access to vertical space, allowing for social distancing etc.; owners of these cats will need to ensure continuous, plentiful access to preferred spaces for their cats. Other cats may rarely or never make use of vertical spaces, preferring hiding places in closets, boxes, covered cat beds, etc. – for these owners, providing ample vertical space would be less important than ensuring the cat had easy access to these hiding places. It is the owner's responsibility to familiarize his or herself with the signs of stress in pet cats (see "Understanding cat body language" above), and to address these signs once identified.

Summary

Appropriate management and environmental enrichment can be very beneficial in preventing the development of behavior problems in domestic cats, and avoiding damage from undesirable but natural feline behaviors. Among the most important elements of knowledge for sustaining successful human–cat relationships appear to be: (1) the importance of providing the resources needed by cats, in abundance (particularly in multi-cat homes), with a primary goal being the reduction of stress levels for resident cats; (2) the ability to read feline body language, particularly the language of stress in cats; and (3) vigilance concerning the physical health of their pets, as medical issues are often linked to behavioral problems in domestic cats.

Sources of Additional Information

Books

Atkinson T. *Practical feline behaviour: Understanding cat behaviour and improving welfare.* Oxfordshire, UK: CABI; 2018:274.

Bradshaw J, Ellis S. *The trainable cat: A practical guide to making life happier for you and your cat.* New York: Basic Books; 2016:352.

Pryor K. *Getting started: Clicker training for cats,* 2nd ed. Waltham, MA: Karen Pryor Clicker Training/Sunshine Books; 2003:85.

Turner DC, Bateson P. *The domestic cat: The biology of its behaviour,* 3rd ed. Cambridge, UK: Cambridge University Press; 2013:288.

Guidelines

Ellis SL, Rodan I, Carney HC, Heath S, Rochlitz I, Shearburn LD, Sundahl E, Westropp JL. AAFP and ISFM feline environmental needs guidelines. *J Feline Med Surg.* 2013;15(3):219–230. doi:10.1177/1098612x13477537.

Hammerle M, Horst C, Levine E, Overall KL, Radosta L, Rafter-Ritchie M, Yin S. 2015 AAHA canine and feline behavior management guidelines. *J Am Anim Hosp Assoc.* 2015;51:205–221.

Herron M, Buffington T. Environmental enrichment for indoor cats. *Compend Contin Educ Vet*. 2010;2010 Dec;32(12):E4.

Horwitz DF, Rodan I. Behavioral awareness in the feline consultation: Understanding physical and emotional health. *J Feline Med Surg*. 20(5):423–436. doi:10.1177/1098612x18771204.

Monroe-Aldridge, et al.AAFP position statement: Environmental enrichment for indoor cats. *JFMS Clinical Practice*. 2011. Available at: https://catvets.com/public/PDFs/PositionStatements/EnviromentalEnhancement-.pdf (accessed July 2020).

Overall KL, Rodan I, Beaver B, Carney H, Crowell-Davis S, Hird N, Wexler-Mitchell E. *Feline behavior guidelines from the American association of feline practitioners*. 2004. Available at: https://catvets.com/guidelines/practice-guidelines/behavior-guidelines (accessed July 8, 2020)

Rodan I, Sundahl E, Carney H, Gagnon A-C, Heath S, Landsberg G, ... Yin S. AAFP and ISFM feline-friendly handling guidelines. *J Feline Med Surg*. 2011;13:364–375.

Websites

Cat School https://www.catschool.co – Videos, product, and online courses for clicker-training your cat.

Food Puzzles for Cats http://foodpuzzlesforcats.com Great source for ideas for commercially available and DIY food dispensing toys for cats.

International Cat Care https://icatcare.org – Information on a wide variety of cat-related topics.

The Indoor Pet Initiative at The Ohio State University's School of Veterinary Medicine https://indoorpet.osu.edu/cats – Resources for pet owners on a number of cat care topics, particularly identifying and avoiding typical stressors, and enrichment for indoor cats. [Also available in Spanish https://indoorpet.osu.edu/pet-owners/cats-spanish]

Videos

"*Body language in cats*" (2013) Cats Protection (UK). Available at: https://youtu.be/bvsfB7sf4QU

"*Getting your cat in the carrier*" Fundamentally Feline (2013). Available at: https://youtu.be/b1wDsJ5snFk

"*How to make sure your cat isn't bored*" Howcast.com (2013) with E'lise Christensen, DVM, DACVB https://youtu.be/-KlmRExaBRM

"*Why do cats act so weird?*" Buffington, T. (2016). Available at: https://youtu.be/sI8NsYIyQ2A. [for the complete interactive TedEd lesson on this topic, see https://ed.ted.com/lessons/why-do-cats-act-so-weird-tony-buffington]

References

1 American Pet Products Association (APPA) *2017-2018 American pet products association national pet owners survey*. Greenwich, CT: American Pet Products Association; 2018.

2 Friedmann E, Thomas S. Pet ownership, social support, and one-year survival after acute myocardial infarction in the Cardiac Arrhythmia Suppression Trial (CAST). *Am J Cardiol*. 1995;76;1213–1217.

3 Kanat-Maymon Y, Antebi A, Zilcha-Mano S. Basic psychological need fulfillment in human-pet relationships and well-being. *Pers Individ Differ*. 2016;92:69–73.

4 Grigg EK. Helping clients facing behavior problems in their companion animals. Ch. 16 In: Kogan L, Blazina C, eds. *Clinician's guide to treating companion animal issues (1st Ed.): Addressing human-animal interaction*. Elsevier;San Diego, CA 2018:281–317.

5 Grigg EK, Donaldson TM. Helping clients cope with grief associated with euthanasia for behavior problems. Ch. 14 In: Kogan L, Erdman P, eds. *Pet loss, grief, and therapeutic interventions: Practitioners navigating the human–animal bond.* Milton Park, UK:Routledge; 2019:236–264.

6 Buller K, Ballantyne KC. Living with and loving a pet with behavioral problems: Pet owners' experiences. *J Vet Behav.* 2020;37:41–47.

7 Salman M, Hutchison J, Ruch-Gallie R, Kogan L, New J, Kass P, Scarlett J. Behavioral reasons for relinquishment of dogs and cats to 12 shelters. *J Appl Anim Welf Sci.* 2000;3(2):93–106.

8 Ellis SL, Rodan I, Carney HC, Heath S, Rochlitz I, Shearburn LD, ... Westropp JL. AAFP and ISFM feline environmental needs guidelines. *J Feline Med Surg.* 2013;15(3):219–230. doi:10.1177/10986 12x13477537.

9 Buffington CT, Bain M. Stress and feline health. *Vet Clin: Small Anim Pract.* 2020;50(4):653–662.

10 Westropp JL, Kass PH, Buffington CA. Evaluation of the effects of stress in cats with idiopathic cystitis. *Am J Vet Res.* 2006;67:731–736.

11 Stella J, Croney C, Buffington T. Effect of stressors on the behavior and physiology of domestic cats. *Appl Anim Behav Sci.* 2013;143:157–163.

12 Stella J, Croney C, Buffington T. Environmental factors that affect the behavior and welfare of domestic cats (*Felis silvestris catus*) housed in cages. *Appl Anim Behav Sci.* 2014;160:94–105. doi:10.1016/j.applanim.2014.08.006.

13 Stella JL, Croney CC. Environmental aspects of domestic cat care and management: Implications for cat welfare. *Sci World J.* 2016;2016 6296315. doi:10.1155/2016/6296315.

14 Buffington CA, Chew DJ, Kendall MS et al. Clinical evaluation of multimodal environmental modification (MEMO) in the management of cats with idiopathic cystitis. *J Feline Med Surg.* 2006;8(4):261–268.

15 Amat M, Camps T, Manteca X. Stress in owned cats: Behavioural changes and welfare implications. *J Feline Med Surg.* 2016;18(8);577–586. doi:10.1177/1098612x15590867.

16 Rochlitz I. A review of the housing requirements of domestic cats (*Felis silvestris catus*) kept in the home. *Appl. Anim. Behav. Sci.* 2005;93, 97–109.

17 Heath SE. Behaviour problems and welfare. In: Rochlitz I., ed. *The welfare of cats.* Dordrecht, The Netherlands: Springer; 2007;91–118.

18 People's Dispensary for Sick Animals (PDSA) (2013) *The State of Our Pet Nation: Pet Animal Wellbeing (PAW) Report 2013 (UK).* Available at: https://www.pdsa.org.uk/media/2579/paw_report_2013.pdf (accessed June 29, 2020).

19 Grigg EK, Kogan LR. Owners' attitudes, knowledge, and care practices: Exploring the implications for domestic cat behavior and welfare in the home. *Animals.* 2019;9(11). doi:10.3390/ani9110978.

20 Bain M, Stelow E Feline aggression toward family members: A guide for practitioners. *Vet Clin North Am: Small Anim Pract.* 2014;44(3):581–597. doi:10.1016/j.cvsm.2014.01.001.

21 Ramon ME, Slater MR, Ward MP Companion animal knowledge, attachment and pet cat care and their associations with household demographics for residents of a rural Texas town. *Prev Vet Med.* 2010;94:251–263.

22 Welsh CP, Gruffydd-Jones TJ, Roberts MA, Murray JK. Poor owner knowledge of feline reproduction contributes to the high proportion of accidental litters born to UK pet cats. *Vet Rec.* 2014;174:118, doi:10.1136/vr.101909.

23 Howell TJ, Mornement K, Bennett PC Pet cat management practices among a representative sample of owners in Victoria, Australia. *J Vet Behav.* 2016;11:42–49.

24 Mariti C, Guerrini F, Vallini V, Bowen JE, Fatjo J, Diverio S, Sighieri C, Gazzano A. The perception of cat stress by Italian owners. *J Vet Behav.* 2017;20:74–84.

25 Elzerman AL, DePorter TL, Beck A, Collin J-F. Conflict and affiliative behavior frequency between cats in multi-cat households: A survey-based study. *J Feline Med Surg.* 2020;22(8):705–717. doi:10. 1177/1098612X19877988.

26 Finke LR Conspecific and human sociality in the domestic cat: Consideration of proximate mechanisms, human selection and implications for cat welfare. *Animals*. 2022;12:298. doi:10.3390/ani12030298.

27 Farm Animal Welfare Council *Farm animal welfare in Great Britain: Past, present and future*. London, UK: Farm Animal Welfare Council (FAWC); 2009.

28 Ellis JJ, McGowan RTS, Martin F. Does previous use affect litter box appeal in multi-cat households? *Behav Processes*. 2017;141(Pt 3):284–290. doi:10.1016/j.beproc.2017.02.008.

29 Carney HC, Sadek TP, Curtis TM, Halls V, Heath S, Hutchison P, ... Westropp JL. AAFP and ISFM guidelines for diagnosing and solving house-soiling behavior in cats. *J Feline Med Surg*. 2014;16(7):579–598. doi:10.1177/1098612x14539092.

30 Horwitz DF, Rodan I. Behavioral awareness in the feline consultation: Understanding physical and emotional health. *J Felin Med Surg*. 2018;20(5):423–436. doi:10.1177/1098612x18771204.

31 Why do cats act so weird? https://youtu.be/sI8NsYIyQ2A (accessed October 3, 2022).

32 Bennett PC, Rutter NJ, Woodhead JK, Howell TJ. Assessment of domestic cat personality, as perceived by 416 owners, suggests six dimensions. *Behav Processes*. 2017;141:273–283. doi:10.1016/j.beproc.2017.02.020.

33 Bradshaw J. Normal feline behaviour: ... and why problem behaviours develop. *J Feline Med Surg*. 2018;20:411–421.

34 Lipinski MJ, Froenicke L, Baysac KC, Billings NC, Leutenegger CM, Levy AM, Longeri M, Niini T, Ozpinar H, Slater MR, Pedersen NC, Lyons LA.. The ascent of cat breeds: Genetic evaluations of breeds and worldwide random-bred populations. *Genomics*. 2008;91:12–21.

35 Atkinson T. *Practical feline behaviour: Understanding cat behaviour and improving welfare*. Oxfordshire, UK: CABI; 2018:274.

36 Driscoll CA, Menotti-Raymond M, Roca AL, Hupe K, Johnson WE, Geffen E, Harley EH, Delibes M, Pontier D, Kitchener AC, Yamaguchi N, O'Brien SJ, Macdonald DW. The near Eastern origin of cat domestication. *Science*. 2007;317:519–523.

37 Leyhausen P. The tame and the wild – Another just so story? In: Turner DC, Bateson P, eds. *The domestic cat: The biology of its behavior*. Cambridge, UK: Cambridge University Press; 1988;57–66.

38 Bradshaw J. Sociality in cats: A comparative review. *J Vet Behav*. 2016;11:113–124.

39 Ramos D, Reche-Junior A, Fragoso PL, et al. Are cats (Felis catus) from multi-cat households more stressed? Evidence from assessment of fecal glucocorticoid metabolite analysis. *Physiol Behav*. 2013;122:72–75.

40 Chin L. *Cat language*. 2015. Available from: DoggyDrawings.net (accessed July 8, 2020).

41 Kessler MR, Turner DC. Stress and adaptation of cats (*felis silvestris catus*) housed singly, in pairs and in groups in boarding catteries. *Anim Welf*. 1997;6(3):243–254.

42 Overall KL, Rodan I, Beaver B, Carney H, Crowell-Davis S, Hird N, ... Wexler-Mitchell E. *Feline behavior guidelines from the American association of feline practitioners*. 2004. Available at: https://catvets.com/guidelines/practice-guidelines/behavior-guidelines (accessed July 8, 2020).

43 Horwitz DF, Neilson JC. *Blackwell's five-minute veterinary consult: Canine and feline behavior*. Ames, IA: Blackwell Publishing; 2007;595.

44 Griffith C, Steigerwald E, Buffington C. Effects of a synthetic facial pheromone on behavior of cats. *JAVMA*. 2000;217(8):1154–1156.

45 Prior M, Mills D. Cats vs dogs: The efficacy of feliway friends™ and adaptil™ products in multispecies homes. *Front Vet Sci*. 2020;10:July 2020. doi:10.3389/fvets.2020.00399.

46 Frank D, Beauchamp G, Palestrini C. Systematic review of the use of pheromones for treatment of undesirable behavior in cats and dogs. *JAVMA*. 2010;236(12):1308–1316.

47 Pachel CL. Intercat aggression: restoring harmony in the Home: A guide for practitioners. *Vet Clin North Am: Small An Pract*. 2014;44(3):565–579. doi:10.1016/j.cvsm.2014.01.007.

48 American Veterinary Medical Association (AVMA) *Position statements*. 2020. Available at: https://www.avma.org/resources-tools/avma-policies (accessed July 8, 2020).

49 Martell-Moran NK, Solano M, Townsend HGG. Pain and adverse behavior in declawed cats. *J Feline Med Surg*. 2018;20:280–288.

50 American Association of Feline Practitioners (AAFP) *Position statement: Declawing*. 2017. JFMS Clinical Practice NP1. doi:10.1177/1098612X17729246.

51 Stella J, Lord L, Buffington T. Sickness behaviors in response to unusual external events in healthy cats and cats with feline interstitial cystitis. *J Am Vet Med Assoc*. 2011;238(1):67–73. doi:10.2460/javma.238.1.67.

52 Grigg EK, Pick L, Nibblett B. Litter box preference in cats: Covered vs. uncovered. *J Feline Med Surg*. 2012;15:280–284.

53 Neilson J Thinking outside the box: Feline elimination. *J Feline Med Surg*. 2004;6:5–11.

54 Vinke CM, Godijn LM, van der Leij WJR. Will a hiding box provide stress reduction for shelter cats? *Appl Anim Behav Sci*. 2014;160:86–93. doi:10.1016/j.applanim.2014.09.002.

55 Zhang L, McGlone JJ. Scratcher preferences of adult in-home cats and effects of olfactory supplements on cat scratching. *Appl Anim Behav Sci*. 2020;227:104997.

56 Turner DC. The ethology of the human–cat relationship. *Swiss Archive Vet Med*.1991;133:63–70.

57 Turner DC. The mechanics of social interactions between cats and their owners. *Front Vet Sci*. 2021;8. doi:10.3389/fvets.2021.650143.

58 Mertens C. Human-cat interactions in the home setting. *Anthrozoös*. 1991;4:214–231. doi: 10.2752/089279391787057062.

59 Heidenberger E. Housing conditions and behavioural problems of indoor cats as assessed by their owners. *Appl Anim Behav Sci*. 1997;52:345–364.

60 Markowitz H. *Enriching animal lives*. Pacifica, CA: Mauka Press; 2011;246.

61 Bender A, Strong E. *Canine enrichment for the real world*. Wenatchee, WA: Dogwise Publishing. 2019;230.

62 Monroe-Aldridge, et al. AAFP position statement: Environmental enrichment for indoor cats. *JFMS Clinical Practice*. 2011. Available at: https://catvets.com/public/PDFs/PositionStatements/EnviromentalEnhancement-.pdf (accessed July 8, 2020).

63 Hall SL, Bradshaw JWS, Robinson IH. Object play in adult domestic cats: The roles of habituation and disinhibition. *Appl Anim Behav Sci*. 2002;79(3):263–271. doi:10.1016/S0168-1591(02)00153-3.

64 Dantas LM, Delgado MM, Johnson I, Buffington CT. Food puzzles for cats: Feeding for physical and emotional wellbeing. *J Feline Med Surg*. 2016;18(9);723–732. doi:10.1177/1098612x16643753.

65 Masserman JH. Experimental neuroses. *Sci Am*. 1950;182:38–43.

66 Herron M, Buffington T. Environmental enrichment for indoor cats. *Compend Contin Educ Vet*. 2010;Dec; 32(12): E4.

67 Tan SML, Stellato AC, Niel L. Uncontrolled outdoor access for cats: An assessment of risks and benefits. *Animals*. 2020;10(2):258.

68 Karsh E, Turner D. The human–cat relationship. In: Turner DC, Bateson P, eds. *The domestic cat: The biology of its behavior*. Cambridge, UK: Cambridge University Press; 1988:159–177.

69 Lowe S, Bradshaw JWS. Responses of pet cats to being held by an unfamiliar person from weaning to three years of age. *Anthrozoös*. 2002;15:69–79. doi: 10.2752/089279302786992702.

70 McMillan FD. Development of a mental wellness program for animals. *J Am Vet Med Assoc*. 2002;220(7):965–972. doi:10.2460/javma.2002.220.965.

71 Vogt AH, Rodan I, Brown M, Brown S, Buffington CA, Larue Forman MJ, ... Sparkes A AAFP-AAHA: Feline life stage guidelines. *J Feline Med Surg*. 2010;12(1):43–54. doi:10.1016/j.jfms.2009.12.006.

72 Yin S *Low stress handling, restraint and behavior modification of dogs and cats.* Davis, CA: Cattledog Publishing; 2009:469.

73 American Pet Products Association (APPA) *2019–2020 American pet products association national pet owners survey.* Greenwich, CT: American Pet Products Association; 2020.

74 Hart BL, Barrrett RE. Effects of castration on fighting, roaming, and urine spraying in adult male cats. *J Am Vet Med Assoc.* 1973;163:290–292.

75 Kustritz MVR. Determining the optimal age for gonadectomy of dogs and cats. *J Am Vet Med Assoc.* 2007;231(11):1665–1675. doi:10.2460/javma.231.11.1665.

76 Bradshaw J. *Cat sense: How the new feline science can make you a better friend to your pet.* New York: Basic Books; 2013:307.

77 Bradshaw J, Ellis S. *The trainable cat: A practical guide to making life happier for you and your cat.* New York: Basic Books; 2016:352.

78 American Veterinary Society of Animal Behavior (AVSAB) *Position statement: The use of punishment for behavior modification in animals.* 2007. Available at: https://avsab.org/resources/position-statements (Accessed June 1, 2013).

79 Hammerle M, Horst C, Levine E, Overall KL, Radosta L, Rafter-Ritchie M, Yin S. 2015 AAHA canine and feline behavior management guidelines. *J Am Anim Hosp Assoc.* 2015;51:205–221.

4

Play Behavior in Cats

Mikel Delgado

Introduction

Cats are natural predators, but they are often described by their owners as "lazy." Unfortunately, that characterization may be either the cause or result of the insufficient provision of exercise by cat owners. Obesity and behavior problems are rampant among domestic cats,[1-3] and cats who are kept indoors-only may be at particular risk (although it should be noted that obesity and behavior problems are still observed in cats with outdoors access).[4,5] Play can be one part of a broad plan to enrich a cat's environment and provide them with exercise, mental stimulation, and social interactions that may be beneficial to their health and welfare. This chapter will review some characteristics of play in domestic cats, with a focus on the empirical evidence. It will also address play-related problems cat owners may experience with their cats, as well as recommendations for advising clients on providing appropriate play interactions for their cats.

What Is Play and Why Play?

There is no consensus among animal behaviorists for a singular definition of play in animals. It is assumed that play is a pleasurable activity that serves no immediate function for an individual. The movements exhibited during play may resemble those of other functional behaviors such as hunting, fighting, or reproduction, but may be exaggerated, inhibited or out of their usual sequence.[6,7] Play behavior is typically categorized based on presentation as falling into one of the following categories: social, object (Figure 4.1), or locomotor.

Although play is often described as being purposeless, there may be multiple functions and benefits to play. The most noted presumed long-term functions of play include motor training, socialization, cognitive benefits, and information gathering.[6] Following Darwin's principles of evolution via natural selection, in order for play behavior to evolve, there should be variability among individuals for playfulness; playful behavior must be in some part heritable; and there must be some fitness advantage for individuals who play.[8] It has been posited that animals must pay a "cost" to play (such as energy expenditure, or giving up hunting time or vigilance to engage in play), and that because of this cost, play must offer significant benefits to animals. However, at least for domestic cats, it appears that the time budget for playful activities and their related metabolic costs are relatively small.[9]

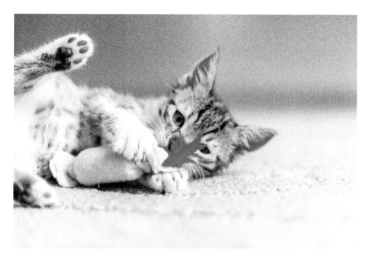

Play is a necessary part of feline enrichment, especially for the indoor-only cat. Photo credit: radub85/Adobe Stock.

Despite this low energetic investment and unclear payoff, cats (and especially kittens) will readily play. We can extrapolate from studies of other species, including humans, what the potential benefits of play are. The commonly cited benefits of play include locomotor training, cognitive training, the development of social relationships, and the ability to learn about and explore one's environment.[10]

It is often assumed that play behavior is training for other "real life" behaviors, such as hunting. Although the play behavior of cats strongly resembles hunting behavior, one study found no differences in the adult prey-related behavior in kittens given the opportunity to play with small objects compared with kittens who were not. This suggests that play opportunities do not improve, and are not necessary, for adult cats to become competent hunters. Experience with actual prey seemed to provide more benefits to later hunting competence.[11–13]

Although play is inexpensive to the individual and may not offer significant direct benefits (i.e., play does not appear to be necessary for cats to develop competency in hunting skills),[11–14] we generally recommend that cat owners play with their cats due to assumed benefits of such activity, including exercise, mental stimulation, and its potentially stress-reducing properties. A problem we will consider throughout this chapter is that there is little research related to play in cats (particularly in adult cats) and little empirical evidence or consensus on how to play with domestic cats in homes.

How Play Develops in Domestic Cats

Most studies of play behavior in cats focus on kittens. Play emerges when kittens begin interacting with littermates or their mother between two and three weeks of age when vision, hearing and motor skills are improving. Although kittens become interested in moving objects by four weeks of age, the activity of littermates is of more interest. Social play peaks between nine and fourteen weeks of age, which is one reason that kittens likely benefit from the presence of littermates at this age.

Object and predatory play emerge and peak later in a kitten's development. Object play appears at around four weeks of age, which coincides with when mother cats begin bringing prey to kittens.

Kittens start to show fewer interactions with littermates and more object play between four and six months of age.[15,16] Kittens prefer to play with small objects such as wine corks, ping pong balls, and the like, presumably because they resemble prey items in their mobility, size, and weight.[17]

There are few studies of play behavior in mature cats, but studies of play that include adults and personal observations by cat owners demonstrate that play is found throughout the lifespan. Cat owners observe social play between adult cats who are on friendly terms, although to date there has been no research specifically focused on this behavior. Adult cats who hunt are observed "playing with their prey," often when they are either less hungry or more fearful of prey animals. Many of the behaviors that appear playful to humans, may in fact be strategic – head bobbing and tentative interactions such as batting may be ways to avoid being bitten or scratched, and may allow hunting cats to test the strength of prey animals.[18]

Although it is assumed that play behavior decreases throughout the lifespan, the onset, rate, or intensity of that decrease is unknown due to a lack of research, and there are likely many individual differences and environmental factors that may contribute. Senior and geriatric cats will continue to play, although the play may be markedly different from that of kittens and young adults. Play bouts may be shorter and of lesser intensity, and it may be more challenging to get older cats engaged in play, as will be discussed later in this chapter.

Body Language during Play

Many behaviors exhibited during play resemble those of both hunting and fighting. An extensive review of the literature summarized the behaviors that had been used to categorize object, predatory and social play.[19] Many behaviors, such as biting, holding, pawing, patting, raking, rearing, or stalking, are exhibited toward an object or a conspecific. Some behaviors have been primarily documented only toward toys or prey, including batting, clutching, chewing, exploration, kicking, kill-biting, licking, mouthing, pinning, sniffing, swiping, and tapping.[17,20] Finally, some behaviors appear to be specific to social play among kittens. These behaviors include back arching, the "belly up" pose, cantering, chasing, crouching, face offs, foot contact, leaping, pouncing, rolling, and wrestling.[21] A "mouth gape" may be a signal between kittens that serves as a play solicitation.[21]

Factors Known to Influence Play in Cats

Play behavior in cats is impacted by several factors. Kittens who do not have littermates direct their play behavior toward their mother. The result is often that the mother avoids her offspring, likely because the play is irritating to her. Conversely, kittens without a mother are more playful with their littermates when compared to litters of kittens with their mothers (Figure 4.2).[22] However, the redirection of play behavior may serve different functions. Lacking playmates, kittens without littermates are likely redirecting that play behavior toward the mother. But kittens without a mother may be increasing play behavior because the absence of maternal care may signal that kittens need to begin hunting at a younger age.[23,24] Maternal deprivation may speed up the developmental processes usually associated with weaning in kittens and this increase in play may be one result.[25]

Once mature and in homes, the play behavior of cats may be either stimulated or inhibited by other animals in the home (including humans). Fear of other animals may increase hiding or withdrawal behavior and reduce playfulness whereas friendly relationships with other animals may stimulate more play and interaction. It is possible that humans who instigate play with their cats

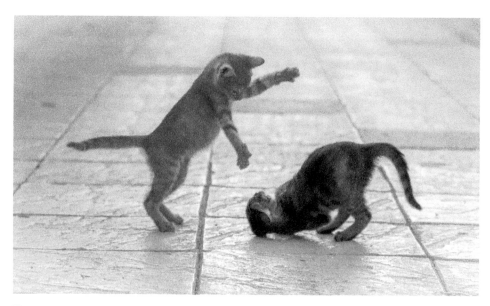

Figure 4.2   Many kitten play behaviors resemble hunting or fighting. Photo courtesy of birgl/Pixabay.

(such as by presenting toys and providing an enriched environment) will observe a higher level of playful behavior throughout their cat's lifespan.

Play is influenced by a cat's hunger; when cats are hungry, they are more likely to play and are more interested in larger, "rat-like" toys; when they are less hungry, they are more likely to engage in play with smaller toys.[26] Cats who are well-fed will still hunt, so although hunting and playing have similar motivations, it is unlikely that hunger is the only factor related to a desire to play. But a cat's willingness to hunt and kill larger, potentially threatening prey (rats versus mice) increases with hunger.[18]

Qualities of toys or play objects affect play responses by cats. Furry-textures, complexity of surface textures, movement, and size all enhance the attractiveness of objects for cats (Figure 4.3).[27,28] Kittens preferred to play with small objects, particularly items that could be moved easily (e.g., corks, ping pong balls).[17] In the same study, kittens initially showed exploratory behaviors toward new objects (e.g., sniffing and touching, moving toward or around the object), then increased playful behavior toward them as the objects became more familiar.

Conversely, adult cats show reduced interaction (habituation) with repeatedly exposure to objects. One study presented cats with the same toy (a faux-fur object on a string) three times with either five, 15- or 25-minute intervals between presentations. Cats consistently showed fewer clutches and bites to the toy by the third presentation, suggesting habituation. On a fourth trial, cats were presented with an identical, differently colored object (which presumably also did not have the cat's odor on it). Cats showed increased responding to the novel toy, and in the case of 5-minute intervals, the responding to the new toy was greater than the response to the first presentation of the original toy.[29] This finding suggests that cats may remain highly motivated to play, despite an apparent decrease in responding to an individual toy.

Novelty and change-ability may therefore represent two key features of toys that maintain a cat's interest in play. Habituation to a non-changing prey item may prevent cats from engaging with a prey animal longer than is useful. Changes in prey, such as bleeding, a decrease in temperature, or the breaking down of skin, fur or feathers, serve as signals to cats that their predation efforts are

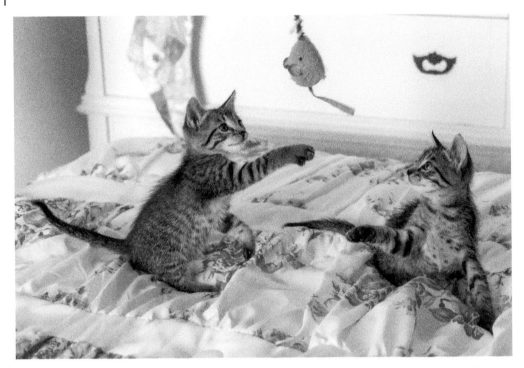

Figure 4.3 When cats are hungry, they are more likely to play with rat-like toys. Photo courtesy of Michelle_Raponi/Pixabay.

successful;[28] a failure to physically damage the object, or a lack of change in these physical properties could signal to the cat that the object is not actually prey, or that the prey animal is too strong and is resisting predation attempts. Thus, a cat can conserve predatory efforts by stopping engagement with an object or prey that does not change in form.

Play and Welfare

In many contexts, animal play is considered a sign of positive welfare. For example, play often indicates a lack of threat or chronic environmental stressors such as hunger, injury, or predation risk.[30] Play has been identified as one of the ten behavioral indicators of feline well-being.[31] Playful behavior in cats is observed less frequently or not at all in conditions associated with stress, including overcrowding,[27] being housed in shelters,[32] and being previously declawed.[33] However, play also increases in some situations that would be considered stressful, such as in kittens experiencing premature maternal separation.[22-24] Therefore, the presence of play cannot be a sole indicator of welfare or lack thereof.

The potential neurochemical effects of play are not well understood. In some animals, social play activates or involves the dopaminergic or cannabinoid systems.[34] Activity, play, and enrichment all likely have generally anxiolytic effects,[35,36] but animals experiencing high levels of stress are less likely to play.[37] Animals under lower levels of stress may be more likely to benefit from opportunities to play and exercise, and in these cases, play may be therapeutic. For example, play is recommended as one part of a multi-modal environmental modification program to treat feline with chronic lower urinary tract signs.[38]

Due to a lack of research, it is unknown whether a lack of play decreases the welfare of cats or even how much play would be required for good welfare. At least in some cats, a lack of play can lead to problems as diverse as increased aggression and obesity.[39] Therefore, play should be modified and tailored to the needs of an individual cat based on guidelines presented later in this chapter. The cat's behaviors during play can be assessed to help determine preferences and ways to encourage positive responses.

Although play may not be necessary for the good welfare of all cats, it engages cats in both cognitive and physical interactions, and can stimulate natural predatory behaviors. Importantly, play should not decrease welfare (for example, by frightening the cat). Play can also provide secondary benefits such as being used as a reinforcer during behavior modification. For cats that do not tolerate a lot of handling or who are not outwardly affectionate, play can be an effective way for owners to interact with and bond with them.

Social Play in Cats

Social play is very important to young kittens, especially during the period between two and four months of age.[15] As our understanding of cat social behavior increases, the importance of family in the formation of colonies becomes more apparent.[40] Many cats, especially when younger, benefit from having the companionship of other cats. Unfamiliar cats who are introduced when young are more likely to have a positive relationship later in life.

Play between adult cats is understudied; one study found that 15% of cat owners reported that their cat played with other cats,[41] but the ages of the cats and the nature of this play was not described. In some cases, social play can serve as a bridge between cats – such as by building the confidence of a shy cat who is friendly toward other cats. In households where there might be an energetic mismatch (e.g., a senior cat with a kitten or teenager), the addition of a cat to serve as a playmate for the more active cat can take some of the pressure off the older or more sedentary cat. Later in this chapter, concerns with discerning play and fighting in socially housed cats, as well as problems related to the management of play in multi-cat households, are addressed.

Working with Clients to Help Them Understand Cats' Play Needs

There is no empirical basis for assessing how much play a cat needs; almost all cat owners in one survey reported that they played with their cats daily.[2] However, the nature of that play was unclear from the survey, and only 39% of respondents reported using "fishing pole toys." The most commonly provided toys were solo toys, such as furry mice, catnip toys, and balls with bells.[2] Another study of cat owners reported 43% of cats played with humans,[41] but again the nature of the play is unclear from the survey questions.

Play should be framed as an opportunity to provide cats with an outlet for a species-typical behavior: hunting. This may help clients better understand why an interactive toy will be more engaging for most cats than a "dead" solo toy. Lacking many empirical studies on what types of play cats respond to best, we can inform our recommendations by looking at the research on felid hunting behavior. Owners can then structure their play sessions to simulate the natural hunting sequence observed in most cats.

General Recommendations for Play with Cats

- **Cats are stalk and rush hunters**: Rather than pursue prey until they are exhausted like some predators (persistence hunters) do, cats depend on their ability to detect prey and approach carefully. Once they are close enough, they will rush at their prey.[42] Cats should be allowed opportunity to watch and slowly approach the toy before pouncing.
- **Short and often**: Short burst activity means that some cats prefer several short play sessions throughout the day, rather than one longer session.
- **Appropriate pacing:** The pace of activity may need to vary; owners should alternate speed of toy movements. Very slow movements of the toy may initially solicit more response.
- **Play needs may be age dependent**: Kittens and younger cats may need or respond to more frequent play or longer play sessions than older cats.
- **Clients should understand the difference between interactive and solo play**: Interactive play requires humans to move the toy for the cat and may be instigated by human or cat; solo play is play that is motivated purely by the cat's activity/interest.
- **What is an "interactive toy?"** Interactive toys include wands or rods with attachments, such as string or wire. These toys often have objects attached at the end, which may resemble prey animals such as bugs, birds, mice, or snakes (Figure 4.4). These toys require human manipulation to move them in a prey-like fashion.

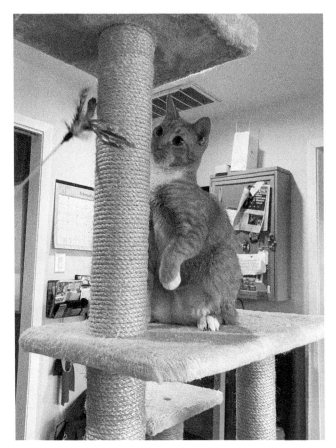

Figure 4.4 Clients should be helped to understand that interactive toys, like wands toys, provide an outlet for the cat's need to hunt. Photo courtesy of Liz Stelow.

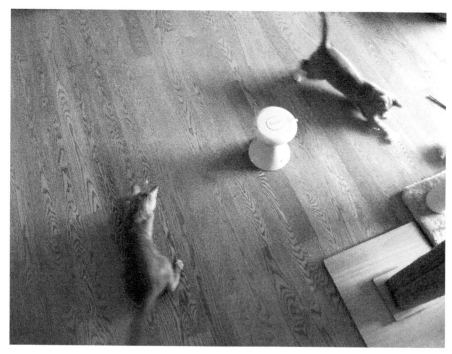

Figure 4.5   Automated toys can provide an outlet for play when owners are busy; but they are no substitute for interactive play. Photo courtesy of Liz Stelow.

- **Prey preferences**: Some cats who hunt are specialists, preferring one prey type, and others are generalists.[43] Similarly, cats may have preferences for toys that resemble specific prey types, such as birds, mice, lizards, and bugs.[38]
- **Safety:** Interactive toys should be locked away when not in use; strings and wires can otherwise present a strangulation or choking hazard. Toys should be inspected routinely for damage or small parts that could be swallowed.
- **Automated and digital toys**: Other types of toys that can stimulate play activity include lasers and automated (battery-operated) toys. There are also tablet or screen-based digital games that some cats may respond to. In general, these toys should be a supplement to interactive play, not a replacement for it (Figure 4.5).
- **A need for physical contact**: Cats should be allowed regular contact with a moving interactive toy. Owners should not "tease" the cat or always keep the toy out of reach of the cat, as clutching and biting the toy are regular features of play in cats. Because laser pointers and other forms of "digital play" do not allow the cat to "catch" the prey, some have posited that they may lead to frustration.[44] Although "light-obsession" has not been documented in cats and some cats respond well to other forms of 2-D stimulation such as videos,[44] it is observed in dogs that are exposed to laser lights.[45]
- **Sensory engagement**: Clients should be encouraged to engage multiple senses during play (vision, hearing, olfaction, touch, etc.) during play, just as cats would utilize when hunting. Interactive toys can be moved under a piece of tissue paper to create a rustling sound, which has been observed to solicit hunting behavior.[27] Catnip or similar olfactory enrichment (silvervine, valerian, honeysuckle) may stimulate some cats to play.[46]

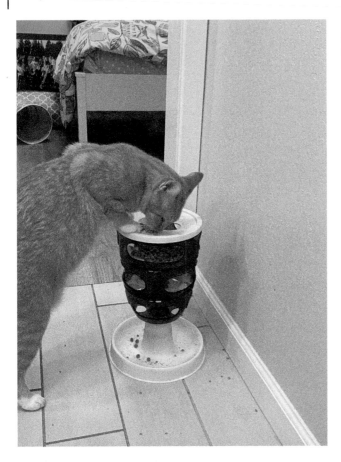

Figure 4.6 Cats can be encouraged to eat from food toys and puzzles as additional mental exercise. Photo courtesy of Liz Stelow.

- **Move toys like prey**: Owners should be encouraged to move toys like prey might move, allowing cats to make occasional contact with toy;[47] mimicking different types of prey, and changing the speed and direction of movements.[48]
- **Rotate toys to prevent habituation and boredom**: Because research has demonstrated that cats habituate to the same toy before they tire of playing,[29] owners should switch out toys both during and between play sessions. Cats should have several toy options available for interactive play.
- **Play on empty stomach**: Cats are more likely to hunt and play when hungry.[26] Owners can schedule play sessions before mealtimes to increase activity/response to toys.
- **Food play**: Cat owners can encourage activity and provide mental stimulation for their cats by encouraging them to "play with their food" via food puzzles (Figure 4.6),[49] by hiding small amounts of food for their cats in different areas of the home to encourage foraging/search behavior, or by tossing individual kibbles for their cat to catch and eat.

Challenges Related to Play Behavior

At your practice, clients may report problems related to play behavior in their cats. Because clients may not readily volunteer information about a cat's play behavior, questions about activity and play can be incorporated into your existing history-taking process. Questions such as "does your cat like to play" or "has your cat's playful behavior changed since your last visit" will prompt clients to ask you questions, and may also reveal issues that suggest further inquiry is needed; for example, a decline in play in an adult cat could indicate a painful condition such as joint degeneration.

Commonly reported problems usually fall into a few categories: lack of interest or difficulty engaging a cat in play; challenges with special-needs cats; aggression or roughness toward humans during play behavior; and play-related problems in multi-cat households. Addressing each type of problem will require understanding the underlying motivation(s), and referral to a veterinary behaviorist may be warranted in some cases. The context under which the behavior concerns, the owner or other cat's response, and level of enrichment/activity provided for the cat may all provide clues as to an appropriate modification plan and solutions.

Lack of Interest in Play

Many owners report that their cat has little interest in play (Figure 4.7); this is more likely to be a concern of owners of adult or elderly cats. In many cases, the play of adult cats looks dissimilar from play in young cats or kittens, and the owner may misinterpret these changes in play behavior as a lack of interest. Alternatively, many owners may find that if they change their play style, that their cats will still engage with interactive toys.

Play for adult cats will primarily be interactive, meaning that the owner will move a toy for the cat. Adult cats often have less interest in small objects that require self-directed play. Owners may also have to change how they move toys, focusing more on small movements of the toy, or by partially hiding the toy under the corner of a rug, towel, or piece of tissue paper. Cats are naturally attracted to certain aspects of prey behavior that elicit hunting behavior, such as fast movement away from them, rustling sounds, and lying in wait at the hiding sight of prey resembling the entryway of a burrow.[27] These features can be replicated in play and may increase the responsiveness of an adult cat that is otherwise challenging to play with.

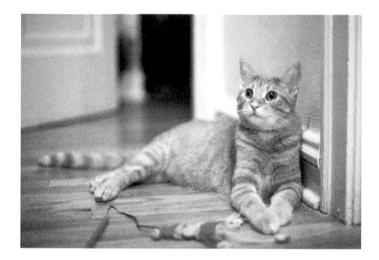

Figure 4.7 Sometimes cats show lack of interest in play. Owners can change their play style to try to engage the cat. Photo credit: Page Light Studios/Adobe Stock.

Special-Needs Cats

The same methods that can be used to encourage play in disinterested cats can also work with older cats, chronically ill cats, or cats with physical limitations. In any case, owners can modify the environment as needed: older cats, cats with missing limbs or with degenerative joint disease will benefit from ramps or steps to allow them to climb, rather than jump, onto elevated surfaces to play. The pacing of play may need to be slower, and the toy may need to be more accessible. The mantra for playing with these cats should be "weaker predator, weaker prey." Many owners interpret a subdued response in special-needs cats as a lack of interest on behalf of the cat. Instead, they should accept that for some cats, just watching or gently batting at the toy is play.

Fearful cats may also prefer quieter, smaller toys, that resemble bugs, rather than larger toys or toys with bells or that make other noises. They may also be more responsive to smaller, less frenetic movements of toys. Shy cats may also prefer to play with some amount of cover, such as while they are in a cubby, cardboard box, or other hiding spot that provides them with a sense of protection.

Aggressive or Rough Behavior toward Humans

Aggressive behaviors (biting, scratching, pouncing) related to play can happen during play, or at other times (such as while the owner is walking around the home, sleeping, or trying to interact with the cat in other ways, such as petting). These behaviors may be undesirable to most cat owners, but encouraged by others.

During play, predatory behaviors should be directed toward a toy. Interactive toys are ideal because they naturally create distance between human body parts, and the object that a cat is biting, clutching, or scratching. Holding a small toy (such as a furry mouse) in one's hand while encouraging the cat to pursue it in a predatory manner may lead to inadvertent bites and scratches. Small toys should instead be tossed, or reserved for the cat to use in self (solo) play. Some cats may follow the movement of the hand instead of the toy on the end of the string/wire; a toy with a longer handle may prevent this. Otherwise, owners may want to wear a glove or hide their hand in their sleeve while directing their cat toward the movement of the toy. Finally, trying a variety of interactive toys will allow owners to find toys that their cat is most responsive to. Their hand may be more attractive than the toy currently being offered.

Roughhousing in the form of using hands as toys, wrestling with a cat, or otherwise provoking a cat to elicit biting or scratching should be discouraged. Many cat owners may encourage this kind of behavior when kittens are small and damage from biting and scratching may be minimal. However, it is believed that in some cats, there are risks to this type of interaction. Some cats may bite and scratch as adults, they may bite harder, or become defensive about other types of interactions.[48] They may direct the biting and scratching toward some individuals in the home, which can be especially problematic in households with young children, immune-compromised adults or individuals on anti-coagulants.

An ounce of prevention is worth a pound of cure in this case, but some cats may still attempt to bite or scratch body parts, even when these behaviors are not encouraged by owners. Cats may pounce on their owner's arms and legs, exhibit stalking behaviors, and ambush or chase their owners. Some cats may also resist an end to a play session, and it may be difficult to get them to calm down after playing with a toy. In response to these types of issues, some owners believe that they should cease play altogether rather than allow the cat to get overly excited. However, a lack of play may just increase frustration and behavior problems if the cat does not have adequate outlets for predatory and playful behaviors.

Prevention and Behavior Modification for Playful or Predatory Aggressive Behaviors

Here are some general guidelines that may be helpful for clients dealing with problematic play or predatory aggression in their cats:

- **Direct all play behavior toward toys**: All playful and predatory behaviors should be directed toward toys, rather than body parts (Figure 4.8).
- **Consistency in handling is important**: All members of the household need to be consistent in respecting a cat's boundaries and not using hands for play.
- **Accept that the cat may not want petting**: Owners often want to pet or handle kittens and cats when the cat would prefer other types of interaction. It is important to recognize that forced handling of cats when they do not want to be touched is a form of flooding that may not only lead to bites and scratches, but can make the cat less likely to appreciate human approaches in the future.[50]
- **Limit petting**: Cats should not be petted during a play session.
- **Avoid chase/hide and seek games**: Activities where owners chase their cats or hide and surprise their cats may elicit some conflicting or negative emotional states, such as fear, in some cats. Although cats may respond to chase games or rough-housing, it may be that they are not being offered other, appropriate types of play and are accepting whatever interaction is available to them.
- **Energy cannot be "squashed"**: Some owners, fearing that play gets their cat too wound up, may cease playing altogether. However, playful and predatory behavior needs an outlet, and a lack of play will likely only make the problem worse.[51]
- **Increase play with interactive toys**: It is implied (although has not been empirically tested) that there is a relationship between increased play opportunities and decreased aggression.[47]
- **Increase cardio activity via vertical space**: Play "effort" can be increased by incorporating vertical space (cat condos/trees/shelving or human furniture) into the interactive play, encouraging cats to climb or jump.
- **Wind down the play**: To end a play session, owners can move the toy slowly to bring the cat's heart rate and excitement level down. This decreases the likelihood that the cat will be left frustrated and consequently redirect toward human body parts.

Figure 4.8   Using hands to play with a cat is a risk factor for human-directed play aggression. Photo credit: photosaint/Adobe Stock.

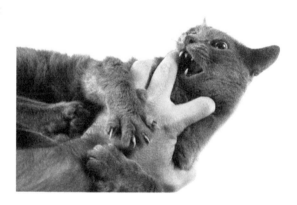

- **End play with a snack**: Much as hunting often ends with a meal, a play session can be ended with food to calm the cat down. Ending play with food also helps the cat build a positive association with the end of play via classical conditioning.

- **Minimize response to aggression to avoid provoking excitement or fear**: If a cat bites or scratches in play, it is advised to avoid having a large physical reaction to the incident. Screaming, yelling, or rapid movement may increase the cat's predatory response, or may make the cat respond in a fearfully defensive manner.[48]

- **"Time out"**: Instead of having a large reaction to bites and scratches, owners should stay calm and leave the room or avoid interaction with the cat momentarily.[48,50] The cat will calm down and will also learn that its behavior leads to a withdrawal of attention (negative punishment in the four quadrants of operant conditioning). The desired outcome is reduced likelihood of biting and scratching in the future. Owners should leave the room rather than trying to move the cat to another room for a "time out," which could lead to further bites or scratches if the cat is aroused.

- **Physical punishment is not helpful**: Scruffing, spanking, nose-tapping, spray bottles, and other types of corrections are not appropriate responses to any behavior problem. These types of responses (positive punishment in the four quadrants of operant conditioning) may increase fear and reactivity, while diminishing the human-animal bond.

- **Distraction**: Some cats can be prevented from playful/predatory pouncing by directing that motivation toward other objects (Figure 4.9). Owners can carry small toys (fuzzy mice, jingle balls, etc.) and toss them away from their body as they move around the house.

- **Differential reinforcement of other behaviors (DRO)**: Training and reinforcement for alternative behaviors than stalking or pouncing on owners can help owners focus on desirable behaviors (e.g., sitting, going to a mat, targeting), increasing the likelihood that a cat will exhibit those behaviors in the future.

- **Kittens/young cats may do best with a playmate with a similar temperament**: Some playfully aggressive cats, especially kittens or young adults, may show noticeable improvement if they have a companion cat of a similar activity/energy level and they are social with other cats.

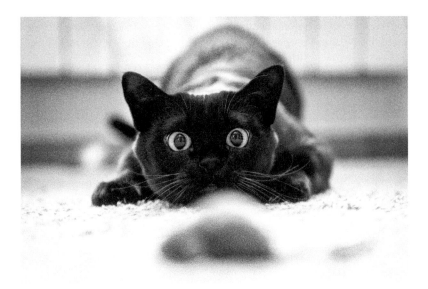

Figure 4.9 Owners can toss a toy to distract a cat from pouncing on them during play. Photo credit: scaliger/Adobe Stock.

Play-related Conflict in Multi-cat Households

Cat owners may have difficulty distinguishing playing from fighting among familiar cats.[52] Play between cats, especially between younger cats, may at times appear quite rough, although generally is significantly more inhibited than when cats fight. During play, injuries are rare, and playing cats are typically able to be distracted by a noise or other activity in the room. Cats who play often take turns chasing each other, whereas fights between cats are often one-sided, consistently with one cat pursuing the other. Play is generally quiet with the occasional small hiss or growl, as opposed to fighting, which often involves shrieking, yowling, or screaming. Most importantly, cats who play show other signs of being "preferred associates,"[40] such as sleeping together or in the same room, allogrooming and rubbing, and exhibiting the "tail up" signal when approaching one another.[40,53] Aggressive behaviors in the absence of friendly signs suggest a more serious problem, that may require the intervention of a veterinary behaviorist or psychopharmaceuticals.

Problems can also arise when cat owners try to play with multiple cats simultaneously. One cat may monopolize an interactive toy, preventing other cats from playing. Owners may interpret this as the other cats being less interested in play, rather than recognizing that one cat is being inhibited by the presence of the other cat.

Addressing Play Concerns in Multi-cat Households

- **Playing or fighting?** Clients may need guidance as to how to distinguish between playing and fighting (Figure 4.10). It is also possible that at times, otherwise friendly cats may have negative interactions, so broader patterns of relations between the cats may need to be assessed.[52] For inter-cat aggression concerns, also see Chapter 11, "Aggression toward other cats," and Chapter 14, "Cat relationships in the home."

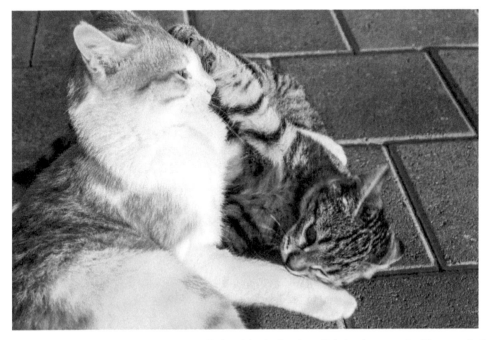

Figure 4.10 It is sometimes difficult to distinguish playing from fighting between familiar cats. Body language and vocal communication can help. Photo courtesy of dimitrisvetsikas1969/Pixabay.

- **Energy mismatch:** Younger cats may be annoying to senior or geriatric cats, especially if they try to solicit play or do not respect the older cat's personal space. Younger cats may need additional mental stimulation and exercise; older cats may need a private refuge/retreat where they can get a break from the younger cat.
- **Play with cats separately while confined**: In cases where one cat monopolizes play, it may be necessary to play with cats in separate areas of the home with a closed door between them. This allows a cat who is inhibited by the behavior of another cat to play freely.
- **Increased and separate resources:** Providing multiple resources in separated areas in the home can reduce competition and tension between co-housed cats.
- **Manage/separate as necessary:** Clients may need to manage problems between cats by separating the cats temporarily, on a daily schedule, or by providing access to safe spaces (such as with a microchip controlled cat door) to one or more cats.
- **Classical counterconditioning**: Positive associations can be made between cats by bringing them together for favored treats.
- **Differential Reinforcement of Other behaviors (DRO):** Training and reinforcement for alternative behaviors than stalking or pouncing on other cats can help owners focus on desirable behaviors (e.g., sitting calmly together), increasing the likelihood that cats will exhibit those behaviors together in the future.
- **Interrupt rough play if necessary:** Owners should supervise any play that seems rough; play can be briefly interrupted by dropping a magazine on the floor or by tossing a toy away from the cats. Aversives, including spray bottles, should be avoided. If cats are difficult to separate or appear to be fighting, a blanket, large pillow or piece of cardboard may be placed between the cats to separate them. Owners should consider that aroused cats may not be safe to handle. Frequent rough play, especially if one cat does not seem to be a willing recipient of play attempts, may require the assistance of a behavior professional.
- **Distraction/prevention:** As with playful/predatory behaviors toward humans, some cats can be redirected away from similar behaviors toward other household cats via distraction (e.g., tossing toys away from the cat being stalked).

Summary

To sum, there are still significant gaps in the study and understanding of cat play behavior. As clinicians, it is important to make recommendations for cat owners that are based in the natural ethology and hunting behavior of domestic cats to the extent possible while recognizing that some of these recommendations may not have an empirical basis at this time. Hopefully, the gaps in our knowledge will be addressed by future research.

Play likely provides many benefits for domestic cats, including providing an important outlet for species-typical behaviors such as hunting. Interactive play may strengthen the cat–human bond and may have anxiolytic effects for cats, while providing exercise and its related health benefits. Play can also be part of a treatment plan for stress-related disorders. Based on studies of other animals, and the existing research on cat play behavior, we can conclude that play likely improves the welfare of most, if not all, cats.

There are several ways for clients to improve their play technique, and to use play for behavior modification in their pet cats. This chapter has also addressed specific ways to counsel clients on problematic play behaviors they may encounter with their cats. Clinicians can also encourage their clients to provide appropriate play for their cats in several ways, including asking questions about play while taking a medical and behavioral history, by having educational handouts available for their clientele, and by selling appropriate interactive toys at their practice.

References

1 Amat M, de la Torre, JLR, Fatjó J, et al. Potential risk factors associated with feline behaviour problems. *Appl Anim Behav Sci.* 2009;121:134–139.
2 Strickler BL, Shull EA. An owner survey of toys, activities, and behavior problems in indoor cats. *J Vet Behav.* 2014;9:207–214.
3 Rowe E, Browne W, Casey R, et al. Risk factors identified for owner-reported feline obesity at around one year of age: Dry diet and indoor lifestyle. *Prev Vet Med.* 2015;121:273–281.
4 Levine E, Perry P, Scarlett J, et al. Intercat aggression in households following the introduction of a new cat. *Appl Anim Behav Sci.* 2005;90:325–336.
5 Colliard L, Paragon BM, Lemuet B, et al. Prevalence and risk factors of obesity in an urban population of healthy cats. *J Feline Med Surg.* 2009;11:135–140.
6 Burghardt GM. On the origins of play. In: Smith PK, ed. *Play in animals and humans.* New York, NY: Basil Blackwell Inc NY; 1984:5–42.
7 Bekoff M, Beyers JA. A critical reanalysis of the ontogeny and phylogeny of mammalian social and locomotor play: An ethological hornet's nest. In: Immelmann K, Barlow GW, Petrinovich L, Main M, eds. *Behavioral development.* Cambridge: Cambridge University Press; 1981:296–337.
8 Darwin C. *The origin of species and the descent of man.* NY, NY: Modern library; 1859.
9 Martin P. The time and energy costs of play behaviour in the cat. *Zeitschrift für Tierpsychologie.* 1984;64:298–312.
10 Bekoff M, Byers JA. *Animal play.* Cambridge, UK: Cambridge University Press; 1998.
11 Caro TM. Effects of the mother, object play, and adult experience on predation in cats. *Behav and Neural Biol.* 1980;29:29–51.
12 Caro TM. The effects of experience on the predatory patterns of cats. *Behav and Neural Biol.* 1980;29:1–28.
13 Caro TM. Relations between kitten behaviour and adult predation. *Zeitschrift für Tierpsychologie.* 1979;51:158–168.
14 Caro TM. Predatory behaviour and social play in kittens. *Behaviour.* 1981;76:1–24.
15 Mendoza DL, Ramirez JM. Play in kittens (*Felis domesticus*) and its association with cohesion and aggression. *Bull Psychon Soc.* 1987;25:27–30.
16 Barrett P, Bateson PP. The development of play in cats. *Behaviour.* 1978;66:106–120.
17 West MJ. Exploration and play with objects in domestic kittens. *Dev Psychobiol.* 1977;10:53–57.
18 Biben M. Predation and predatory play behaviour of domestic cats. *Anim Behav.* 1979;27:81–94.
19 Delgado M, Hecht J. A review of the development and functions of cat play, with future research considerations. *Appl Anim Behav Sci.* 2019;214:1–17.
20 Egan J. Object-play in cats. In: Bruner JS, Jolly A, Sylva K, eds. *Play: Its role in development and evolution.* NY, NY: Penguin; 1976:161–165.
21 West M. Social play in the domestic cat. *Am Zool.* 1974;14:427–436.
22 Bateson P, Young M. Separation from the mother and the development of play in cats. *Anim Behav.* 1981;29:173–180.
23 Bateson P, Martin P, Young M. Effects of interrupting cat mothers' lactation with bromocriptine on the subsequent play of their kittens. *Physiol Behav.* 1981;27:841–845.

24 Bateson P, Mendl M, Feaver J. Play in the domestic cat is enhanced by rationing of the mother during lactation. *Anim Behav*. 1990;40:514–525.

25 Martin P. An experimental study of weaning in the domestic cat. *Behaviour*. 1986;99:221–249.

26 Hall SL, Bradshaw JWS. The influence of hunger on object play by adult domestic cats. *Appl Anim Behav Sci*. 1998;58:143–150.

27 Leyhausen P. *Cat behaviour*. New York, NY: Garland; 1979.

28 Hall SL, Bekoff M, Byers JA. Object play by adult animals. In: Bekoff & Byers, ed. *Animal play*. Cambridge, UK: Cambridge University Press; 1998:45–60.

29 Hall SL, Bradshaw JWS, Robinson IH. Object play in adult domestic cats: The roles of habituation and disinhibition. *Appl Anim Behav Sci*. 2002;79:263–271.

30 Held SDE, Špinka M. Animal play and animal welfare. *Anim Behav*. 2011;81:891–899.

31 Fraser AF. *Feline behaviour and welfare*. Oxfordshire, UK: CABI; 2012.

32 Moore AM, Bain MJ. Evaluation of the addition of in-cage hiding structures and toys and timing of administration of behavioral assessments with newly relinquished shelter cats. *J Vet Behav*. 2013;8:450–457.

33 Duffy DL, de Moura RTD, Serpell JA. Development and evaluation of the Fe-BARQ: A new survey instrument for measuring behavior in domestic cats (*Felis s. catus*). *Behav Process*. 2017;141:329–341.

34 Trezza V, Vanderschuren LJ. Cannabinoid and opioid modulation of social play behavior in adolescent rats: Differential behavioral mechanisms. *Eur Neuropsychopharmacol*. 2008;18:519–530.

35 Guszkowska M. Effects of exercise on anxiety, depression and mood. *Psychiatria Polska*. 2004;38:611–620.

36 Haug LI. Canine aggression toward unfamiliar people and dogs. *Vet Clin North Am: Small Anim Pract*. 2008;38:1023–1041.

37 Klein ZA, Padow VA, Romeo RD. The effects of stress on play and home cage behaviors in adolescent male rats. *Dev Psychobiol*. 2010;52:62–70.

38 Westropp JL, Delgado M, Buffington CAT. Chronic lower urinary tract signs in cats: Current understanding of pathophysiology and management. *Vet Clin: Small Anim Pract*. 2019;49:187–209.

39 Heath SE. Behaviour problems and welfare. In: Rochlitz I ed. *The welfare of cats*. The Netherlands: Springer Dordrecht; 2007:91–118.

40 Crowell-Davis SL, Curtis TM, Knowles RJ. Social organization in the cat: A modern understanding. *J Feline Med Surg*. 2004;6:19–28.

41 Shyan-Norwalt MR. Caregiver perceptions of what indoor cats do "for fun". *J Appl Anim Welf Sci*. 2005;8:199–209.

42 Beaver BV. *Feline behavior*. St Louis, MO: Elsevier Health Sciences; 2003.

43 Dickman CR, Newsome TM. Individual hunting behaviour and prey specialisation in the house cat Felis catus: Implications for conservation and management. *Appl Anim Behav Sci*. 2015;173:76–87.

44 Ellis SLH, Wells DL. The influence of visual stimulation on the behaviour of cats housed in a rescue shelter. *Appl Anim Behav Sci*. 2008;113:166–174.

45 Luescher UA, McKeown DB, Halip J. Stereotypic or obsessive-compulsive disorders in dogs and cats. *Vet Clin North Am: Small Anim Pract*. 1991;21:401–413.

46 Bol S, Caspers J, Buckingham L, et al. Responsiveness of cats (*Felidae*) to silver vine (*Actinidia polygama*), Tatarian honeysuckle (*Lonicera tatarica*), valerian (*Valeriana officinalis*) and catnip (*Nepeta cataria*). *BMC Vet Res*. 2017;13:70.

47 Ellis SL, Rodan I, Carney HC, et al. AAFP and ISFM feline environmental needs guidelines. *J Feline Med Surg.* 2013;15:219–230.

48 Rodan I, Heath S. *Feline behavioral health and welfare.* St Louis, MO: Elsevier Health Sciences; 2015.

49 Dantas LM, Delgado MM, Johnson I, et al. Food puzzles for cats: Feeding for physical and emotional wellbeing. *J Feline Med Surg.* 2016;18:723–732.

50 Overall K. *Manual of clinical behavioral medicine for dogs and cats.* St Louis, MO: Elsevier Health Sciences; 2013.

51 Hetts S. *Pet behavior protocols: What to say, what to do, when to refer.* Lakewood, CO: AAHA press; 1999.

52 Elzerman AL, DePorter TL, Beck A, et al. Conflict and affiliative behavior frequency between cats in multi-cat households: A survey-based study. *J Feline Med Surg.* 2019. doi: 10.1177/1098612X19877988.

53 Cafazzo S, Natoli E. The social function of tail up in the domestic cat (*Felis silvestris catus*). *Behav Process.* 2009;80:60–66.

5

Feeding Behavior of Cats

Katherine Albro Houpt VMD PhD

Introduction

Feeding a cat is often a pleasurable experience for owner and cat alike. This chapter delves into the whys and how of normal feline feeding as well as the clinical problems of obesity, pica, hyperphagia, and anorexia.

What's Normal

Many cats regulate their food intake to match their exercise level. They often follow a cycle of play/exercise – eat a small meal – sleep/rest. For feral or a free-fed cat, meals can happen 8–20 times per day.

Cats prefer to eat alone.

What's Normal but Unacceptable:

Because cats eat round the clock, some get into the habit of waking their owners during the night or early in the morning to be fed. While this is part of the cat's normal feeding routine, the owners can be less than happy about it.

A cat's disinterest in different types of food offered by the owner can create some tension and label that cat as "picky," when it is simply typical cat resistance to new food categories.

Predatory behavior can be unacceptable to owners if other pets or wildlife are being harassed.

What's Abnormal but Often Acceptable?

Some cats, whether free-fed or meal fed, eat more than they need to maintain their energy. These cats tend toward obesity.

Offering one food bowl for multiple cats can create competition, and often a lower-ranked cat with less access to resources.

Owners may overlook pica, unless it causes an obstruction.

Some cats show signs of hyperphagia – constantly being hungry. They may steal food or be aggressive around food they find. Typically, there is a history of food deprivation at some point in that cat's life.

Obesity is a diagnosis among indoor cats and can cause many health problems. It may be acceptable to owner until those health problems arise and must be addressed.

Understanding the Physiological Controls of Feeding

Some of the early experiments on the control of food intake were performed on cats. Cats with lesion in the lateral hypothalamus stopped eating, whereas those with lesions in the ventromedial hypothalamus become obese. We now know that there are not specific "centers" in the brain for feeding, but rather a complex interaction of neurotransmitter and signals from the body that lead to hunger or satiety.

A variety of factors influence feeding in cats. Glucoreceptors that suppress feeding in cats appear to be present in the liver.[1] Gastric factors, particularly gastric fill, can suppress feeding and the hormone ghrelin can stimulate it. Changes within the intestinal, tract, such as an increase in osmotic pressure and release of the hormones cholecystokinin (CCK), Cholecystokinin-pancreozymin and bombesin, a peptide related to CCK, suppress food intake of cats[2,3] due to their effect on brain neuropeptides. The neuropeptides involved are NPY (Neuropeptide Y), AGRP (agouti-related protein) orexin (hypocretin) and MCH (melanin-concentrating hormone) which stimulate feeding and alpha melanocyte stimulating hormone (MSH), corticotropin releasing hormone (CRH), thyrotropin releasing hormone (TRH), cocaine and amphetamine-regulated transcript (CART) and interleukin-1 which inhibit feeding.[4] Leptin is a hormone that is released from fat cells and it acts on the brain to reduce food intake through the system just described.

There is a colony of cats at the University of Zurich that has a genetic predisposition to obesity. The genotyping analysis identified markers in the regions of the chromosome D3 containing melanocortin receptor 4 (*MC4R*) and neuropeptide Y receptor 1 (*NPY1R*). The obesity is a result of consuming more energy even as kittens, not of using less energy.[5]

There has not been a complete study of the effect of temperature on food intake in cats, but one demonstration showed that cold environmental temperature, rather than changes in brain or body temperature, affects feeding. This early study found that cats drinking milk not only show a decline in brain temperature but also cease to eat.[6] If brain temperature was the factor affecting feeding, one would expect the cat to eat even more as its brain temperature fell.

Reproductive hormones affect body weight. Ovariohysterectomized and castrated cats have a lower metabolic rate,[7] and if the cat is fed all it wants of a very palatable food and is not very active, obesity can result.

Defense of Body Weight

The most important determinant of body weight in cats appears to be cyclical in nature. Cats lose and gain body weight in cycles of several months' duration.[8–10] Food intake was least in the summer months (e.g. June to August), and greatest during the months of late autumn and winter (e.g. October to February), with intermediate intake in the spring (e.g. March to May) and early autumn (e.g. September). For this reason, it has been difficult to demonstrate defense of body weight. There have been two studies in which it appeared that when their diet was diluted, cats did not eat more and, therefore, lost weight.[11,12] In both studies, the diet, a dry food, was diluted with a dry diluent, either kaolin or cellulose. The cats actually ate a smaller volume than they ate of the undiluted food, indicating that it was unpalatable. In contrast, when cats' food is diluted with water, they do compensate by increasing the volume of intake and maintaining a constant caloric intake.[13] Because the cats were consuming more of a diet when it was diluted with water, their water intake was increased. A watery cat food may be used to increase water intake when clinically indicated, that is, in cats with urolithiasis or hypernatremia.[14]

Can Cats Count?

Cats demonstrate numerosity (counting ability) both with non-food items and with food items. Cats will choose three mice over one mouse as food items.[15-17] Cats can also discriminate quantities.[18] Cats' satiety is not achieved simply by the number of calories consumed. Cats will eat more of a preferred food even when they are not hungry, but will not eat a less-preferred food unless they are hungry.[19]

Cats also show anti-apostatic behavior in that they will choose the less-abundant food over the more abundant one, presumably a behavior that evolved to enhance their ability to acquire all the necessary nutrients.[20] When presented with a choice between a food frequently made available to them and one that is rarely offered, cats will choose the scarcer one, even if both foods are dry commercial cat food. Because cats' prey is usually small rodents they consume many small meals a day and this pattern persist even when food is available ad libitum.

Cats learn to avoid foods that make them sick.[21] This ability, termed taste aversion, may be responsible for some of the difficulty veterinarians find in coaxing sick cats to eat.

Waking Owners

There are serious feline behavior problems such as house soiling and aggression, but there are also less serious problems that still threaten the cat–human bond. The most common non-serious behavior problem of cats is waking their owners very early in the morning. If the cat has access to the bedroom he may paw at the owner, lick their hair or, as a last resort, knock things off the dresser or bedside table. If he is barred from the bedroom he may scratch at the door or, most commonly, meow. Some owners have resorted to setting up a spray outside the bedroom door to punish the cat if he approaches. This usually serves only to make the cat meow a little farther away. When addressing any behavior problem, it is best to try to determine the cat's motivation. In most cases of early rising cats, it is hunger. Cats in the wild are crepuscular animals so the cat may start its day when the sun is about to rise, which in the summer in northern latitudes can be quite early. This type of nocturnal meowing should be differentiated from the hyper-vocalization that occurs in older cats suffering from cognitive dysfunction.[22] Feeding the cat a large meal just before bedtime should help because the animal will be satiated until its owners wake. Playing with the cat after that last meal – cats are likely to want to play after they eat – may also help the cat to rest at night. This post prandial play seems to be similar to their behavior toward their prey. The cat will catch and release its prey several times and, even after the prey is dead, flinging it into the air and pouncing on it.[23]

The solution that has worked for most owners is to provide a device that opens on a timer so that the cat has access to the food only after 0400h, for example. In the best case scenario, the cat transfers its meowing to the kitchen where the cat tries to "wake" the timer by meowing.

Hyperphagia

Cats that are constantly hungry are rare, despite what owners of obese cats may claim. These hyperphagic cats will scavenge for food – stealing food from human plates, opening packages and even fishing bacon from a hot frying pan. Some of these cats will growl while eating and chase off any other cat (or even a human) who attempts to approach their food. A thorough history usually reveals that these cats were malnourished at some point in their life – usually as kittens. Other situations of extreme hunger arise when a cat is abandoned in a house or is in a hoarding situation in which there are many, many cats and very little food. The easiest way to deal with these cats is to allow them to feed free choice. Gradually increase the kibble available in their bowls and feed a high fiber diet to reduce the risk of obesity. Food dispensing toys will allow the cat to exercise at the same time that it is obtaining food.[24] Specific serotonin reuptake inhibitors (SSRI) have anorexia as a side effect which can be taken advantage of to reduce the ravenous cat's appetite.

When Cats Eat

Cats eat many small meals (twelve) per day when given free access to food, but unlike dogs, cats eat both in the light and in the dark.[25] One might argue that this intake pattern is not natural, yet the caloric intake per meal is approximately equal to that contained in one mouse.[26] A feral cat with good hunting skills might easily catch twelve mice (or three rats) per day.[27] Most owners provide two meals a day. Free choice feeding is one way of letting the cat have many meals a day, but would be contraindicated if the cat is obese (see below). Providing food dispensing toys, of which there are many available commercially, allows to cat to "hunt" for its food. One very easy, but messy, solution is to simply broadcast the kibble around a room for the cat to find. A commercially available system is called the Hunting Feeder ®(No Bowl®). It consists of half a dozen plastic mice with hollow bodies into which kibble can be inserted. The mice can then be hidden around the house and the cat will have to expend calories locating each mouse and expend more energy trying to free the kibble from the mouse. (See Figure 5.1 and Video 5.1).

Where Cats Eat

Most cats are fed in the kitchen because of the proximity to bowls, can openers, and refrigerators. One problem with this is the effect on low-ranking cats in a multi-cat household. Although cats rarely fight over food as dogs do, they would eat alone in a natural situation. This natural behavior should be encouraged by feeding cats in different rooms or at different levels (floor, table, shelf) so that all the cats can eat without tension or anxiety.

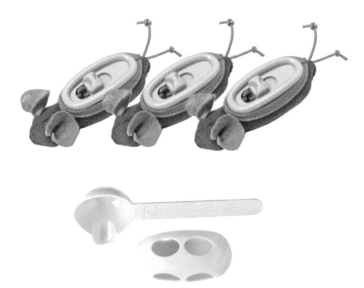

Figure 5.1   The Hunting (No Bowl) Feeder® Courtesy of https://docandphoebe.com/.

Bowl Position

Some years ago owners of dogs at risk of gastric bloat were persuaded to buy raised feeding stands for their dogs in hopes of preventing the disease. That was not effective and, in fact became a risk factor for gastric bloat because owners of dogs at risk fed them from raised bowls. Recently raised feeding bowls for cats have been advertised to prevent backaches in cats. Because cats lie down to eat their prey that is probably the natural situation. Owners should provide bowls that do not impede the cat's whiskers. Saucers work well. Clean dishes and a clean surface under the bowl appear to be important.

Determining Feline Food Preferences: *Palatability*

Palatability is defined as the momentary and subjective orosensory pleasantness of food consumption. Cats are notoriously finicky. This reflects the strong influence of palatability on food intake in cats. There is one striking peculiarity of cats: they do not prefer sucrose as most animals do because of a deletion in the sweet receptor gene.[28,29] Cats do not show a sucrose preference for aqueous solutions of sugar, but they do prefer sucrose in salt solutions.[30] Most cat owners realize that cats find sweet fatty food such as ice cream or pumpkin pie to be very palatable. Cats will not eat diets containing medium-chain triglycerides or hydrogenated coconut oil.[31] This may be because they break the triglycerides down to fatty acids in their mouths (cats possess lingual lipase) and are peculiarly sensitive to bitter tastes. They will avoid as little as 0.1 percent or 0.000005 M quinine. The amino acid taste units are sensitive to sodium chloride (NaCl), but their threshold to salt is much higher (>0.05 M) than in other species. This may explain why cats appear to have no salt "hunger" even when sodium deficient.[32] As carnivores, a sodium deficiency is unlikely to occur in the natural situation.[33]

Cats prefer fish to meat and prefer novel diets to familiar ones.[25] Cat-food manufacturers no doubt take advantage of both of these feline preferences. If the new diet is not innately more palatable than the familiar one, the cat will, after a few days, begin to choose the familiar food. Cats prefer fish to rabbit flavor and both are preferred over orange flavor but, no matter the flavor, cats chose a protein to fat ratio of 70 to 30.[34] Cats seem to prefer tuna to beef flavor and will work harder in an operant conditioning session to obtain it.[35] It must also be borne in mind that preference order can be influenced more by the processes involved in the manufacture of the diets than by the taste of the diets.[36]

Experience may modify the choice of a novel food. Farm cats avoid dry food, which is difficult to ingest, whereas pet cats avoid raw beef.[37] Determining feline preferences is of particular interest to cat food producers. They use two different approaches; the two choice Preference test and the single choice Liking test in which the amount of food consumed in a preset timed single choice test is measured.[38] Preferences depend on the aroma, taste, and also the temperature, texture, and consistency of the food. The shape of the dry food pellet – star shaped, cubical, or spherical can be important. Spray-dried plasma, yeast products, choline chloride, and hydrolyzed proteins are the commonly used palatability enhancing food additives in cat diets.

Appearance, aroma, texture, and flavor are sensory characteristics that are important in determining cat food acceptability. Sometimes humans are used to assess which food cats might find palatable. Human sensory analysis can include description of sensory properties.[39] More direct testing can assess acceptance or preference testing by pet owners, and food or attitude-related testing through questionnaires. Analysis by pets is usually focused on choice, consumption, or behavioral characteristics of the pet or the research cat before, during, and after eating.

Instrumental analysis, such as gas chromatography, mass spectroscopy, and high pressure liquid chromatography, electronic noses and tongues; other methods to measure volatile compounds, acids, sugars, peptides and protein analysis; and instrumental texture analysis are available to aid in sensory research.

Sensory analysis has two main types of methods: analytical (descriptive and discrimination) and consumer (acceptance, preference, consumption, and qualitative testing). Pet food appearance, aroma, flavor, and texture can be characterized using humans and instruments, while preference or consumption can be measured using either animals or humans.

Overall, when judging a food the pet or its owner will assess the food for an amazing number of characteristics: color or lightness, size uniformity of pellets, oily, size, and surface roughness or smoothness for appearance; burnt, cardboard, caramel, chicken, cooked, fish, grain or cereal, liver, meaty, metallic, methionine, offaly, oxidized oil or painty, prawn, pungent, rancid or oxidized, soy, spice, vegetable, vitamin, bitter, salty, sour, and sweet for odor and flavor attributes; cohesiveness, firmness, fracturability or brittleness, gritty, and hardness for texture attributes. Other attributes are cohesiveness of mass, chewiness, fibrous, firmness, graininess, gritty, hardness, initial crispness, mouthcoat, oily mouthfeel, roughness, powdery, springiness, and viscosity. There are also the effects of processing, such as extrusion and baking, packaging, ingredient effects, and formulation on sensory characteristics. Kibble shape and size are important factors for palatability as well.

Preference implies that a choice is to be made between sample foods and this is typically conducted using a two-bowl test. The two-bowl test includes which sample is sniffed or tasted first, reflecting the olfactory perception and attractiveness; the amount of food consumed; the ratio (A/B) of food consumed; the percentage of food intake (A/(A+B)); and the preference ratio (quantity of food A consumed over the total of food distributed).[38]

A one-bowl test is used to measure acceptability of a food sample. Important factors would include amount consumed as well as intake ratio in case several foods are compared using a consecutive feeding plan. The two-bowl test would often be conducted using kennel or laboratory cats, while the one-bowl test is more suitable for pet cats in their home environments. Other environmental factors such as living conditions, number and age of people living in a household, other pets in household, should be considered.

Cats find medium-chain fatty acids unpalatable.[30] Texture importance was shown by Nijland et al. (2009).[40] Those authors found that when extruded, diets that contain vegetable ingredients become more palatable.

When major categories of food are considered, cats are neophobic. If a cat has had only dry food for most of its life it may not eat canned food and vice versa. This is called the primacy effect. The longer cats had been fed a dry diet the less willing they were to eat a canned diet.[41] Owners of kittens should be sure to provide both canned and dry food to kittens to forestall food refusals later in the cat's life. The preference for novelty extends only to similar foods – canned cat food of various flavors. Obviously, the primacy effect and novelty effect are incompatible but both can be demonstrated by varying innate palatability.[35,42]

Observation of cats' behavior can be an indication of palatability. Cats may react to a food they do not want to eat by scratching the floor as if to bury it. Cats lick their noses after encountering unpalatable food, but groom their face (licked paw over ear) after eating palatable food.[43] They spend less time sniffing highly palatable food but do not consume it any more quickly.[44] Cats can influence – by their behavior – feeding time, quantity, and type of food served.[45]

Persuading cats to take medication is difficult. One approach is to "hide" medication in food. Cats in their own homes were video-recorded while they ate one of three foods: a favored food (FF), a non-flavored food (NFF) and the flavored food containing a mini-tablet (TFF). Five behavioral patterns differentiated FF from NFF; "flick ears backwards," "lick nose, not eaten," "flick tail" and

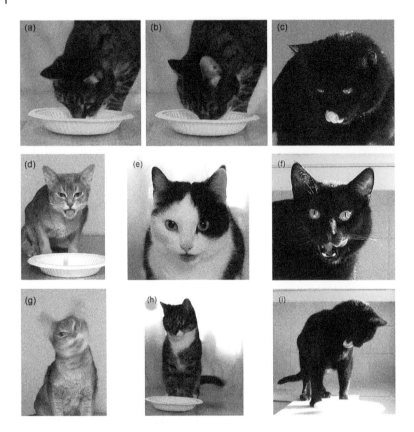

Figure 5.2 Facial expressions of cats while eating. Examples of eight behavioral indicators in still images captured from video clips. (a, b) "Flick ears backwards," which involves a rapid ear movement from position (a) to position (b) and back. (c) "Lick nose." (d) "Drop item"; the cat drops the piece of food and/or the mini-tablet hidden inside it, from the mouth. (e) "Smack"; the behavior pattern involves "smacking" the tongue with the mouth partly open, accompanied by rapid movements of the mouth that are not chewing. (f) "Flick lip." (g) "Shake head." (h) "Flick tail"; the behavioral pattern involves moving the tail sideways in rapid, wide sweeps. (i) "Groom body." Reprinted from Savolainen, S., Telkänranta, H., Junnila, J., Hautala, J., Airaksinen, S., Juppo, A., Raekallio, M., Vainio, O., 2016. A novel set of behavioral indicators for measuring perception of food by cats. Vet J. 216, 53 -58. Reproduced from Savolainen et al., (2016), ELSEVIER. https://docandphoebe.com/

"groom body" were more frequent with NFF, whereas "lick lips" was more frequent with FF. One indicator, "drop item," was more frequent with TFF than FF.[46] (Figure 5.2. Cat facial expressions).

Predation

Cats were probably domesticated originally because of their hunting ability; they could keep grain storage areas rodent free, but this same behavior can be very undesirable. True wild cats (*Felis silvestris*) are larger than feral domestic cats (*Felis catus*) and the former may occasionally eat the latter, but both consume mostly voles and other small rodents. The feral cats eat a more varied diet than wild cats because they will also consume household food.[47]

The extent of predation by cats is much larger than originally thought because early studies relied on the cat bringing its prey back to its home. Newer techniques, such as a cameras mounted on the cat's collar, have made estimates much more accurate. Only twenty percent of prey are brought back to the house; other prey is consumed or simply left at the killing site. In general, cats kill mostly rodents; only 25% of their victims are birds. When cats hunt they usually walk to a spot, possibly following mouse urine trails, and wait until a mouse appears and then pounce. When stalking, the cat will pause just before pouncing, the mouse will not notice the cat behind it; but the bird, with more peripheral vision, sees the cat and flies away. That is the reason why the cat makes three times as many attempts to catch a bird as a rodent. This is reflected in the statistics that cats kill 2.4 billion birds and 12.3 billion rodents per year in the USA[48] Predation by cats is a problem especially in places where cats are not endemic such as Australia and on islands where ground-nesting birds are especially easy prey for cats. Feral cats have more impact on wildlife than owned cats so providing food for those cats would help reduce their predation rate.

There are several ways to reduce predation by owned cats. Belling the cat is not too effective, but several bells or a bib attached to the cat's collar can inhibit the cat's ability to catch and kill. Keeping the cat indoors, at least during the periods when its most vulnerable prey is active, is effective. Kittens raised with a rat in the same cage do not kill rats,[49] but it would be difficult to expose a kitten to multiple types of prey in that manner.

Obesity

Feline obesity was a rare presentation a generation ago, when more cats were allowed outdoor access and cat food was not as palatable. There has been an astonishing increase of feline obesity from 6–12% of cats in 1972[50] to 25% of cats in 1994[33] to 40% in 2019.[51] Consequently, there has been considerable interest in factors that place a cat at risk of obesity. Factors linked statistically to obesity in cats are indoor living, being fed a prescription diet or a dry-food-only diet, and neutering.[52–54] Male sex, body weight around 15 weeks of age and being born during the increasing photoperiod were significantly associated with being overweight at 9 years.[55]

Neutering is a risk factor because metabolic rate drops in both male and female cats after gonadectomy and owners should be warned that this is a critical time to monitor the cat's weight carefully.[7,52,56] The animal will need less food to meet its energy requirements.

There is a relation of owner factors to feline obesity. Nijland et al. (2009)[40] looked at overweight dogs and cats in the Netherlands and tried to determine if animal obesity is related to owner obesity. These authors found that overweight dogs are likely to have overweight owners. This association was not proven for cats, though. This may depend on the age of the owner, as a different study conducted by Heuberger et al. (2011)[57] determined that cats of older people were more likely to be overweight than cats of younger owners.

Human personality traits include: Openness; Conscientiousness; Extraversion; Agreeableness; Neuroticism. Agreeableness in the personality of the owner was associated with a higher level of owner reported satisfaction with their cat, and with a greater likelihood of owners reporting their cat as being of a normal weight. Higher owner Neuroticism was associated with overweight cats.[58] In another study it was found that Conscientiousness decreases the risk of feline obesity, but surprisingly so does indulgence.[51]

The solution to feline obesity would seem easy; feed the cat less. Veterinarians have found that it is very difficult to convince owners to do that. Owners are afraid the cat will no longer like them or feel that the logistics of dealing with a fat cat in a multi-cat household is too difficult. Cats of different degrees of adiposity should be fed in different places. For example, the thinner cat can have access to its food free choice inside a cage or through a door, the opening of which is too small for the heavy cat to pass through. (See Figure 5.3; Video 5.2) In other cases, feeding the lighter cat on

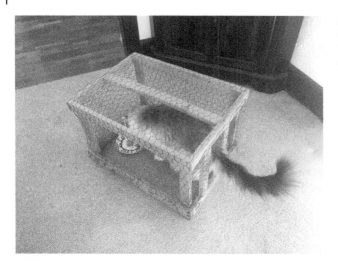

Figure 5.3 Feeding cage. The small opening will allow the slim, but not the obese cat to enter. Small dogs will also be deterred.

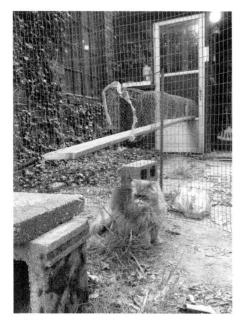

Figure 5.4 Catios homemade. The cat exits house through tunnel.

a high shelf can prevent the fatter cat from gaining access. One can even make use of an electronic cat flap that will open only for the cat wearing the proper magnet on its collar.

There are several weight control diets on the market and these can be effective IF the owner feeds the correct amount. Fat cats lost weight on both maintenance and high fiber diets when the owners fed only the proper amount. Supplying the owners with a 1/3 cup measuring devise led to weight loss. In the same study owners reported that their cats were MORE affectionate on the restricted diet. They apparently interpreted the increased meowing and rubbing as affection rather that misery.[59] An earlier study found that sending the owners individually packaged meals for the cat led to more weight loss in their obese cats, but providing a cup did not.

Indoor living is a risk factor for obesity, but access to the outdoors exposes the cats to a myriad of risks including being hit by a car, attacked by a wild predator or a dog, catching a disease from another cat or fighting with another cat. There are some compromises that can be made. One is to keep the cat indoors at night. This can also reduce predation on nocturnal wildlife and has been used in Australia to help save marsupials who have evolved no anti-predator behavior because there were no predators before humans arrived on the continent. Cats can be contained within fences as long as the top of the fence turns in on itself thus preventing the cat from escaping by climbing the fence. The Purrfect® fence is an example of that type of enclosure, although one can construct a cat-proof enclosure with chicken wire. Bird netting over the enclosure is necessary to keep the cat in as well as keeping the birds out. The generic term for such enclosures is "catio." One with grass growing inside can help with pica problems (Figure 5.4, Video 5.3.)

Another solution is an electronic fence. Use of electronic fences in which the animal is taught that if he goes beyond the line where a warning beep is sounded, he will be shocked, is controversial. Owners will be reassured that Kasbaoui et al. (2016)[60] found that cats confined by these "invisible" fences are not physiologically stressed. Of course, the electronic fence does not deter other animals from coming in to attack the resident cat and some prey may wander inside the perimeter.

Pica

The definition of pica is consumption of non-food items. When the diagnoses of cat behavior problems were analyzed pica was the problem in only 4% of the cats, while the most common diagnoses were house soiling and aggression.[61] Despite the rarity of pica it is important to be able to diagnose and treat it because it can be life threatening. There are two main types of pica. Cats that eat fabric primarily or preferentially wool and those that eat other objects, like plastic or wood. The former is most frequently seen in Siamese cats. The behavior is often termed wool sucking and a few cats may actually suckle on the fabric, but most chew the fabric with their molars while tilting their heads. The cats exhibit a preference for knitted objects, but when deprived of those things they will chew on woolen clothing, cotton towels, or even upholstery. Shoes, laces, strings, and thread are also ingested. Siamese breeders tried to prevent the wool sucking from arising by delaying weaning of kittens until 12 weeks. Early weaning and small litter size was associated with wool sucking in Birmans, but not Siamese.[62] (See Figure 5.5 and Video 5.4). Many cats will chew on photographs or cardboard but these behaviors rarely lead to obstruction or other illnesses). (See Video 5.4).

The reason that pica can be life threatening is that cats that eat indigestible objects may become obstructed and need surgery. Unfortunately, the same cat may become obstructed again and the costs may be more than the owners can afford. Treatment with high doses of SSRIs is

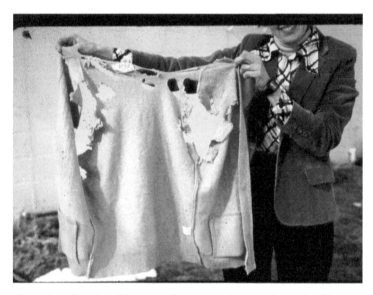

Figure 5.5   Sweater after overnight exposure to a wool-chewing Siamese cat.

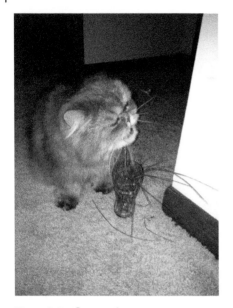

Figure 5.6   Grass eating.

recommended, but the success rate is low. Access to grass can be helpful. See Figure 5.6. Some cases of pica in dogs are associated with upper gastrointestinal disease, but this does not seem to be the case in cats. One management practice that lowers the risk of pica is free choice feeding.[63] Obesity is less of a health risk to these cats than obstruction.

Anorexia

Anorexia is one of the first sign of many feline diseases, especially kidney failure, and neoplasia.[64] Tumor necrosis factor is one of the products of a neoplasia that reduces appetite. Treatment of anorexia is difficult, but owners should be encouraged to offer highly palatable food such as chicken and tuna. There is often a conflict between which diets would be best for cats with kidney disease (low protein) and what the cat will actually eat. Pet food manufacturers have responded to this problem by improving the palatability of their products, but if, despite offering the most palatable "renal" diet, the cat will not eat the therapeutic diet, a food the animal will eat should be provided.

Cats may alter their food choice if a preferred meat is present but unavailable (tuna inside a sealed bowl) they will choose the food closest to the sealed bowl. The presence of the "phantom" food influences their choice.[65] This could be used to entice cats to eat the healthy diet because the unhealthy, but palatable, diet is next to it.

The drug mirtazapine can be used to stimulate appetite and can be compounded as a transdermal. Its mode of action is antagonism of central pre-synaptic alpha$_2$ receptors that inhibit norepinephrine release. Blocking those receptors results in more norepinephrine release and a consequent increase in appetite.[66] Another feline appetite stimulant, capromorelin, has been developed; it is a selective ghrelin agonist.[67]

Acknowledgments

The author wishes to thank Charles Houpt for supplying most of the figures and videos.

References

1 Russek M, Morgane PJ. Anorexic effect of intraperitoneal glucose in the hypothalamic hyperphagic cat. *Nature*. 1963;199:1004–1005.
2 Bado A, Rodriguez M, Lewin J, Martinez J, Dubrasquet M. Cholecystokinin suppresses food intake in cats: Structure-activity characterization. *Pharmacol Biochem Behav*. 1988;31:297–303.
3 Bado A, Lewin MJ, Dubrasquet M. Effects of bombesin on food intake and gastric acid secretion in cats. *Am J Physiol*. 1989;256:R181–R186.

4   Swartz MW, Woods SC, Porte D, Seeley RJ, Baskin DG. Central nervous system control of food intake. *Nature*. 2000;404:661–671.

5   Ghielmetti V, Wichert B, Rüegg S, Frey D, Liesegang A. Food intake and energy expenditure in growing cats with and without a predisposition to overweight. *J Anim Physiol Anim Nutr*. 2018;102:1401–1410. doi:10.1111/jpn.12928.

6   Adams T. Hypothalamic temperature in the cat during feeding and sleep. *Science*. 1963;139:609–610.

7   Root MV, Johnston SD, Olson PN. Effect of prepuberal and postpuberal gonadectomy on heat production measured by indirect calorimetry in male and female domestic cats. *Am J Vet Res*. 1996;57:371–37.

8   Randall W, Swenson R, Parsons V, Elbin J, Trulson M. The influence of seasonal changes in light on hormones in normal cats and in cats with lesions of the superior colliculi and pretectum. *J Interdiscip Cycle Res*. 1975;6:253–266.

9   Kappen KL, Garner LM, Kerr KR, Swanson KS. Effects of photoperiod on food intake, activity and metabolic rate in adult neutered male cats. *J Anim Physiol Anim Nutr*. 2014;98:958–967. doi:10.1111/jpn.12147.

10 Serisier S, Feugier A, Delmotte S, Biourge V, German AJ. Seasonal variation in the voluntary food intake of domesticated cats (*Felis Catus*). *PLoS ONE*. 2014;9(4):e96071. doi:10.1371/journal.pone.0096071.

11 Hirsch E, Dubose C, Jacobs HL. Dietary control of food intake in cats. *Physiol Behav*. 1978;20:287–295.

12 Kanarek RB. Availability and caloric density of the diet as determinants of meal patterns in cats. *Physiol Behav*. 1975;15:611–618.

13 Castonguay TW. Dietary dilution and intake in the cat. *Physiol Behav*. 1981;27:547–549.

14 Carver DS, Waterhouse HN. The variation in the water consumption of cats. *Proc Anim Care Panel*. 1962;12:267–270.

15 Uller C, Jaeger R, Guidry G, Martin C, Chacha J, Szenczi P, González D, et al. Revisiting more or less: Influence of numerosity and size on potential prey choice in the domestic cat. *Anim Cogn*. 2003;19:879–888. doi:10.1007/s10071-020-01351-w.

16 Bánszegi O, Urrutia A, Szenczi P, Hudson R. More or less: Spontaneous quantity discrimination in the domestic cat. *Anim Cogn*. 2016;19:879–888. doi:10.1007/s10071-016-0985-2.

17 Chacha J, Szenczi P, González D., et al. Revisiting more or less: Influence of numerosity and size on potential prey choice in the domestic cat. *Anim Cogn*. 2020. doi:10.1007/s10071-020-01351-w.

18 Pisa PE, Agrillo C. Quantity discrimination in felines: A preliminary investigation of the domestic cat (*Felis silvestris catus*). *J Ethol*. 2009;27:289–293. doi:10.1007/s10164-008-0121-0.

19 Van den Bos R, Meijer MK, Spruijt BM Taste reactivity patterns in domestic cats (*Felis silvestris catus*). *Appl Anim Behav Sci*. 2000;69:149–168.

20 Church SC, Allen JA, Bradshaw JWS. Anti-apostatic food selection by the domestic cat. *Anim Behav*. 1994;48:747–749.

21 Fox RA, Corcoran M, Kenneth R, Brizzee KR. Conditioned taste aversion and motion sickness in cats and squirrel monkeys. *Can J Physiol Pharm*. 1990;68(2):269–278. doi:10.1139/y90-041.

22 Horwitz DF, Neilson JC. *Blackwell's five-minute veterinary consult clinical companion: Canine and feline behavior*. Oxford, UK: Blackwell Publishing; 2007.

23 Leyhausen P. *Cat behaviour*. New York, NY: Garland STPM Press; 1979.

24 Dantas L, Delgado MM, Johnson M, Buffington CA. Food puzzles for cats: Feeding for physical and emotional wellbeing. *J Fel Med Surg*. 2016;18:723–732. doi:10.1177/1098612X16643753.

25 Mugford RA. External influences on the feeding of carnivores. In: Kare MR, Maller O, eds. *The chemical senses and nutrition*. New York, NY: Academic Press; 1977:25–50.

26 Fitzgerald M, Turner DC. Hunting behavior of domestic cats and their impact on prey populations. In: Turner DC, Bateson P, eds. *The domestic cat: The biology of its behaviour*, 2nd ed. Cambridge, UK: Cambridge University Press; 2000:151–176.

27 Turner DC, Bateson P. *The domestic cat. The biology of its behaviour.* New York, NY: Cambridge University Press; 1988.

28 Li X, Li W, Wang H, Cao J, Maehashi K, Huang L, Bachmanov AA, Reed DR, Legrand-Defretin V, Beauchamp GK, Brand JG. Pseudogenization of a sweet-receptor gene accounts for cats' indifference toward sugar. *PLoS ONE.* 2005;1(1):e3.

29 Beauchamp GK, Maller O, Rogers JG. Flavor preferences in cats (*Felis catus* and *Panthera* sp.). *J Comp Physiol Psychol.* 1977;91:1118–1127. doi:10.1037/h0077380.

30 Bartoshuk LM, Harned MA, Parks LH. Taste of water in the cat: Effects on sucrose preference. *Science.* 1971;171:699–701.

31 MacDonald ML, Rogers QR, Morris JG. Aversion of the cat to dietary medium-chain triglycerides and caprylic acid. *Physiol Behav.* 1985;35(3):371–375.

32 Yu S, Rogers Q, Morris JG. Absence of a salt (NaCl) preference or appetite in sodium-replete or depleted Kittens. *Appetite.* 1997;29:1–10. doi:10.1006/appe.1996.0088.

33 Bradshaw JWS, Goodwin D, Legrand-Défrétin V, Nott HMR. Food selection by the domestic cat, an obligate carnivore. *Comp Biochem Physiol Part A: Physiol.* 1996;114(3):205–209. doi:10.1016/0300-9629(95)02133-7.

34 Hewson-Hughes AK, Colyer A, Simpson SJ, Raubenheimer D. Balancing macronutrient intake in a mammalian carnivore: Disentangling the influences of flavour and nutrition. *R Soc Open Sci.* 2016;3. doi:10.1098/rsos.160081.

35 Stasiak M. The effect of early specific feeding on food conditioning in cats. *Dev Psychobiol.* 2001;39:207–215. doi:10.1002/dev.1046.

36 Hullar I, Fekete S, Andrasofszky E, Szocs Z, Berkenyi T. Factors influencing the food preference of cats. *J Anim Physiol Anim Nutr.* 2001;85:205–211. doi:10.1046/j.1439-0396.2001.00333.x.

37 Bradshaw JWS, Healey LM, Thorne CJ, Macdonald CD, Arden-Clark C. Differences in food preferences between individuals and populations of domestic cats *Felis silvestris catus*. *Appl Anim Behav Sci.* 2000;68:257–268.

38 Tobie C, Péron F, Larose C. Assessing food preferences in dogs and cats: A review of the current methods. *Animals.* 2015;5(1):126–137. doi:10.3390/ani5010126.

39 Pickering GJ. Optimizing the sensory characteristics and acceptance of canned cat food: Use of a human taste panel. *J Anim Physiol Anim Nutr.* 2009;93:52–60. doi:10.1111/j.1439-0396.2007.00778.x.

40 Nijland ML, Stam F, Seidell JC. Overweight in dogs, but not in cats, is related to overweight in their owners. *Public Health Nutr.* 2009;13(1):102–106. doi:10.1017/S136898000999022X. Epub 2009 Jun 23. PubMed PMID: 19545467.

41 Hamper BA, Rohrbach B, Kirk CA, Lusby A, Bartges J. Effects of early experience on food acceptance in a colony of adult research cats: A preliminary study. *J Vet Behav.* 2012;7:27–32.

42 Stasiak M. The development of food preferences in cats: The new direction. *Nutr Neurosci.* 2002;5:221–228. doi:10.1080/1028415021000001799.

43 Hanson M, Jojola SM, Rawson NE, Crowe M, Laska M. Facial expressions and other behavioral responses to pleasant and unpleasant tastes in cats (*Felis silvestris catus*). *Appl Anim Behav Sci.* 2016;181:129–136. doi:10.1016/j.applanim.2016.05.031.

44 Becques A, Larose C, Baron C, Niceron C, Feron C, Gouat P. Behaviour in order to evaluate the palatability of pet food in domestic cats. *Appl Anim Behav Sci.* 2014;216:53–58. doi:10.1016/j.tvjl.2016.06.012.

45 Salaun F, Le Paih L, Roberti F, Niceron C, Blanchard G. Impact of macronutrient composition and palatability in wet diets on food selection in cats. *J Anim Physiol Anim Nutr*. 2017;101:320–328. doi:10.1111/jpn.12542.

46 Savolainen S, Telkänranta H, Junnila J, Hautala J, Airaksinen S, Juppo A, Raekallio M, Vainio O. A novel set of behavioural indicators for measuring perception of food by cats. *Vet J*. 2016;216:53–58. doi:10.1016/j.tvjl.2016.06.012.

47 Biró Z, Lanszki J, Szemethy L, Heltai M, Randi E. Feeding habits of feral domestic cats (*Felis catus*), wild cats (*Felis silvestris*) and their hybrids: Trophic niche overlap among cat groups in Hungary. *J Zool*. 2005;266:187–196. doi:10.1017/S0952836905006771.

48 Loss SR, Wil T, Marra PP. The impact of free-ranging domestic cats on wildlife of the United States. *Nature Commun*. 2013;4:1396. doi:10.1038/ncomms2380rch.

49 Kuo ZY. The genesis of the cat's responses to the rat. *J Comp Psychol*. 1930;11:1–35.

50 Anderson RS. Obesity in the dog and cat. *Vet Annu*. 1973;14:182–186.

51 Wall M, Cave NJ, Vallee E. Owner and cat-related risk factors for feline overweight or obesity. *Front Vet Sci*. 2019;19(6):266. doi:10.3389/fvets.2019.00266. eCollection 2019.

52 Rowe E, Browne W, Casey R, Gruffydd-Jones T, Murray J. Risk factors identified for owner-reported feline obesity at around one year of age: Dry diet and indoor lifestyle. *Prev Vet Med*. 2015;121(3–4):273–281. doi:10.1016/j.prevetmed.2015.07.011. Epub 2015 Jul 31.

53 Scarlett JM, Donoghue S, Saidla J, Wills J. Overweight cats: Prevalence and risk factors. *Int J Obes Relat Metab Disord*. 1994;18(Suppl 1):S22–S28.

54 Larsen JA. Risk of obesity in the neutered cat. *J Fel Med Surg*. 2017;19(8):779–783.

55 Cave NJ, Bridges JP, Weidgraaf K, Thomas DG. Nonlinear mixed models of growth curves from domestic shorthair cats in a breeding colony, housed in a seasonal facility to predict obesity. *Anim Physiol Anim Nutr*. 2018;102:1390–1400. doi:10.1111/jpn.12930.

56 Hoenig M, Ferguson DC. Effects of neutering on hormonal concentrations and energy requirements in male and female cats. *Am J Vet Res*. 2002;63:634–639. doi:10.2460/ajvr.2002.63.634.

57 Heuberger R, Wakshlag J. Characteristics of ageing pets and their owners: Dogs v. cats. *Brit J Nutr*. 2011;106:S150–S153.

58 Finka LR, Ward J, Farnworth MJ, Mills DS. Owner personality and the wellbeing of their cats share parallels with the parent–child relationship. *PLoS ONE*. 2019;14(2):e0211862. doi:10.1371/journal.pone.0211862. eCollection 2019.

59 Levine ED, Erb HN, Houpt KA. Owner's perception of changes in behaviors associated with dieting in fat cats. *J Vet Behav*. 2016;11:37–41.

60 Kasbaoui N, Cooper J, Mills DS, Burman O. Effects of long-term exposure i.e. an electronic containment system on the behaviour and welfare of domestic cats. *PLoS ONE*. 2016;11(9):e0162073. doi:10.1371/journal.pone.0162073.

61 Bamberger M, Houpt KA. Signalment factors, comorbidity, and trends in behavior diagnoses in cats: 736 cases (1991–2001). *JAVMA*. 2006;229:1602–1606.

62 Borns-Weil S, Emmanuel C, Longo J, Kini N, Barton B, Smith A, Dodman NH. A case-control study of compulsive wool-sucking in Siamese and Birman cats (n = 204). *J Vet Behav*. 2015;10:543–548. doi:10.1016/j.jveb.2015.07.038.

63 Demontigny-Bédard I, Beauchamp G, Belanger MC, Frank D. Characterization of pica and chewing behaviors in privately owned cats: A case-control study. *J Fel Med Surg*. 2015;18:652–657.

64 Johnson LN, Freeman LM. Recognizing, describing, and managing reduced food intake in dogs and cats. *J Am Vet Med Assoc*. 2017;251(11):1260–1266. doi:10.2460/javma.251.11.1260.

65 Scarpi D. The impact of phantom decoys on choices in cats. *Anim Cogn*. 2011;14(1):127–136.

66 Quimby JM, Lunn KF. Mirtazapine as an appetite stimulant and anti-emetic in cats with chronic kidney disease: A masked placebo-controlled crossover clinical trial. *Vet J.* 2013;197:651–655.

67 Wofford JA, Zollers B, Rhodes L, et al. Evaluation of the safety of daily administration of capromorelin in cats [published online ahead of print Oct 22, 2017]. *J Vet Pharm Ther.* 2018;41:324–333. doi:10.1111/jvp.12459.

6

Eliminative Behaviors

Jeannine Berger and Wailani Sung

Introduction

In the United States, approximately 3.2 million cats are placed in animal shelters. Approximately 860,000 shelter cats are euthanized each year.[1] Cats at the highest risk of being relinquished are cats that exhibit inappropriate elimination.[2] Another study that involved 12 shelters reported that 37.7% of the cats were relinquished due to house-soiling.[3] In many shelters, the classification as a "house-soiler" may be an immediate reason a cat is euthanized without being given any further medical evaluation or a chance for adoption. A recent study performed at the San Francisco SPCA indicated that cats diagnosed with undesirable elimination had a 91.8% adoption rate compared to a 94.9% adoption rate for cats without elimination issues.[4] This indicates that house-soiling cats with an appropriate medical work up and behavioral intervention can be successfully adopted. In order to address undesirable elimination causes in domestic cats, it is crucial to have a clear understanding of the elimination behavior patterns of cats living in conditions free from human intervention. Using that information, we can apply it to owned cats that have adapted their elimination behavior patterns to indoor life. Clinicians need to be able to diagnose the nature of the behavior (marking versus inappropriate urination/defecation) then rule out any medical causes. Once the problem can be correctly identified, then it can be successfully addressed in most cases.

This chapter presents normal feline eliminative behaviors and behaviors for which cats are presented to veterinarians, diagnostic plans, and treatment options. A summary of these behaviors are presented as Table 6.1

What Is Normal for an Indoor Cat?

Feline elimination behavior is an innate behavior. It has been documented in kittens as young as five to six weeks of age. When these five- to six-week-old kittens were placed on loose substrate, the kittens automatically exhibited similar patterns of elimination as an adult cat.[5] Kittens housed indoors will leave their nest and choose a site for elimination. If they are not provided with a litter box containing an appropriate substrate, they will use another part of the room in which they are located.[6] Kittens have an innate preference for loose substrate. When cats are provided with the appropriate substrate, they will limit their eliminations to that specific substrate.

Clinical Handbook of Feline Behavior Medicine, First Edition. Edited by Elizabeth Stelow.
© 2023 John Wiley & Sons, Inc. Published 2023 by John Wiley & Sons, Inc.
Companion Website: www.wiley.com/go/stelow/behavior

Table 6.1 Elimination Behavior.

What is normal?	What is normal but often unacceptable?	What is abnormal but often accepted?	What is abnormal and typically unacceptable?
Innate behavior to eliminate in manipulatable substrate	Elimination on preferred substrates outside of the litter box	Urinating small amounts, straining, hematuria. Not digging or covering in the litter.	Stranguria, Vocalization, Laying down during urination
Digging, squatting over the depression in the substrate, eliminating and covering afterwards	Elimination in areas of the house where a litter box has not been provided	Not defecating for days, mild constipation	Anuria
Individual preferences for substrates and the cleanliness of the little box		Kittens eliminating outside of the litter box or using another substrate for elimination	Polyuria/Polydipsia
Using a communal latrine area (litter box) inside the house		Vocalization prior to, during or after elimination	Hematuria
			Constipation/Obstipation
			Urine marking inside the home
			Defecation outside the litterbox in areas of the house commonly frequented by the cat

The typical elimination sequence for a domestic cat starts with an approach to the area containing the cat's chosen substrate. The cat may or may not sniff prior to digging with both forepaws to create a shallow depression. Figure 6.1 The cat will then squat low over the substrate and deposit urine. Urine is eliminated in a strong stream with the tail held stiffly in a caudal direction.[7] When finished, the cat will turn around and using one forepaw, pull the surrounding substrate over the voided urine and walk away. The cat may use alternating forepaws to cover in two different directions. Squat urinating has been seen in kittens, juveniles, and adult females. Afterwards, the felines cover the deposited urine with soil or litter. In owned cats living indoors, it was found that cats that did not have elimination behavior issues spent more time in the litter box manipulating the litter compared to cats with a history of eliminating outside the litter box.[8]

A similar elimination sequence is repeated in defecation although there is more elevation in the squat position as the cat deposits feces. Indoor cats may have their movements in the litter box restricted by space or lack of substrate when they stretch their forelegs out to cover their eliminations. Therefore, owners may witness cats pawing at the wall or floor in the immediate proximity of the litter box.

Feral cats or cats with outdoor access may or may not cover after their eliminations. Lack of covering may occur more frequently when the cats eliminate away from their core area. The core area

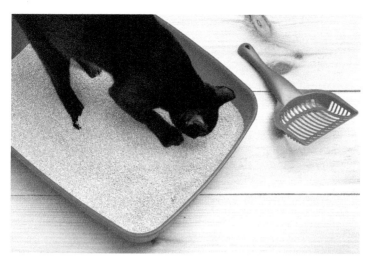

Figure 6.1   Cats that are comfortable in their litter boxes spend more time digging before eliminating and covering afterward. ELENA / Adobe Stock

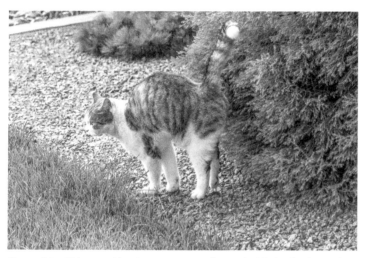

Figure 6.2   Urine marking is common species-typical behavior in outdoor cats. It is less accepted indoors. ELENA / Adobe Stock

is an area in which the cat spends the majority of the time; where it eats, sleeps, and conducts social interactions. Cats that live in colonies use a communal latrine within the core area where feces are covered. Covering feces is suspected to be a strategy that cats use to reduce their risk of exposure to parasites. Exposed feces are typically found further away from the core area of activity.[9]

Marking Behavior in Outdoor Cats

Urine deposited on horizontal or vertical surfaces signals a cat's presence in a territory. Spray marking is commonly used by intact male cats within their territories. The cat backs up to an object and urine is forcibly ejected onto a vertical surface, backwards and upwards (Figure 6.2).[7,10] The tail is held vertically in a rigid position and may quiver as urine is ejected. The cat may or may not tread its hind legs during this activity. The force of the ejected urine can cover a surface area typically one to two feet above the ground.[7] The objects sprayed tend to be distinct such as a fence post, hay bale, side of a building, or a patch of tall grass.

Tom cats tend to spray more when courting females than during hunting excursions. They spray less frequently when they are within the vicinity of other cats.[10,11] Mature male cats tend to spray more often than females.[11] The purpose of spray marking is to announce the tom cat's presence to the females in the area, to reassure himself, and as a signal to other males in the vicinity. However, the deposited urine is not a deterrent to other cats. It is a social communication that conveys information regarding the potential age and physical health of the depositor, and how recently the tom cat was there. The communication is conducted through the presence of volatile compounds in the urine, thereby providing the investigating cat with an opportunity to avoid potential conflict by moving out of the area, if the deposit is fresh.

The use of spray marking during agonistic encounters between males with adjacent territories is supportive of the hypothesis that it is an "honest signal" of a male's prey-catching ability. The odor of tom cat urine is due to the presence of sulfur-containing breakdown products of felinine. Felinine is biosynthesized from cysteine and methionine. Muscle meat is the main dietary source of cysteine and methionine. Therefore, the stronger the odor is, the greater the indication that the male is a good hunter.

Female cats can also spray urine, as well as neutered cats. In feral colonies, both males and females have increased rates of spraying during times of estrus, indicating there is a seasonal pattern.[10] Spraying is part of the feline courtship behavior. Both male and female cats sniff vertically sprayed urine marks longer than urine deposited on a horizontal surface.

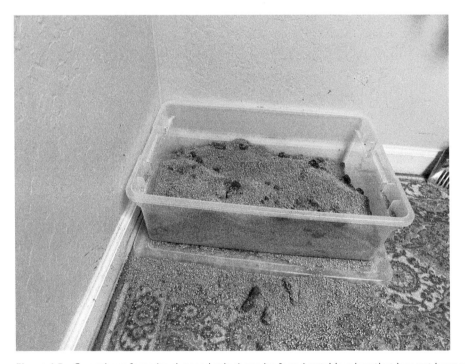

Figure 6.3 Sometimes feces (or clumped urine) can be found outside a box that has not been scooped recently (Figure 6.3). This can happen when cats try to cover their waste and should not be confused with a cat intentionally defecating outside the box.

Marking Using Feces

Within its core area, farm cats use a communal latrine in locations with loose substrate such as turned soil, gravel, sand, or hay. Cats bury their feces within the core area.[11] However, some feces may be exposed within the core area as a result of the cat not burying them at all, or being exposed by another cat's attempt to bury. One study found that heavier male cats in the colony tended to bury their feces at sites closer to the core area than lighter cats.[12] Cats sniff the area in which they bury their feces, but not after feces have been left exposed.

Away from the farmyard, piles of feces can be found on exposed, conspicuous sites.[10] There has been speculation that unburied feces may be used as territorial markers.[11] This is an interesting theory because domestic cats do spend more time sniffing the feces of unfamiliar cats, compared to their own feces or the feces of familiar cats.[13] Therefore, feces do provide some information to other cats in the vicinity. There has been variable data reported by several studies of different cat populations. However, there is no conclusive evidence that cats commonly use feces for marking. If feces are found outside a litter box, as in Figure 6.3, it may have been accidentally pushed out due to an overloaded litter box.

What Is Normal but Often Unacceptable?

Cats are ideal pets to keep indoors due to their natural preference for elimination in a latrine location within their core area. It is normal for cats to eliminate in loose substrates that can be easily manipulated. Such substrates can include soil, sand, leaves, and litter (in the home). When the litterbox is full due to use by multiple cats in the household, infrequent cleaning, and/or an inadequate number of available litter boxes, some cats may prefer to eliminate in an area of their choosing. Remember, in the wild, it is normal for cats to eliminate throughout their entire territory.

Often, owners have a tendency to place litter boxes in obscure places believing litter boxes to be unsightly and malodorous. When the litter box is placed in an area far from where the cat spends the majority of its time (core area), or contains litter that the cat objects to, the cat may choose other areas or substrates of elimination. It may choose a location that is within or closer to its core area for easy access. Such locations are preferred over a litter box that is placed on a different level of the house, the basement or in a dark closet.

Placement of a litter box in a non-preferred location, such as by doors that may open unexpectedly or next to noisy appliances or air vents, can contribute to the cat's choice of using another, in the cat's view more appropriate location. Often, these areas humans consider inappropriate and consequently are cleaned immediately unlike the "hidden" litter box itself; inadvertently encouraging the cat to use the newly chosen area further.

Some cats have or develop individual preferences for using certain substrates or locations in the home. Elimination may be found on specific materials such as area rugs, carpeting, bedding, the laundry basket or items left on the floor. Some cats may prefer to eliminate in the soil of potted plants. This may indicate a natural preference for soil. Another factor that may contribute to the choice of an alternate location is by offering a non-preferred substrate in the litter box, such as scented litter or large granular material (pellets or crystals). Some cats may eliminate outside the litter box due to personal preference. They may favor separate litter boxes for each type of elimination. If not given the option of two different litter boxes, they may choose to urinate on one substrate and defecate on another, regardless of whether or not that substrate is in the litter box.

Marking: Cats can deposit urine either vertically or horizontally to convey messages to other members of the household. For the indoor cat, urine marking is associated with stress, whether it is internal or due to conflict with other household members. The amount of urine deposited horizontally is typically a smaller amount compared to the amount of urine voided in a litter box. Small amounts of urine are also vertically deposited. Urine is usually deposited by exit and entry points, as well as on furniture or other objects in prominent locations. Urine can be found in areas of social significance within a household.[14] When there is conflict with outside cats, urine is typically deposited on the boundaries of the house. A study by Hart and Cooper found that neutering all of the cats that sprayed did not resolve the spraying behavior in all cats but a significant number of spraying behavior was resolved by neutering.[15]

What Is Abnormal but Often Accepted?

There are various situations in which a cat may exhibit undesirable elimination but the owner tolerates it. Even though it is an innate behavior for kittens to eliminate in manipulatable substrate or in a latrine area, many owners will put up with "accidents." The owners are tolerant due to the kitten's age and think that the kitten was unable to hold urine or feces long enough to make it to the litter box. They may also think they have not figured out the right substrate to use yet. However, a kitten consistently eliminating outside the litter box indicates a problem that needs to be addressed right away.

Some owners have occasionally found urine or feces deposited in their sink or bath tub. The owners may be disgusted, but since it is an area that is easy to clean, they may not try to figure out why their cat is not consistently eliminating in the litter box.

Cat owners may think that spending a lot of time squatting in the litter box is normal behavior. The cat may be voiding small amounts of urine or straining to urinate or defecate. The cat keeps digging or turning around in the litter box because he feels the continuous urge to urinate but he may only be able to urinate a small amount or not at all. Small amounts of urine deposited frequently in the litter box or other locations often goes unnoticed by cat owners. This is especially true when owners are not using clumping litter. The owners may not notice that the cat is voiding small amounts when they clean the litter box. Non-clumping litter does not form a solid removable mass indicating the number of eliminations.

Cats that do not have enough litter in the litter box may paw at the wall or floor next to the litter box. Owners may consider their cat very fastidious about their behavior in the litter box. While there is individual variation in the time spent manipulating litter, many owners may not realize that this may be an indication of an inadequate amount of litter in the litter box.[16]

Hematuria frequently goes unnoticed when a cat eliminates in the litter box unless there is an obvious sanguineous coloration to the urine and it is noted in the litter. It is more easily noticed when cats urinate on light-colored fabric or on hard surfaces, or when a blood clot is present in the urine.

Some owners do not realize that cats should be defecating daily. They may think one to two defecations per week are normal. Cat owners may notice when a cat vocalizes prior to, during or after elimination, but may not think it is out of the ordinary. They do not make the connection that the vocalization may be a "cry" for help. It is not normal for cats to vocalize when they eliminate and may indicate pain.

Many owners also do not realize the significance of a cat racing out of the litter box after elimination. Or, for long-haired cats, the significance of finding a trail of stool in a linear pattern outside the litter box. This frequently occurs when stool may be caught on the long fur around the perianal region. When the cat moves, it may feel the sensation of the stool hanging or dangling on his fur. This can be startling to cats. They may run out of the litter box with stool dropping behind them. This phenomenon may also occur when a cat is straining to defecate and feels pain during the process. They may run out of the litter box with feces being deposited along the way due to the extra exertion during departure. Afterwards, cats often avoid using the litter box when they associate pain with urination or defecation in that location or on that substrate.

What Is Abnormal and Typically Unacceptable?

Cat owners are frequently upset about multiple episodes of elimination outside the litter box and in certain locations around the house. Many cat owners have a low tolerance when their cats elimi-nate on their personal items such as bed, bedding, pillow, furniture, rug/carpeting, shoes, or clothing. Cats suffering from medical conditions that cause polyuria and polydipsia often void large amounts of urine frequently in the litter box. When the litter box is not kept clean, the cat may elim-inate in other areas around the house. For example, if there is an urgent need and the litter box is located too far away or on another level of the house, the cat may choose a more convenient loca-tion. This is often noted in cats with diabetes mellitus, chronic kidney disease, or in older cats.

It is certainly abnormal and unacceptable for cats to strain during urination or defecation, inside or outside of the litter box. Straining indicates a difficulty and/or discomfort regarding a natural body function. Cat owners must be educated as to why it is a life-threatening situation when their male cat is unable to urinate within a 24-hour period. Owners need to be made aware that male cats can experience urinary obstructions due to cystic calculi (Figure 6.4). Female cats can

---

What is normal?

Innate behavior to eliminate in manipulatable substrate
Digging, squatting over the depression in the substrate, eliminating and covering afterwards
Individual preferences for substrates and the cleanliness of the litter box
Using a communal latrine area (litter box) inside the house

What is normal but often unacceptable?

Elimination on substrates outside the litter box
Elimination in areas of the house where a litter box has not been provided
Urine marking inside the house

What is abnormal but often accepted?

Urinating small amounts, straining, hematuria
Not defecating for days, mild constipation
Kittens eliminating outside of the litter box or using another substrate for elimination
Vocalization prior to, during, or after elimination

What is abnormal and typically unacceptable?

Stranguria
Anuria
Polyuria/Polydipsia
Hematuria
Constipation/Obstipation

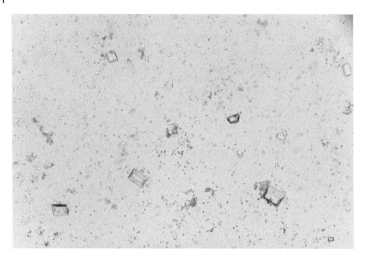

Figure 6.4 A cat with a previous history of urinary tract inflammation and associated pain while urinating may develop litter box aversion.

certainly become obstructed due to urinary calculi, but it is a far less common condition for female cats due to the gender-specific anatomy of the urinary tract. Cats unable to defecate may become obstipated and need enemas, or to be fully sedated to have the fecal material manually extracted. Repeated episodes of constipation/obstipation may potentially lead to the development of a more severe medical condition such as megacolon.

How to diagnose: The history/background of the problem.
The goal of taking a thorough history is for the clinician to be able to develop a complete behavioral and medical problem list. Communication skills, as well as knowledge about how and what to ask during an appointment, are critical as behavior appointments can be very lengthy if not approached with focused, specific questions. A good history will allow the clinician to identify all of the problems and create a list of differentials. With all of the information in hand, the clinician can then decide what kind of further diagnostics is needed to reach a diagnosis. The questions may vary depending on what type of problem will be addressed; however, the general framework provided here will allow a clinician to create a complete behavior problem list for house soiling.

Basic Information

History taking is a basic, necessary skill for all practicing veterinarians. Specifically, within behavioral medicine, compiling a complete history and detailing the findings of behavioral observations are the main aspects for reaching a diagnosis. Hence, a large portion of any behavior appointment is dedicated to getting the complete history. To abbreviate the process of history taking, many veterinary behaviorists require the clients to fill out a history form and will review the information prior to or during the meeting with the client and the patient. This process is helpful in that it asks more specific questions related to the presenting complaint.

Basic information is similar to a medical appointment with regards to the signalment of the patient. It identifies the patient by age, gender, breed, and weight. This data can affect the diagnosis, the differential diagnosis and even the prognosis.

Basic information also includes any information about the patient's physical health, current and past medical conditions, and the patient's diet. It may also include any recent changes, current and past medications (including herbal or other supplements), travel history, and number of human and animal household members. It is important to finish your data gathering by performing a complete physical examination and any ancillary diagnostic or laboratory tests that are indicated based on the history.

Environmental Information

In the exploration phase of the history, it is common practice to start with the presenting complaint. The client should be asked to describe the perceived problem with the patient. It is useful to gather as much information as possible about the specific complaint. This helps to later determine triggers that elicit the unwanted behavior. It is often helpful to encourage the client to be as specific as possible (e.g. when used clothing is left on the floor, the cat urinates on it or when the owner is away for over three days, urine is found on the closet floor upon their return). It also helps to determine when the unwanted behavior does NOT occur. For example, the client may say, "My cat used the litter box regularly until I bought a new type of litter." The goal is to ask questions that help determine the situations or circumstances that may have caused the behavior to change. Open-ended questions are preferred in the beginning stages of an interview so as not to "lead" the client in a specific direction, and to get better information about the problem.

It is useful to gather information about the patient and the family's daily schedule such as feeding times, sleeping locations and exercise routine. Even with feline patients, questions regarding any training background can be useful. For example, what tricks or cues does the cat know, and what training methods were used to train or disrupt the unwanted behavior when caught in the act? The use of confrontational techniques used in the past can directly affect your differentials and diagnosis.

Environmental information also includes type and size of living space, type and location of resting places, feeding and watering locations, time spent inside and outside, in addition to litter and litter box type, size, location, and hygiene schedule. As shown in Figure 6.5, not all litter box types are equally appealing to all cats. A drawing of the layout of the living space, a video tour of the house, or photographs of any relevant areas are convenient ways for the owner to present this information when a house call is not possible.

With elimination issues, it is critical to gather any information on other animals in the household, especially animals that directly share the litter box or animals that have access to the litter box location. Any positive or negative interactions between the patient and other animals or people in the home should be documented, as any stressful social exchanges can cause a change in elimination behavior.

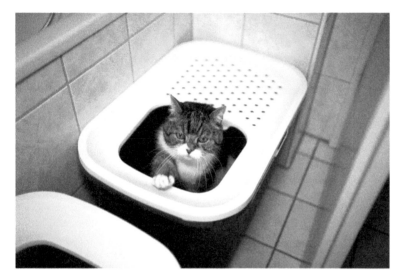

Figure 6.5   The size, type, and location of litter boxes, as well as the substrate type, should be part of a thorough history. Not all cats are comfortable with all types of boxes. Photo courtesy of Designer.

Owners may or may not be immediately aware of an elimination problem. They may never observe the patient in the process and only find "evidence" after the fact, especially if there are multiple cats in the home. Hence, video observation can be very helpful to learn more about the elimination behavior inside and outside the litter box, as well as to identify the culprit.

During this stage, a clinician will ask questions about the cat's body language before, during, and after the elimination. This information may be a verbal description from the client through direct observation or via observation of a video and/or pictures. In most cases, it is helpful to place a camera near the litter box so as not to disturb the cat during elimination. Observations of the posture and any eliminatory behaviors are often helpful in determining the diagnosis and rule out any differentials. Further information on the amount of urine, the location, and the substrate on which the elimination occurs needs to be gathered. It is critical to know if the patient is using the litter box at all. The frequency of elimination, as well as any additional facts in conjunction with litter box use or undesirable elimination bouts, will be helpful in coming to a diagnosis.

Summary of History

History taking should be completed by reviewing the information with the client. Reciting back to the owner the important points which led the clinician to creating the problem list is very helpful so as to clear up any misunderstandings or identify missing items. Review the client's goals and

Table 6.2 Summary of information needed for a thorough elimination history

Basic Information

Pet's name, age, reproductive status, breed, weight
Household members (people and animals)
Medical history including previous behavioral assessments
Acquisition: age, source, known conditions at previous home

Environmental Information

Daily activities
Feeding routine: diet, how/where fed, appetite, behavior when other cats present at source
Litter box and hygiene information: number, locations, substrates, cleaning schedule and routine
Household members using the same litter boxes or having access to the litter box area
Enrichment: toys, interactive play time, window perches, trees/shelves, outdoor time, liners, type of litter

Incident Information

Frequency, amount of urine, location, placement of elimination (horizontal and/or vertical)
Behavior before, during and after elimination inside and outside litter box including body language, position (standing or squatting), vocalization, behavior entering and exiting the litter box
Outcomes of management that owner has tried (change in litter, location, etc.)
Making a house map and marking the locations of previously soiled areas

Owner Information

Level of bond with the cat – their relationship
Goals and how success is defined
Willingness and ability of owner to implement treatment/management plan sometimes for life
Resources and willingness to perform further medical work up
Risk/tolerance assessment (How severe does the owner perceive the situation?)

expectations for the consultation. Many problems have been ongoing for years and a change in environment, routine or social events might elicit the consult. This is especially important when there is a long problem list as addressing each and every problem is likely not possible in the initial appointment. It allows the clinician to discuss the priorities of the problem being addressed. Often the client's priorities and the clinician's assessment of the severity of the problem may not be the same. By summarizing the important points, the clinician will be able to find discrepancies and avoid non-compliance or frustration. It is useful, either during or after taking the history, to encourage the client to ask any questions he/she may have. It is helpful to recognize and acknowledge a client's limitations to carry out a suggested treatment plan (e.g. emotional, environmental, financial and time restrictions; other family member's views). A client's commitment to compliance should be acknowledged and understood for a more complete understanding of the prognosis. A summary of the questions to be explored with clients is presented as Table 6.2.

Before you determine a diagnosis, make sure you have ruled out any underlying medical problems that may cause a cat to avoid or miss its litter box.

Medical Differentials

Degenerative: Loss of vision, osteoarthritis
Developmental: Lissencephaly, hydrocephalus, cerebellar hypoplasia
Anomalous: ectopic ureters
Metabolic: Uremic encephalopathy, hepatic encephalopathy, hyperthyroidism
Neoplastic: Intracranial neoplasia, cerebral infarct
Neurologic: Psychomotor or partial seizure, peripheral neuropathy
Nutritional: Renal calculi, cystic calculi
Infectious: Bacterial cystitis
Inflammatory/Pain: Feline interstitial cystitis, arthritis
Toxins: Ingestion of lilies, ingestion of marijuana
Traumatic: Brain injury, causes of pain, injuries to the lower spinal cord or pelvis

Once you have ruled out underlying medical causes, then refer to the decision tree.

Potential Behavioral Motivations

In cases where it has been determined that the cat does not have a clear aversion or preference, you will need to explore other factors that contribute to a cat's litter box usage. It is important to determine the cat's motivation for its behavior in order to deliver the best treatment plan and prognosis for the situation. We first need to examine intrinsic and extrinsic factors.

Intrinsic factors would include the cat's natural preferences and experiences. Cats have an innate behavior of using granular substrate in which to eliminate. Some cats will use whatever substrate we provide them in the litter box; granular litter, pellets, crystals, etc. Some cats are more selective in what they will use in the litter box. A cat may use a certain substrate for a discrete period of time but may elect to find an alternative option in which to eliminate that is located outside of the litter box. Typically, it is not one factor the cat is responding to but a cumulative effect of additional factors such as not liking the substrate, the litter box not being cleaned often, the litter box being located far away or in a high traffic location, or the litter box being too small Figure 6.6, or a bout of diarrhea or an undiagnosed UTI. Any one of these factors, or combination of factors, coupled with a cat's preference for another substrate may contribute to the cat's decision to latrine on the new, preferred substrate.

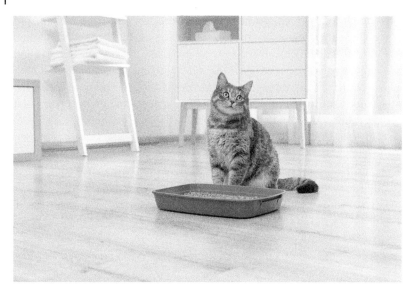

Figure 6.6 Example of too small a box. Litter boxes can be too small for a cat to use comfortably and may cause the cat to eliminate elsewhere. Large, shallow storage bins often make comfortable litter boxes.

When we examine extrinsic factors, we look at interactions between cats and members of the household, such as family members, other cats, and other kept species. We also need to examine factors that are outside of the cat's control such as litter box placement, substrate offered, size of the litter box, litter box style (covered vs. uncovered) and how often the litter box is cleaned. We need to provide ideal conditions to encourage the cat to continue using the litter box. We will also need to address any negative dynamics occurring in the household such as being bothered by the dog while the cat is in the litter box, people walking past the cat while the cat is in the midst of elimination, or the prevention of litter box access by feline housemates.

A factor that owners need to be aware of is that cats in multiple-cat household may be more likely to exhibit undesirable elimination issues. One study found that there was a higher number of male cats and cats from multi-cat households that were reported for urine marking. In this particular study, the owners reported the causative factor was agonistic interactions with other cats inside and outside the home. A newer study found that the presence of at least one other cat in the household was associated with a higher frequency of undesirable urination. Owners should think carefully before adding another feline to the family. Owners with multiple cats need to be counselled to closely monitor interactions between the cats in their household to ensure everyone is getting along. They need to provide adequate places for the cats to retreat from each other, spots in which they can hide and elevated places so as to avoid interacting with other cats. These households need to have multiple litter boxes placed in various locations so that cats do not compete over the same litter box.

Barcelos et al., also found a six-fold increase in the risk of marking and two-fold increase in undesirable urination, also referred to as latrine behavior (Figure 6.7).[17] In households where cats had access to the outside, the cats had a higher rate of marking behavior but a lower frequency of latrine behavior inside the home. Owners that allow their cats outdoor access may decrease the risk that their cats will eliminate in undesirable places inside the home but may increase the risk that their cats will mark inside the house. Owners need to know the advantages and disadvantages of allowing their cats to remain indoors completely or allowing outside access. Indoor cats need to be kept in an enriched environment. Cats with outdoor access need to be carefully monitored to ensure they do not mark inside the house.

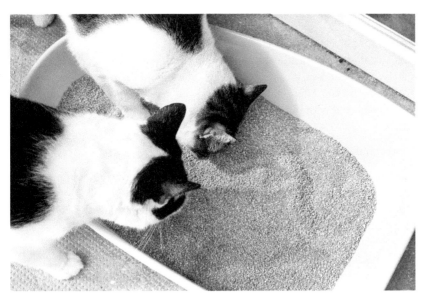

Figure 6.7   Cats in multi-cat households are more likely to have undesirable elimination issues, especially when not immaculately cleaned.

Intact cats have a higher rate of urine spraying compared to gonadectomized cats. Spaying and neutering cats can decrease the expression of sexually related behaviors such as roaming, fighting, mating, and urine spraying. However, neutering does not completely prevent spraying in all cats. Hart and Cooper determined that about 10% of 134 male cats and 5% of 152 female cats that were prepubertally gonadectomized continued to urine spray as adults.[15] It is still important to counsel owners that gonadectomy can reduce spraying in 90% of male and 95% of female cats.

Bamberger and Houpt's retrospective study reviewed 736 cats presented to their behavior practice over a ten-year period and noted 128 cats presented for marking behavior and 128 cats for spraying.[18] It was unclear whether the cats were separated into mutually exclusive groups, but male cats were identified in 75% of the cases. Barcelos et al.'s study (2018) did not find a gender difference, but noted that cats with a marking history were on average older (median nine and a half years) than cats that exhibited latrine behaviors (median five years) or no periuria (median four years).[17] This information indicates that male cats may be more likely to spray and should be closely monitored, especially as they get older.

Barcelos et al. (2018) also found when a cat defecated outside the litter box, the odds of urinating outside the litter box in the home were five times higher.[17] This would be a clear indication that undesirable bouts of defecation need to be addressed right away to prevent the cat from escalating its urination behavior.

How to Treat Elimination Issues

Clearly distinguish urine spraying from undesirable urination/toileting based on the history provided to you and/or any video evidence. Typically, urine marking consists of small amounts of urine deposited on vertical surfaces. The marking cat will continue to use the litter box to void its bladder. Urine marking cats also exhibit a distinct pattern of backing up and spraying urine on vertical surfaces. Undesirable urination or toileting consists of large amounts of urine deposited on horizontal surfaces. (refer back to decision-making graph.)

Marking

Marking behavior occurs more often in intact cats and cats with access to the outdoors.[17] Urine marking typically occurs in prominent locations in the house. Marking can also occur in exit and entry points, such as doors and windows, if there is conflict with neighborhood cats. Urine is typically used to mark inside the house. There is inconclusive evidence that stool may be used for marking. Marking can be comorbid with intact cats, multiple-cat households, anxiety, aggression, and confinement distress.

Treatment for conditions should involve the following basic plan:

1) Alter an intact cat. Spaying/neutering an intact cat can reduce marking behavior by 90–95%[15]
2) Restrict access to the outdoors or limit access just to your property (e.g. backyard only).
3) Restrict access to locations where the cat has previously marked
4) Resolve conflict between cats in the household
5) Use remote deterrents to keep neighborhood cats out of your yard or coming up to the house
6) Provide more resources, such as feed/water stations, perches, and litter boxes, so as to avoid potential confrontations
7) Separate "warring" cats until a behavior treatment plan is implemented

To treat soiling/toileting, as well as marking behavior, you need to identify a primary trigger causing the behavior. Based on the owner's provided history, you should be able to use the grid below to help you determine the underlying motivation for the cat's behavior to eliminate outside the litter box. This grid can also be used in cases of undesirable defecation.

Diagnosis Grid for Soiling/Toileting

	Aversion	Preference
Substrate	Q1: Never in the litter box?	Q2: Always on what substrate?
Location	Q3: Never uses litter box in that particular location?	Q4: Always uses a specific location for soiling?

Explanation:

Aversion: Never or rarely uses that substrate or location
Preference: Has a preference for a certain location or substrate (may not be offered substrate)
Location: Where do you find urine/feces? Consistently in one place? Or does it vary locations due to social significance?
Substrate: In what substrate do you find urine/feces? Consistent similar substrate? Or does it vary?

Litter Box Avoidance (Eliminations Outside the Litter Box)

When cats experience pain or fear upon urination or defecation, they may consequently form a negative association with the litter substrate, the litter box or even the location of the litter box.

This may lead to an aversion to one, all, or a combination of those factors. It may take time to determine which factor (or combination of factors) affects the cat's behavior.

In order to determine the type of aversion, you want to offer the cat a new substrate in the previously used litter box in the previously used location. If the cat then starts to use the new substrate, then we have identified that the substrate was the problem. However, if the cat continues to avoid the litter box, continue to rule out other factors.

Offer the old substrate in a previously used litter box but place it in a new location. If the cat uses the box, then we know the substrate was not the problem nor was the shape of the litter box, but rather the location.

If the cat continues to avoid the new substrate in a similarly shaped litter box in a new location, offer the cat the new substrate in a differently shaped litter box in a new location. If the cat has developed an aversion to the litter box itself, then the cat may continue to not use the box, despite the new substrate and a new location.

Once you think you may have discovered the reason of the aversion, you can test against it and bring the factor back to see if the hypothesis stands. However, owners are often not willing to "challenge" the cat after resolution. Also keep in mind that it is not uncommon for cats to have multiple aversions based on negative associations.

General treatment for this condition should involve the following basic plan:

1) Provide an adequate number of litter boxes plus one additional for the number of cats living in the household.
2) Keep the litterboxes immaculately clean. Some households may benefit from multiple cleanings per day. Clean the empty box with mild dish soap weekly?
3) Place the litter boxes in quiet, and easily accessible locations for the cat.
4) Place the litter boxes on each floor in a multi-leveled house.
5) Set up pet gates to ensure cats are not disturbed by other animals while trying to eliminate.
6) Provide comfortably large litter boxes.

Treating Q1: Substrate Aversion

Treatment for this condition should involve the following basic plan:
  Substrate trial

1) Place two identical litter boxes side by side. Place current substrate in one litter box and a new substrate choice different from the original one in the second litter box. Figure 6.8.
2) Observe litter box usage either via video camera or by recording the urine or feces left in each box. Figure 6.9.
3) After one week, switch the location of the first substrate with the litter box containing the second substrate.
4) If the cat prefers the new substrate, more deposits will be noted in the new litter box. The cat will also use the litter box with that particular substrate even if the location of the litter box has changed.
5) Remove the previous litter substrate and provide the preferred substrate in all litter boxes.
6) You may have to repeat the process with a second new choice to test the new choice against an even better option. See Q2.

Treating Q2: Substrate Preference

Treatment for this condition should involve the following basic plan:
Substrate trial

1) Limit the cat's access. The cat should be confined in an area with no access to her preferred substrate and only allow easy access to the desired substrate. Alternatively, preferred substrates should all be removed such as picking up carpets or not leaving cloth on the floor.

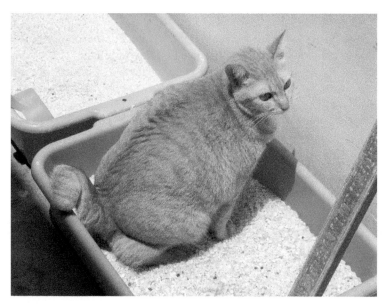

Figure 6.8 To test for substrate preference or aversion, place two identical litter boxes side by side and put the original substrate in one and a novel (but likely desirable) substrate in the other. Monitor to see which the cat uses.

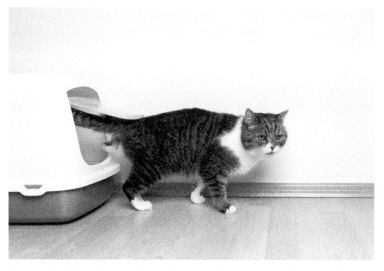

Figure 6.9 If a cat is avoiding a litter box, it's necessary to find out what aspect of it is displeasing. Photo courtesy of Designer.

2) Place two identical litter boxes side by side. Place a new substrate in one litter box and the old substrate in the second litter box.
3) Observe litter box usage either via video camera or by recording the urine or feces left in each litter box.
4) After one week, switch the location of the first substrate with the litter box containing the preferred substrate.
5) More eliminations will be deposited in the litter box of the cat's choice. If there is equal distribution, continue with a third litter substrate.
6) If you have exhausted all conventional litter substrates and the cat still has a preference of the contraband substrate (i.e. carpeting, area rug, clothing, etc.), then you will need to offer the preferred contraband substrate and perform a litter conversion.
7) Substrate conversion is performed over the course of several weeks where the preferred substrate is offered in a litter box. Every week, add in 10% of the substrate the cat used in the trials.

Treating Q3: Location Aversion

Treatment for this condition should involve the following basic plan:
  Move the location of the litter box
  Typically, the litter box needs to be moved to another location and the cat will immediately use the litter box. No litter preference trial is needed. Relapse happens often when owners move the box back in the location they prefer.

Treating Q4: Location Preference

Treatment for this condition should involve the following basic plan:
  Provide a litter box in the preferred location
  Once a litter box is provided in the cat's preferred location, the cat consistently eliminates in the litter box. Relapse happen often when owners move the box back in the location they prefer.
  In a multiple cat household, there are other factors to consider. We need to accurately identify the culprit. Confinement of the suspected cat can change the social dynamic and eliminate the problem completely. If there is conflict and competition between two or more cats, confining one of the culprits may reduce the conflict enough that a reduction or cessation in marking or periuria results. In the past, it has been recommended to either inject fluorescein stain subcutaneously or administer orally to the cat and then use a black light to determine which cat's urine will fluoresce green. However, there are no clear guidelines on how to use this technique. Drawbacks also include not knowing the half-life of the stain and the metabolism/elimination rate. Another option for inappropriate defecators was to feed brightly colored non-toxic crayon shaving to the cat. The deposited stool would then need to be carefully inspected to look for the colored crayons. The disadvantage would be if the cat partially used the litter box for defecation, and also the clearance time of the crayons through the gastrointestinal tract. In this modern age, there are many remote camera options that allow us to watch the cats live or record and download the content later to identify the culprit.

Surgery, Medications, and Other Related Therapies

All sexually intact cats that are spraying should be gonadectomized. Gondectomy is effective in reducing urine spraying in 90% of male cats and 95% in female cats.[15]

Cystic calculi should be surgically removed whenever possible. If surgery is not possible, then the cat should be placed on the appropriate prescription diet to dissolve the calculi and prevent a future recurrence of the condition. Special diets can also be used to address crystalluria.

Role of the Owner in Prevention

If the cats are provided with the following conditions, they are more likely to eliminate in the litter box:[19]

- Clean the litter box on a frequent schedule
- Provide enough litter boxes for the number of cats in the household
- Place the litter box in a location that is easily accessible by the cat
- Provide adequately sized litter boxes (86 × 39 cm)[20]

Since we limit our cat's use of the toileting area to the size of the litter box that we provide, it is important that the litter box is kept immaculately clean. On average, a cat urinates 2.1 times per day, which means cleaning should occur at a minimum once a day. A cat with abnormal urination patterns eliminates 2.9 times per day.[21] Ideally, the more cats in the household, the more often the litter box should be cleaned. Some cats may have a preference for cleanliness and a particular litter box. If the preferred litter box has been used by another cat, the fastidious cat may choose another location that is not acceptable to the owner.

The common recommendation is to provide at least one more litter box beyond the number of cats in the household. This means if you have four cats, the household should contain five litter boxes. The litter boxes should be placed in quiet locations outside of high traffic areas. Remember, cats are not only predators to small prey but also prey to many larger predators. Therefore, cats also display prey animal behaviors. They are vulnerable, especially during elimination, where there are 10–20 seconds in which they may not be as vigilant and cannot move as quickly if they spot or are threatened by a predator. Therefore, they may be sensitive to movement and noise while they eliminate. The litter boxes should be spaced so that cats that are not getting along can choose litter boxes located in other areas of the house to avoid conflict. This also limits the need to compete over one litter box.

Cats were found to show a preference for larger (86 × 39 cm) litter boxes over regular-sized (56 × 38 cm) litter boxes.[20] It is important to provide a litter box with adequate space for the cat to get in, turn around, dig and cover after elimination. Cats have individual preferences; some cats may prefer covered litter boxes, whereas others may prefer open litter boxes.[21] It is important to provide different options for the cats and allow them to choose.

Management

Tools and Household Enrichment

Indoor cats, which evolved to live an outdoor lifestyle, can show increased stress from the pressures of overcrowding, insufficient mental stimulation, and lack of physical activity. Studies have shown that increasing the activity levels and providing environmental enrichment for indoor cats can decrease their stress.[22] There are simple ways to enrich a cat's indoor environment. Toys are an obvious method, both self-play toys (those that the cat can play with, without owner involvement) and interactive toys (those that are usually handled, at least in part, by people). Any positive inter-action with a cat is a form of enrichment; exceptions are teasing a cat or playing with inappropriate toys or objects, such as hands or toes.

Incidence of Medical Diagnoses in Feline Elimination Problems

Most of the cats that spray or exhibit undesirable elimination receive the most basic work up which consists of a physical examination, urinalysis and urine culture or fecal test (if the cat has undesirable defecation). Tynes et al.'s case-controlled study evaluated urinary tract disease in gonadectomized urine-spraying cats.[23] The study included 58 gonadectomized cats (47 males and 11 females) with urine-marking behavior (e.g. marking on vertical sur-faces) and 39 (26 males and 13 females) with no undesirable urination issues. A cystocen-tesis and urinalysis were performed on all cats. The comparison between the two groups revealed no differences associated with urine marking. Based on this study, urinalysis was determined to be an appropriate test to rule out lower urinary tract disease.

Frank et al. performed a more thorough medical work up on 34 urine-spraying cats which consisted of a physical examination, complete blood count, biochemistry profile, urinalysis, urine culture, urine cortisol : creatinine ratios and abdominal radiographs.[24] In Frank et al.'s study, 13 patients (38%) had abnormalities or crystalluria.[24]

Ramos et al. found that out of 23 healthy appearing cats that exhibited inappropriate latrine-related behavior, nine (39.1%) had underlying medical conditions.[25] Medical condi-tions were also found in six control cats (26.1%). The difference was not significant between case and control cats (Pearson's $\chi2$ test, P = 0.365). The medical conditions found in cats with undesirable urination behavior included: renal insufficiency, leukocytosis, leukocytosis plus bladder plug, bladder lithiasis, bladder plug and hepatic disease. The medical condi-tions found in the control cats were: leukemia, bladder diverticulum, renal insufficiency, bladder lithiasis, abdominal liquid, and hepatic disease plus urinary infection.

The majority of cats that exhibited marking or undesirable urination did not have evi-dence of urinary tract disease. But keep in mind that more diagnostic tests may be needed to rule out medical conditions in refractory cases.

Many self-play toys dispense food, which motivate the cat to play with the toy, and perhaps take their focus away from another cat in the house or other stressor. The basic principle is that the toy is filled with dry kibble or treats, and the cat learns to manipulate the toy to release the food out of a hole. Self-play toys that do not dispense food are not nearly as exciting for the average cat. Some examples of simple food-dispensing toys are: toilet paper tube filled with kibble and ends folded over; dried water bottle filled with kibble; or a cleaned and dried plastic yogurt container with a hole cut in the lid and filled with food. Commercial food-dispensing toys are also available.

Interactive toys help strengthen the bond between owners and their cats. Both can have a great time playing with wand-type toys with strings, feathers, and fabric attached. These wand-type toys provide an opportunity for the cat to engage in activities such as chase, pounce, and bite in a manner that is safe for people as the cat's claws and teeth are kept away from the owner. Some cats enjoy playing with laser pointers, chasing the point of light around the house. Low-cost (or no-cost) toys are often the cat's preferred toys. Some suggestions are wadded-up paper or foil balls and plastic rings from milk jugs. Not every toy is right for every cat; for instance, ingestion of plastic can lead to intestinal blockage and string can easily become a linear foreign body. Care must be taken to ensure that the toys are safe and serve their enrichment purpose.

In a multi-cat household, it is important that the cats are provided with multiples; multiple litter boxes spread throughout the house, multiple levels for the cats to perch, multiple toys, beds, and feeding stations. Providing multiple options will help reduce competition and conflict when cats that are not getting along encounter each other. It is easier for the cats to retreat and go to another location where there is no risk of conflict.

For more details, please refer to the Chapters on stress management and environmental enrichment.

Confinement (Avoidance)

Cats may need to be temporarily or permanently restricted from assessing certain substrates or certain parts of the house. The cat may be allowed into the restricted area under close supervision. Access may be allowed for short periods of time as part of the behavior modification exercise.

Behavior Modification

Behavior modification exercises can be used to address the underlying motivations that contribute to the cats' undesirable behaviors. Important concepts to learn for behavior modification in cats are clicker training, and desensitization and counter-conditioning. Clicker training or marker-based training is an easy technique of capturing and reinforcing behaviors in cats. It is used to reinforce behaviors that cats already perform but can also be used to teach new behaviors. The clicker, also known as a marker, produces a clicking noise which is paired with high-value treats. Other rewards that can be used are verbal praise and physical attention, such as petting or scratching the cat. Repeated pairings of the click and reward are first performed before the clicker can be applied. Once the cat has learned the association between the click and treat, you are ready to use a clicker to mark and reinforce desirable behaviors.

Desensitization (DS) and counter-conditioning (CC) are the hallmarks of most behavior modification plans. DS is the gradual exposure of a trigger stimulus below the level of an animal's avoidance, its threshold. Counter-conditioning (CC) pairs a particular stimulus with something that is rewarding for that animal, thus causing the formerly negative-inducing stimulus to now induce a positive emotional response. We can reinforce a behavior that is incompatible with the currently established undesirable behavior pattern. For cats that spray, we would clean the spray area with an enzymatic cleaner to remove all traces of urine odor. Then, rub catnip or apply a catnip spray to induce the spraying cat to perform allomarking behavior instead of urine spraying. Another approach would be to place high-value treats or food in the previously sprayed areas to reinforce an incompatible behavior. This would allow the cat to form the association of this area as the feeding area instead of the area where urine marks should be applied.

DS/CC can be used to treat several feline problem behaviors, including inter-cat directed aggression and litter box aversion. If the spraying or toileting behavior is caused by inter-cat conflict, it is important to address this issue. Cats that are aggressive toward their feline housemates usually respond well to this process. We start by teaching cats alternate and incompatible behaviors to perform when presented with the triggers. We use clicker training to reinforce appropriate behavior. The cats are provided with a safe haven where it has learned to go for relaxation and security. Owners are educated to move slowly in the DS/CC process and set reasonable goals. The cat is either offered food or played with while the other cat is present at a comfortable distance. Playing with the cat using manipulatable toys (e.g. wadded-up paper balls or food-filled toys) and wand-type toys offers the owner a way to positively interact with the cat while building a positive association (CC) in the presence of the other cat with which it has conflict. The goal is that distance between the cats gradually decreases with subsequent sessions and the cats learn to tolerate each other's presence.

For cats that have formed a negative association with the litter box, clicker training can be applied with desensitization. The click/marker is given when the cat approaches within a designated proximity of the litter box. The cat is reinforced several times for being near to the litter box. Then, reinforce the cat for taking one step closer to the litter box until, over multiple sessions, the cat willingly enters the litter box. Another approach is to incorporate a target stick and provide a target for the cat to approach. Over multiple sessions, the target is moved closer to the litter box until the cat willing steps into the litter box. Marker-based training can also be used to capture when the cat enters the litter box on its own and to capture elimination behavior in the litter box.

Medications and Other Related Therapies

Medications can be an important part of treating cats with marking or undesirable urination. Selective serotonin reuptake inhibitors (SSRIs) and tricyclic antidepressants (TCAs) have been used to reduce anxiety and the frequency of undesirable spraying or toileting behavior.

Fluoxetine hydrochloride is a strong inhibitor of serotonin reuptake. The primary metabolite is norfluoxetine. Possible side effects include sedation, vomiting, diarrhea, sedation, changes in urinary frequency, excitement, and changes in appetite.[26] Fluoxetine inhibits the cytochrome liver enzyme: CYP2C9, CYP2D6, CYP2C19, and CYP3A4. This means that any medication that is eliminated through these enzymes may remain at elevated levels. Pryor et al.[27] examined the effect of fluoxetine on spraying cats. The dosage of fluoxetine used in the study ranged from (1 mg/kg [0.45 mg/lb], PO, q 24 h to 1.5 mg/kg [0.68 mg/lb], PO, q 24 h. At the end of eight weeks, the cats in the treatment group had a > 70% reduction in spraying.

Clomipramine is the most serotoninergic-specific tricyclic antidepressant. The primary mechanism of action is preventing serotonin reuptake in the CNS. Its active metabolite, desmethylclomipramine, inhibits norepinephrine reuptake.[26,28] Possible side effects include urinary retention, constipation, sedation, changes in appetite, and mydriasis.[26,28]

King et al. conducted a study for spraying cats.[29] The group of 67 neutered cats were randomly assigned to be treated with a placebo or with clomipramine at a dosage of 0.125 to 0.25 mg/kg (0.057 to 0.11 mg/lb), 0.25 to 0.5 mg/kg (0.11 to 0.23 mg/lb), or 0.5 to 1 mg/kg (0.23 to 0.45 mg/lb), PO, every 24 hours for up to 12 weeks. The results showed clomipramine significantly reduced the frequency of urine spraying in cats. The recommendation from the study was to start spraying cats on the initial dosage of clomipramine at 0.25 to 0.5 mg/kg, PO, every 24 hours.

In a study conducted by Landsberg and Wilson,[27] spraying cats were only administered clomipramine ranging from 0.30 to 0.83 mg/kg (mean 0.54 mg/kg) orally once daily. The result was a reduction in spraying in 23 of 25 cats and a ≥ 75% reduction in 20 cats. Clomipramine doses ranging from 0.25–1.3 mg/kg every 24 hours have also been shown to be effective in several studies.[27,28]

Both fluoxetine and clomipramine also work in cats with undesirable or urinary toileting behavior to reduce anxiety. Cats treated with either medication also saw a reduction in their spraying behavior.[30]

Buspirone is a serotonin 1A partial agonist. Its mechanism of action is blocking presynaptic and postsynaptic serotonin-1A (5-HT$_{1A}$) receptors. It also has an affinity for the D2-dopamine receptors.[26] The anxiolytic effects are due to the action of the neurons in the dorsal raphe. Hart et al. found a > 75% reduction in 55% cats treated for urine spraying or marking when buspirone was administered.[31] (Hart et al., 1993). In this particular study, only half of the cats treated with buspirone resumed spraying when buspirone administration was discontinued after two months of treatment.

While clinical trials addressed urine spraying/marking issues, anxiolytic medications have been used to effectively treat cases in which anxiety was determined to be an underlying factor in the undesirable eliminative behavior.

Pheromone Therapy

Treatment with commercially available feline facial pheromone analogue is also efficacious in treating spraying and undesirable eliminations. Frank et al. (1999) noted that 14 out of 24 cat households reported a decreased frequency of spraying when the pheromone was used.[24] The frequency of urine-spraying cats in one study decreased from a mean frequency of 14.2 times/week to 4.2 times/week by the fourth week of treatment.[32]

When to Seek Help from the Specialist

After a thorough history taking and medical work up has been performed and any underlying medical conditions have been treated or ruled out, refer to the diagnosis grid to help guide treatment. When there is a refractory case, it should be referred to a board-certified veterinary behavior specialist (DACVB.org).

Prevention

SEE OTHER CHAPTERS
REGULAR VET CARE

Summary

Rule out medical problems first
Prevention – offer the ideal litter and litter box options and elimination outside the litter box is less likely to occur
Appropriate management – in most cases, the easy fix is to give the cat what it needs
No reason to surrender a cat
Normal elimination behavior but in undesirable location for the owners can be a challenge

References

1 ASPCA. *Pet Statistics*. Pet Statistics; 2018.
2 Patronek GJ, Glickman LT, Beck AM, McCabe GP, Ecker C. Risk factors for relinquishment of cats to an animal shelter. *J Am Vet Med Assoc*. 1996;209(3):582–588.

3 Salman MD, Hutchison J, Ruch-Gallie R, Kogan L, New JC, Kass PH, Scarlett JM. Behavioral reasons for relinquishment of dogs and cats to 12 shelters. *J Appl Anim Welf Sci*. 2000;3(2):93–106. doi:10.1207/s15327604jaws0302_2.

4 Liu S, Sung W, Welsh S, Berger JM. A six-year retrospective study of outcomes of surrendered cats (Felis catus) with periuria in a no-kill shelter. *J Vet Behav*. 2021;42:75–80. doi:10.1016/j.jveb.2020.12.002.

5 Bateson P. Behavioural development in the cat. In: Turner DC, Bateson P, eds. *The domestic cat: The biology of its behaviour*, 3rd ed. Cambridge: Cambridge University Press; 2014:11–26.

6 Hart BL, Hart LA. Normal and problematic reproductive behaviour in the domestic cat. In: Turner DC, Bateson P, eds. *The domestic cat: The biology of its behaviour*, 3rd ed. Cambridge: Cambridge University Press; 2014:27–36.

7 Beaver BV. *Feline behavior: A guide for veterinarian, second edition*. St. Louis, MO: W.B. Saunders Company; 2003.

8 Sung W, Crowell-Davis SL. Elimination behavior patterns of domestic cats (Felis catus) with and without elimination behavior problems. *Am J Vet Res*. 2006;67(9). doi:10.2460/ajvr.67.9.1500.

9 Macdonald DW, Apps PJ, Carr GM, Kerby G. Social dynamics, nursing coalitions and infanticide among farm cats, Felis catus. *Ethology*. 1987;28(Suppl):66.

10 Bradshaw JWS, Casey RA, Brown SL. *The behaviour of the domestic cat*, 2nd ed. Boston, MA: CABI Publishing; 2012.

11 Feldman HN. Methods of scent marking in the domestic cat. *Can J Zool*. 1994;72(6):1093–1099. doi:10.1139/z94-147.

12 Ishida Y, Shimizu M. Influence of social rank on defecating behaviors in feral cats. *J Ethol*. 1998;16(1):15–21. doi:10.1007/BF02896349.

13 Nakabayashi M, Yamaoka R, Nakashima Y. Do faecal odours enable domestic cats (Felis catus) to distinguish familiarity of the donors? *J Ethol*. 2012;30(2):325–329. doi:10.1007/s10164-011-0321-x.

14 Herron ME. Advances in understanding and treatment of feline inappropriate elimination. *Top Companion Anim Med*. 2010;25(4):195–202. doi:10.1053/j.tcam.2010.09.005.

15 Hart BL, Cooper L. Factors relating to urine spraying and fighting in prepubertally gonadectomized cats. *J Am Vet Med Assoc*. 1984;184(10):1255–1258.

16 McGowan RTS, Ellis JJ, Bensky MK, Martin F. The ins and outs of the litter box: A detailed ethogram of cat elimination behavior in two contrasting environments. *Appl Anim Behav Sci*. 2017;194(November 2016):67–78. doi:10.1016/j.applanim.2017.05.009.

17 Barcelos AM, McPeake K, Affenzeller N, Mills DS. Common risk factors for urinary house soiling (periuria) in cats and its differentiation: The sensitivity and specificity of common diagnostic signs. *Front Vet Sci*. 2018;5(May):1–12. doi:10.3389/fvets.2018.00108.

18 Bamberger M, Houpt KA. Signalment factors, comorbidity, and trends in behavior diagnoses in cats: 736 cases (1991–2001). *J Am Vet Med Assoc*. 2006;229(10):1602–1606.

19 Guy NC, Hopson M, Vanderstichel R. Litter box size preference in domestic cats (Felis catus). *J Vet Behav: Clin Appl Res*. 2014;9(2):78–82. doi:10.1016/j.jveb.2013.11.001.

20 Dulaney DR, Hopfensperger M, Malinowski R, Hauptman J, Kruger JM. Quantification of urine elimination behaviors in cats with a video recording system. *J Vet Intern Med*. 2017;31(2):486–491. doi:10.1111/jvim.14680.

21 Beugnet VV, Beugnet F. Field assessment in single-housed cats of litter box type (covered/uncovered) preferences for defecation. *J Vet Behav*. 2020;36:65–69. doi:10.1016/j.jveb.2019.05.002.

22 Buffington CAT, Westropp JL, Chew DJ, Bolus RR. Clinical evaluation of multimodal environmental modification (MEMO) in the management of cats with idiopathic cystitis. *J Feline Med Surg*. 2006;8(4):261–268. doi:10.1016/j.jfms.2006.02.002.

23 Tynes VV, Hart BL, Pryor PA, Bain MJ, Messam LLM. Evaluation of the role of lower urinary tract disease in cats with urine-marking behavior. *J Am Vet Med Assoc*. 2003;223(4):457–461. doi:10.2460/javma.2003.223.457.

24 Frank DF, Erb HN, Houpt KA. Urine spraying in cats: Presence of concurrent disease and effects of a pheromone treatment. *Appl Anim Behav Sci*. 1999;61:263–272.

25 Ramos D, Reche-Junior A, Mills DS, Fragoso PL, Daniel AGT, Freitas MF, Cortopassi SG, Patricio G. A closer look at the health of cats showing urinary house-soiling (periuria): A case-control study. *J Feline Med Surg*. 2018;1–8. doi:10.1177/1098612X18801034.

26 Crowell-Davis SL, Murray TF, de Souza Dantas LM. *Veterinary psychopharmacology*. Hoboken, NJ: John Wiley & Sons; 2019;103–128.

27 Pryor PA, Hart BL, Bain MJ, Cliff KD. Causes of urine marking in cats and effects of environmental management on frequency of marking. *J Am Vet Med Assoc*. 2001;219(12):1709–1713. doi:10.2460/javma.2001.219.1709.

28 Landsberg GM, Wilson AL. Effects of clomipramine on cats presented for urine marking. *J Am Anim Hosp Assoc*. 2005;41(1):3–11. doi:10.5326/0410003.

29 King JN, Steffan J, Heath SE, Simpson BS, Crowell-Davis SL, Harrington LJM, Weiss A-B, Seewald W. Determination of the dosage of clomipramine for the treatment of urine spraying in cats. *J Am Vet Med Assoc*. 2004;225(6):881–887. doi:10.2460/javma.2004.225.881.

30 Hart BL, Cliff KD, Tynes VV, Bergman L. Control of urine marking by use of long-term treatment with fluoxetine or clomipramine in cats. *J Am Vet Med Assoc*. 2005;226(3):378–382. doi:10.2460/javma.2005.226.378.

31 Hart BL, Eckstein RA, Powell KL, Dodman NH. Effectiveness of buspirone on urine spraying and inappropriate urination in cats. *J Am Vet Med Assoc*. 1993;203(2):254–258.

32 Ogata N, Takeuchi Y. Clinical trial of a feline pheromone analogue for feline urine marking. *J Vet Med Sci*. 2001;63(2):157–161. doi:10.1292/jvms.63.157.

7

Pain and Sickness Behaviors

J. L. Stella and C. A. Tony Buffington

In a nutshell:

What to know before diagnosing and treating pain and sickness behaviors in cats:

- Our understanding of acute and chronic pain in all mammals is rapidly evolving, along with the available treatments.
- Pain, sickness, anxiety, and fear can have similar presentations:
  - Resistance to being touched or moved
  - Increased heart and respiratory rates
  - Dilated pupils
  - Increased licking/grooming of specific body parts
  - Increased vocalization
  - Increased hiding behaviors
  - Toileting outside the litter box
  - Decreased food consumption
  - Decreased socialization with family members.
- Diagnosis of pain is based on history, thorough physical examination, and diagnosis of disease processes with possible pain components.
  - History:
    - Probe for a history of sudden or gradual behavioral or "personality" changes suggesting pain or illness. Each cat is unique, so "changes" are more relevant measures of pain than a list of current abilities or propensities.
    - Ask about previous injuries, and surgeries performed elsewhere, that might inform the current presentation.
  - Physical Exam (if pain or illness is suspected):
    - Observe body language and facial expressions.
    - In cats above middle age, perform a through orthopedic and neurologic examination, remembering that imaging abnormalities may not equal pain.
  - Diseases with known pain components include FIC, osteoarthritis, orofacial pain, inflammatory GI processes (including stomatitis), advanced dental disease, urolithiasis, and others.
- Treating pain can be both important and challenging in cats.
  - Make environmental changes to support painful or sick cat's comfort (see "Behavioral approaches to helping cats..." below).
  - Pharmaceutical pain control options are limited due to the cat's metabolic peculiarities.
  - Use body language and facial grimace scores to assess effectiveness of treatment.

Clinical Handbook of Feline Behavior Medicine, First Edition. Edited by Elizabeth Stelow.
© 2023 John Wiley & Sons, Inc. Published 2023 by John Wiley & Sons, Inc.
Companion Website: www.wiley.com/go/stelow/behavior

Introduction

This chapter describes behavioral assessment and approaches to management of acute pain, chronic pain, and sickness behaviors. Chapters like this usually begin, appropriately, with definitions. In the case of pain however, a recent discussion of the definition suggested by the International Association for the Study of Pain (IASP)[1] ran to 6700 words,[a] nearly the length allotted to this chapter. For our purposes, the traditional IASP definition of acute pain, *"An unpleasant sensory and emotional experience associated with actual or potential tissue damage, or described in terms of such damage,"*[b] will serve. We can define "described" as "inferred from the patient's history, behavior[2,3] and the context of the evaluation," since we care for pets "as if" they were in pain based upon our observations even though they cannot self-report their state. Of course, many humans (infants, the obtunded, etc.) also cannot self-report, and even for those who can, their reports can only be believed, not independently validated by any specific "biomarker," so the situation really isn't that different across species. Definitions for the different kinds of chronic pain are presented later.

Acute Pain

A number of recent publications, including a book,[4] have addressed acute pain recognition and management in cats since the early studies of Lascelles et al.[5] Clinicians are encouraged to look for the presence of pain (and fear and anxiety)[6]) as part of every physical examination.[7-9] Robertson[8] has proposed three questions to guide assessment of acute pain in cats after surgery or injury:

1) (To what extent) Is the cat demonstrating normal behaviors?
2) Are any of the cat's normal behaviors lost?
3) Has the cat developed any new behaviors?

These questions should be answerable by anyone who comes into contact with hospitalized cats so that no cats "slip through the cracks" and suffer pain without recognition and appropriate care. For those with less training and experience, alerting a clinician or technician that "something doesn't look right" may be enough until the person can receive training in pain assessment.

Assessing acute pain usually includes determining its location, duration of pertinent signs and behaviors, and intensity.[7] Acute pain behaviors in cats can be evaluated using a range of behavioral (Table 7.1) and physiological variables (Table 7.2).[7,10-12] Changes in physiological parameters are neither consistent nor specific to pain however.[8] They also can occur in the presence of fear and anxiety, which of course also imply implementing appropriate care to resolve these emotional states to normalize the cat's physiology to the extent possible.

Two validated acute pain assessment scales for cats (Table 7.3) are available: the UNESP-Botucatu Multidimensional Composite Pain Scale (UNESP-Botu-catuMCPS),[13-15] and the Glasgow Composite Measures Pain Scale – Feline (CMPS-Feline).[16] One can use these scales to record baseline data for comparison with post-intervention behavior whenever possible; published forms for this process are available.[17]

---

a Interested readers can find it here.

b Provided by IASP here.

Table 7.1   Behavioral parameters/body postures suggesting acute pain/threat.

Behaviors	Normal	Acute pain/threat
Posture	Relaxed	Immobile – hunched or tense
Attitude/demeanor	At front of cage inquisitive, engaged by surroundings	Withdrawn, indifferent
Facial expression	Relaxed	Narrow palpebral fissure, flattened ear position, bunched and flattened whiskers against the face
Self-care	Eating, drinking grooming, and eliminating normally	Not eating, drinking, grooming, or eliminating
Vocalization	Purring, none	Crying out, groaning, defensive aggression (hissing, growling, spitting, tail twitching, ear flicking, scratching, biting), purring, none
Activity	Stretches on rising, explores cage, purring, kneading, rubbing, etc.	Inactive or hesitant movements, attempts to avoid handlers
Interest in food/water	Yes	No
Eliminations	Yes	No
Attention to the wound	Ignores	Looks at and/or licks wound
Interaction with people	Interested, friendly approach to caregivers	Avoids
Response to touch, pressure, and palpation	Welcomes or at least does not avoid	Avoids, defensively aggressive

Table 7.2   Physiological parameters suggesting acute pain/threat that can be assessed include.

Increase in:	*Presence of*:
● Pupil diameter	● "Sweaty" paws
● Respiratory rate	● Excessive shedding
● Temperature	● Flushing
● Heart rate	● Anxious lip-licking
● Blood pressure	

Limitations to Acute Pain Assessment

Each of the validated tools has limitations. They can be time-consuming to complete, and both have been validated for (presumably) otherwise healthy cats after ovariohysterectomy, so their utility for other pain states is yet to be demonstrated. Behaviors observed in cats with acute pain also overlap with those of cats that perceive the presence of threats, such as presentation to shelters[18] or veterinary practices,[17] and so must be considered in the context of the patient's individual history and presenting complaints. Moreover, differences in age, demeanor,[19] any disease processes present, the nature and extent of necessary interventions (including drug therapy) can occur, so patients need to be evaluated and re-evaluated as individuals. Pain scales also serve as tools to inform, not replace, one's clinical judgment about the cat's state and treatment decisions.

Table 7.3   Assessment categories of validated pain scales.

UNESP-Botucatu Multidimensional Composite Pain Scale[13]	Glasgow Composite Measures Pain Scale – Feline[16]
Subscale 1: Pain expression	
Miscellaneous behaviors:	Observer's impression of the cat
A. Lying quietly, moving tail	
B. Contracts & extends pelvic limbs ± trunk muscles	
C. Eyes partially closed	
D. Licks or bites wound	
Reaction to palpation of surgical wound	Attention to wound
Reaction to palpation of abdomen/flank	Response to palpation of wound or painful area
Vocalization	Vocalization
Subscale 2: Psychomotor change	
Posture	Posture
Comfort	Facial expression: ear and whisker position (Figure 7.1)
Activity	Response to assessor when stroked
Attitude	
A. Satisfied	
B. Uninterested	
C. Indifferent	
D. Anxious	
E. Aggressive	
Subscale 3: Physiological variables	
Arterial blood pressure	
Appetite	

To address some of these limitations, Evangelista et al. recently reported development and validation of a Feline Grimace Scale (FGS) to detect naturally occurring acute pain in cats.[20] Thirty-five client-owned cats with acute pain conditions (excluding those with diseases or conditions that could affect facial expressions, or that had received drugs or analgesics within 24 hours of presentation, were excessively shy or feral, or required immediate treatment) and 20 healthy control cats from a teaching colony at the investigators' university were video-recorded undisturbed in their cages as part of a prospective, case-control study. Painful cats then received analgesic treatment and were videoed again after one hour. Four observers, blinded to the groups and time when the images were obtained, independently scored 110 images of the painful and control cats for five facial features: head position, ear position, orbital tightening, muzzle tension, and whisker changes. FGS scores were higher in painful than in control cats, which strongly correlated with another validated instrument.[21] Good overall inter- and intra-rater reliability and excellent internal consistency also were reported. The FGS also detected response to analgesic treatment (scores after analgesia lower than before). The authors concluded, despite the small sample size and validation

Question 4

    a) Look at the following caricatures. Circle the drawing which best depicts the cat's ear position?

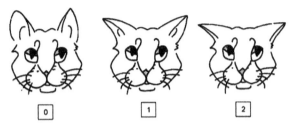

b) Look at the shape of the muzzle in the following caricatures. Circle the drawing which appears most like that of the cat?

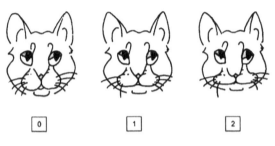

Figure 7.1 Facial expression; ear and whisker position. Glasgow Composite Measures Pain Scale – Feline.[16] John Wiley & Sons.

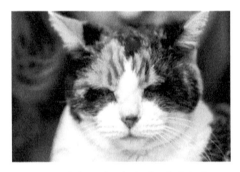

Figure 7.2 Pain scales, including facial grimace, may be useful in identifying painful cats and assessing the extent of their pain. Andriy Blokhin / Adobe Stock

using experts with years of experience working with cats, that the FGS was a valid and reliable tool for acute pain assessment in cats. They acknowledged that it is unknown, and deserves further investigation, how reliability would be affected by novice raters, and have made a Feline Grimace Scale Training Manual available for this purpose.

Shipley et al.[22] recently reported preliminary appraisal of the reliability and validity of a "Colorado State University Feline Acute Pain Scale," which uses psychological and behavioral signs of pain, facial expressions, and body posture and palpation responses to create a numerical pain score. The scale had moderate-to-good inter-rater reliability when used by expert veterinarians to assess pain intensity or the need to reassess analgesic plan after ovariohysterectomy in cats. Unfortunately, the validity fell short of current guidelines for correlation coefficients, necessitating further refinement and testing to improve its performance before further implementation.

McLennan et al.[23] recently provided discussion of some conceptual and methodological issues relating to pain assessment, including development and utilization of pain facial expression scales (Figure 7.2). They offered guidance for developing valid, reliable facial expression scales, as well as how to use them in clinical practice; their clinical recommendations are presented in Table 7.4.

Table 7.4   Best practices for using facial expression scales in clinical practice.[23] With permission of Elsevier.

- Train personnel with detailed protocols.
- Place protocols in key areas where pain assessment will be required.
- Consider continued training and inter- and intra-observer testing to ensure uniformity in scale implementation.
- Carry out multiple observations over time alongside other behavioral and physiological measures.
- Record scores and display near to patients to monitor progress and effectiveness of treatment.
- Use in combination with other validated indices.
- Do not use in patients with head injuries/trauma.

Behavioral Approaches to Helping Cats Showing Acute Pain or Sickness behaviors[24–26]

{Pharmacological approaches to helping cats in acute pain are available elsewhere.[4,27–29]}

Cats tend to form attachments to places rather than to other animals, so confinement in places where they don't feel safe can adversely affect their behavior, physiology, and recovery. Fortunately, effectively enriching these spaces can mitigate these effects.[18,24,30] Enriched conditions permit cats to cope with their surroundings and feel "safer" in their "space." Factors both inside and outside their cage can affect the welfare of cats housed in veterinary facilities.[25,30]

Inside the cage, cats need these resources to cope (Figure 7.3):

a) **A place to hide** – Cats hide to escape threats and to keep warm; place these at the back of the cage to help the cat feel safer. Objects to scratch and to perch on also can be helpful.[31]
b) **Bedding** – Cover the bottom of the cage completely, bare surfaces can be cold and uncomfortable. Bedding with the cat's and owner's scent also may help the cat feel more comfortable. Change bedding only when soiled (rather than daily); most cats prefer familiar bedding.
c) **Food and water** – Provide the cat's usual food if feasible, and put food and water near the back of the cage, as close as possible to its hiding place, to help the cat feel safer.
d) **Litter box** – Place at the front of the cage, since cats use it less frequently than (and only after) they use eating and drinking bowls. Provide the cat's usual litter if feasible.
e) **Door** – Cover as much of the door of the cage as possible to reduce unnecessary stimulation.

Factors outside the cage also can be stressful for confined cats;[18,32] these factors and how to optimize them include:

a) **Lights** – Put on a timer for predictable lighting from day to day if natural light is not available, or turn lights on and off manually at the same time each day. Do NOT turn lights on and off each time someone goes in and out of the space where cats are kept.
b) **Sound** – Minimize (<60 dB – quiet conversational level – can be measured with smartphone apps). Provide music (played softly) cat specific if possible (e.g. https://www.musicforcats.com).[33] There is little research into the effects of white noise on cat stress. It may be useful during especially loud periods of the day to dampen the impact of unpredictable noise with the following caveats:
   i)   Prioritize efforts to decrease the source of the noise or to house cats in quieter areas.
   ii) Ensure the volume is set to below 60 dB.

Reducing our feline patient's stress:
The right way to set up a cage

1. **Select a top cage** - cats feel safer when they are close to our level. Top cages also help you avoid leaning over the patient, which can be threatening to cats.
2. **Cover the bottom of the cage completely.** Bare metal is cold, loud and uncomfortable. Use cage pads to completely cover the bottom of the cage.
3. **A hiding box (or the cat's carrier)** gives patients both a place to hide in and a place to rest on.
4. **Bowls.** Put food and water bowls close to the opening of the hiding box, and as far away from the litter box as possible without interfering with access to the hiding box.
5. **Litter box.** Put the litter box in front of the hiding box and away from bowls. Use a generous amount of litter, enough for the cat to paw without "hitting bottom".
6. **Cover the cage door.** Place a cage pad over the cage door when your patient arrives in the ward to reduce stressful stimulation. Apply 10 sprays of Feliway* onto the pad, wait ~30 seconds for the alcohol to dissipate, then place the pad over the lower 2/3 of the cage to block their view, and so you can still observe them. Binder clips are available if the pad slips.
7. **Enrichment** - feel free to add personal items from home, toys and catnip as you see fit so our patients can enjoy their stay as much as possible!

*NEVER SPRAY FELIWAY SPRAY DIRECTLY ONTO THE CAT OR INTO THE CAGE WHILE THE CAT IS IN IT.

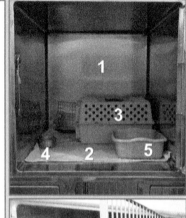
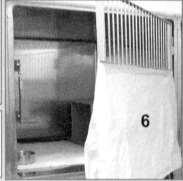

Figure 7.3 Poster of cage set-up recommendations. René Descartes' Traite de l'homme (Treatise of Man).

iii) Place white noise generator near the room door or source of the noise to be masked, not close to an individual cage or housing unit.

iv) Use only intermittently and as needed.

v) Closely monitor cats' behavioral response to use of white noise generators, reassessing use as indicated.

c) **Odors** – Minimize smells from dogs, other cats, perfumes, alcohol (from hand rubs), cigarettes, cleaning chemicals (including laundry detergent), air fresheners, etc.; all can be aversive and stressful, especially to cats confined in a cage where they can't move away from the odors.

d) **Temperature:** Cats prefer warm, 85–100 degrees F, temperatures.[34] Provide bedding that allows cats to "cocoon" to retain warmth if they choose to do so.

e) **Daily routine:** Perform cleaning, feeding, and treatment procedures at the same time each day, preferably by the same person, to increase predictability. Return cage furnishings to the same place after spot-cleaning, and house cats in the same cage throughout their stay.

f) **Low stress handling**[35] – Use these techniques to maximize the cat's perception of safety, predictability, and control. Add extra attention like brushing or playing from a familiar, dedicated person whenever possible.

Behaviors signaling that something may be wrong with caged cats include "resting" in litter boxes, and cages that show no use since the last cleaning or are in disarray. Sickness behaviors also are cause for concern. These include variable combinations of vomiting, diarrhea or soft feces, no eliminations in 24 hours, urinating or defecating out of the litter box, anorexia or decreased appetite, lethargy, and not grooming, which will be discussed later in this chapter.[36]

Acute Pain Resources

How Do I Know if My Cat Is in Pain? https://catfriendly.com/feline-diseases/signs-symptoms/know-cat-pain

2022 AAHA/AAFP Pain Management Guidelines for Dogs and Cats[37]

UNESP-Botucatu Multidimensional Composite Pain Scale https://static1.squarespace.com/static/56c72d078259b517148247e6/t/579dc74744024362eb01bdbc/1469957961939/UNESP+Botucatu+Multidimensional+Composite+Pain+Scale.pdf

Glasgow Composite Measures Pain Scale – Feline (CMPS-Feline).[16] https://www.newmetrica.com/acute-pain-measurement

Fear Free practice[6] https://fearfreepets.com

Cat-friendly practice[38] https://catvets.com/cfp/cfp

Domestic Cat Demeanour Scoring System – https://journals.sagepub.com/doi/suppl/10.1177/1098612X13509081/suppl_file/Annex1.pdf

Chronic Pain (CP)

Acute pain drives behavior in the service of survival. Pain perception usually occurs in the presence of states that threaten physical integrity and survival. Unfortunately, pain can outlive its usefulness, becoming chronic and maladaptive. Pain perception has qualities of both intensity and affect. Intensity describes the physical unpleasantness of the perception, whereas affect describes the feelings that accompany pain perception. These perceptions drive motor activities (withdrawal) and behaviors (guarding) directed toward avoiding continued exposure to the sensory inputs that resulted in the perception, and to protect the individual to permit healing. Acute pain usually results from input from sensory neurons that respond to noxious (nociceptive) stimuli (Figure 7.4), which has influenced thinking about pain for centuries.

In 1979, Patrick Wall,[40] one of the fathers of the gate theory of pain,[41] recognized that the time had come to shift from thinking about pain solely based on the origin of the input and the destination of the output to considering the dynamic stability of the entire interconnected system. He recognized that nociceptive input was but one of many factors evaluated during ongoing analysis of the external and internal environments necessary to permit a response that increased the probability of survival.

Nociceptive input to the central nervous system (CNS) may result in perceptions of immediate unpleasantness, as well as in appraisals of the meaning of the input.[3,42] These appraisals weigh the long-term implications of the presence of the pain state, based on one's genetic and epigenetic history, memory of past events, the environmental context, and imagination of future possibilities (expectation). Complex interactions between amplifying and inhibitory neuronal networks in the central nervous system also influence pain perception,[43] as do emotional, hormonal, and external environmental influences.[44,45]

The situation becomes even more complex with chronicity, when CP can become a disease in its own right.[46] Moreover, perception of environmental threat ("stress") can exacerbate clinical signs in a variety of CP states, including feline interstitial cystitis (FIC),[42] and exposure to chronic or repeated threats, such as chronic restraint or repeated forced swimming in rodents.[47] In contrast, exposure to acute stress (threat) can inhibit pain perception, called "stress-induced analgesia,"[44,47] possibly in part through corticotropin-releasing factor (CRF_2) and oxytocin receptor signaling.[48]

Most human and animal patients with CP are managed in primary care. Approximately 20–55% of human primary care consultations are for pain,

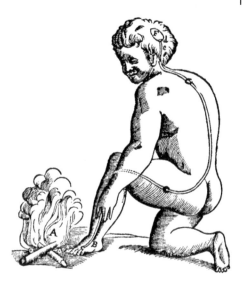

Figure 7.4   Historical illustration of the "labeled line" pathway from nociceptor to painful perception.[39] René Descartes' Traite de l'homme (Treatise of Man).

of which roughly half are for CP. If the figures are anything like this in primary veterinary care, understanding how CP is classified may improve the quality of care for this problem.

Chronic Pain Definitions

A systematic classification coding system for CP in human beings was developed for the first time in the 11th Revision, the International Classification of Diseases, (ICD-11), in 2018.[c] The current (2019) IASP Classification of common CP conditions is presented in Table 7.5.[d]

For many years CP was defined as pain that persists past normal healing time[49] and hence lacks the acute warning function of physiological nociception. Because this definition was difficult to verify in some pain conditions, the IASP currently defines CP as pain that lasts or recurs for longer than 3 months in humans.[46,50] They define primary CP pain in one or more anatomical regions that is associated with emotional distress that interferes with daily life. They differentiate three different kinds of common CP conditions; nociceptive (actual or threatened tissue damage causing the persistent activation of peripheral nociceptors), nociplastic (altered nociceptive function), and neuropathic (disease or lesion of the somatosensory system). In contrast, they consider secondary CP to reflect pathology associated with some other disease (e.g., cancer, some cases of osteoarthritis).

In 2016, the term "nociplastic" pain was proposed as a mechanistic descriptor for chronic pain states not characterized by obvious activation of nociceptors or neuropathy, "but in whom clinical

---

c https://www.who.int/classifications/icd/en.

d https://www.iasp-pain.org/advocacy/definitions-of-chronic-pain-syndromes. Accessed February 22, 2022.

Table 7.5 IASP Classification of common, clinically relevant chronic pain conditions.[50] Adapted from[44]

Name	Description
1) Chronic primary pain	Chronic pain in one or more anatomical regions that persists or recurs for longer than 3 months, and that is characterized by significant emotional distress (anxiety, anger/frustration or depressed mood) or functional disability (interference in daily life activities and reduced participation in social roles). Chronic primary pain is multifactorial: biological psychological and social factors contribute to the pain syndrome. The diagnosis is appropriate independently of identified biological or psychological contributors unless another diagnosis would better account for the presenting symptoms.
2) Chronic secondary musculoskeletal pain	Persistent or recurrent pain that arises as part of a disease process directly affecting bone(s), joint(s), muscle(s), or related soft tissue(s); may be spontaneous or movement-induced, and is limited to nociceptive pain. It does not include pain perceived in musculoskeletal tissues but not arising therefrom, such as the pain of compression neuropathy or somatic referred pain.
3) Chronic secondary visceral pain	Persistent or recurrent pain originating from internal organs of the head/neck region and the thoracic, abdominal, and pelvic cavities.
4) Chronic secondary headache or orofacial pain	Secondary pain caused by chronic headache and orofacial conditions, include chronic dental pains and temporomandibular disorders.
5) Chronic postsurgical or posttraumatic pain	Pain persisting after surgery or other trauma, where the initiating events and normal healing times are known.
6) Chronic cancer-related pain	Pain caused by the cancer itself (by the primary tumor or by metastases) or by its treatment (surgery, chemotherapy, and radiotherapy)
7) Chronic neuropathic pain	Pain caused by a lesion or disease of the somatosensory nervous system, which may be peripheral or central, and spontaneous or evoked by sensory stimuli (hyperalgesia and allodynia).

and psychophysical findings suggest altered nociceptive function."[51] According to the IASP, nociplastic pain might be involved in symptoms reported by patients with fibromyalgia, nonspecific musculoskeletal pain, and visceral pain disorders such as irritable bowel syndrome, and interstitial cystitis.[51] "In addition, patients suffering initially from nociceptive pain, such as osteoarthritis, may develop alterations in nociceptive processing manifested as altered descending pain inhibition accompanied by spread of hypersensitivity. In such cases, variable combinations of nociceptive and nociplastic input contribute to their pain."[51]

Examples of some common chronic pain conditions in people and domestic cats are presented in Table 7.6. The fact that many of those described in people have not (yet) been described in cats is not meant to imply that they do not occur in cats – just that their occurrence has not been identified to our knowledge at the present time. Certainly animal models of some of the conditions in people exist, but the relevance of models based upon injuries inflicted on healthy animals to naturally occurring diseases is not always obvious.[52]

Behavioral signs of chronic pain can be subtle, non-specific, and progress slowly. Owners may report the appearance of new and the disappearance of any combination of the behaviors described in Table 7.7.[53,56,57]

Table 7.6 Examples of chronic pain conditions in people and domestic cats. Adapted from[44]

Name	Examples in people	Examples in cats
1) Chronic primary pain	a) Widespread pain (e.g., fibromyalgia) b) Complex regional pain syndromes c) Headache and orofacial pain (e.g., chronic migraine or temporomandibular disorder) d) Visceral pain (e.g., irritable bowel syndrome or interstitial cystitis (IC)) e) Musculoskeletal pain (e.g., nonspecific low-back pain)	a) Not described b) Not described c) Orofacial pain d) Feline IC[53] and (some cases of) inflammatory bowel disease e) Not described
2) Chronic secondary musculoskeletal pain	a) Rheumatoid arthritis b) Symptomatic osteoarthritis (OA) c) Spasticity after spinal cord injury d) Rigidity in Parkinson disease	a) Not described b) OA c) Similar d) Not described
3) Chronic secondary visceral pain	a) Inflammatory e.g., esophagitis, gastritis, pancreatitis b) Vascular e.g., thrombosis, hypercoagulability, aneurysm c) Mechanical e.g., e.g., lithiasis, stenosis, traction of a viscus	Similar
4) Chronic secondary headache or orofacial pain	a) Trauma or injury b) Vascular c) Infection d) Dental e) Neuropathic	Similar
6) Chronic postsurgical or posttraumatic pain	Many	Many
7) Chronic cancer-related pain	Many	Many
8) Chronic neuropathic pain	See Scholz, et al.[54]	See Epstein[55]

Table 7.7 Behavioral changes observed in cats with chronic pain. Adapted from[53,56,57]

Behavior	Description
Movement	• Less fluid than usual • Less time spent moving, playing, or exploring • Intensity and vitality decreased (activity intolerance) • Jumps on to or down from elevated surfaces in stages rather than directly
Eating behaviors	• Decreased or increased food intake
Elimination behaviors	• Difficulty getting into or out of the litter box • Difficulty getting into or out of normal elimination postures • Urination or defecation outside of the litter box

(Continued)

Table 7.7 (Continued)

Behavior	Description
Grooming behaviors	• Reduced grooming frequency or duration of grooming bouts • Difficulty in positioning for grooming • Reduced scratching behavior • Excessive grooming due to pain or abnormal sensory sensitivity, which can result in self-induced alopecia
Social behaviors	• Less willing to interact with people and other pets • More hiding • Avoids being stroked or handled
Exploratory behaviors	• Less interest in the environment (e.g., playing, going outside, greeting owners and other pets, jumping onto or between elevated surfaces, sniffing objects, looking under furniture) • Seeks out warm, comfortable resting areas
Sudden vocalizing or agitation	• Suddenly vocalizes or runs, either spontaneously or during attempts to pet or stroke the cat* • Suddenly becomes fixated on a particular part of its body and starts licking it intensively for no obvious reason • Normal behavior may resume shortly after these episodes

*Muscle spasms or skin twitches along the back after being stroked could indicate hypersensitivity.

Chronic Pain Scales

Three owner-based and one veterinarian-based chronic OA pain scales currently exist.[53] These include the Feline Musculoskeletal Pain Index (FMPI), the Client Specific Outcome Measures (CSOM), and the Montreal Instrument for Cat Arthritis Testing for Use by Caretaker (MI-CAT[C]) for clients, and the Montreal Instrument for Cat Arthritis Testing for Use by Veterinarian (MI-CAT[V]) for clinicians (links to scales provided in the Resources section). The owner-based scales were developed to permit evaluation of the cat in its usual context to avoid the confounds associated with transportation and evaluation in a clinical environment. These scales are still undergoing validation, and currently are considered "living documents," subject to ongoing studies to further validate them.[53] Whether or not these or other scales will be incorporated into primary practice will depend on the outcome of these studies.

For comparison with scales used in human medicine, a recent study compared standardized response means, standardized effect sizes, and receiver operating curve analyses to assess change between baseline and 3-month assessments in 250 participants from a randomized clinical effectiveness trial of collaborative telecare management for moderate to severe and persistent musculoskeletal pain between 2-, 3-, 4-, and 11-item scales.[58] They reported that some measures were better able to detect changes than were others, and that post hoc analyses suggested that differences in content or rating scale structure (number of response options or anchoring language) did not adequately explain the observed differences in the detection of change. To the author's knowledge, current veterinary scales have not yet been tested for such sensitivity to change over time.

Health-related Quality of Life (HRQoL) Scales[53]

Scales for both general HRQoL[59–61] and specific conditions[62,63] have been developed and partially validated for cats. The generic scales could be used for chronic pain, but to date have not been sufficiently developed to be incorporated into daily clinical practice. They include (links to scales provided in the Resources section):

- VetMetrica[60] – is web-based, and initial evidence supports its use in cats with OA.[64] It consists of 20 items divided into 3 domains (vitality, comfort, and emotional wellbeing), and currently is available for use in clinical practice and research by paid subscription.
- Feline QoL measure[61] consists of 16 items divided into 2 domains (healthy behaviors and clinical signs). It has been evaluated in healthy cats, but is not yet available.
- Cat HEalth and Wellbeing (CHEW),[65] consists of 33 items in 8 domains including physical (mobility, eyes, coat, fitness, and appetite), mental and emotional (emotions and energy), and social functioning (engagement) domains.

As with the pain scales, whether or not these or other scales will be incorporated into primary practice remains to be seen.

Clinical Assessment of CP

Montiero et al.[53,56] have proposed a step-by step approach to evaluation of chronic pain (please consult the references for additional details).

- Schedule sufficient time, especially for initial consultations.
- Obtain details of patient's environment and daily routine. Recent behavior changes may be particularly significant. Environmental,[66] pain and/or HRQoL scales can be used to obtain additional information.
- Perform low-stress physical examination using feline-friendly handling techniques; carefully observe body language and facial expressions, palpate joints and long bones if OA is suspected, conduct neurological examination when neuropathic pain is suspected. NB: Withdrawal, avoidance, vocalization, etc. during palpation of specific body parts can indicate pain, but lack of behavioral response does not exclude pain presence in a shy/fearful cat.
- Observe the cat moving or assess home videos of the cat provided by the owners.
- Consider laboratory tests to investigate identified signs of concomitant diseases (secondary CP). Imaging may aid the diagnosis of some conditions, e.g., OA, stones, and cancer, but may not correlate with clinical signs of pain.

Sickness Behaviors

Sickness behaviors (SB)[67] are well-documented physiological and behavioral responses to infection that has been found in species across the animal kingdom, including zebrafish,[68] rodents,[69] dairy cattle,[70] cats,[36] and humans.[71] Common SB across species include fever, anorexia, inactivity, and decreased social contact.

Psychological stress also can result in SB, via stress response system (SRS)-induced release of corticotrophin-releasing factor (CRF), which activates the sympathetic nervous (SNS) and immune

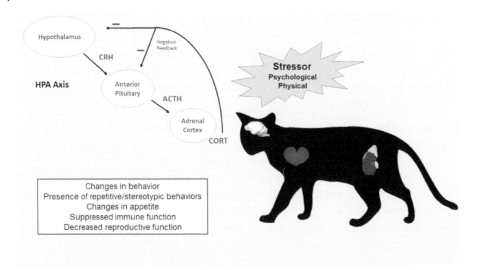

Figure 7.5   Depiction of the stress-induced activation of the HPA-axis and associated behavioral and physiologic responses.

systems, resulting in pro-inflammatory cytokine release.[72,73] This cascade has been linked to SB, mood symptoms, and pathologic pain (Figure 7.5).[74,75]

The associated behavioral response includes suppression of self-care behaviors such as feeding, social contact, and grooming to support processes that conserve energy to boost immune function to fight pathogens,[75,76] along with increased vigilance when exposed to psychological threats.[77,78] These psycho-neuro-immunologic changes are evolutionarily conserved, adaptive, normal responses that helps individuals survive by motivating the animal to change its behavior.

The motivational drive of SB should be considered in welfare assessments, as well as other motivators, such as fear, hunger, and thirst. Seeking rest, withdrawing from the environment, and caring for one's self are evolutionarily adaptive responses to infection that are as normal as arousal and escape are in response to a threat.[79] However, when this motivational state is caused by chronic environmental disturbances that exceed the animal's coping capacity, it is a sign of impaired welfare and should be addressed. Impaired welfare can be considered a chronic imbalance between positive and negative experiences; decreased perception of control and increased perception of threat resulting in chronic activation of the SRS.[80] It is now assumed that, similar to humans, chronic exposure to environmental stressors can induce mental suffering in animals with or without physical health problems.[80]

Clinical Signs of Sickness Behaviors

The most common SB responses to stress in domestic cats include decreased appetite, vomiting of hair, food, or bile, eliminating outside of litter pans, decreased social interactions, decreased grooming behavior, and an increase in the frequency and intensity of attempts to hide (Figure 7.6).[18,30,36,81]

We found increased SB in response to environmental stressors in laboratory-housed cats, which included transient (one-week) discontinuation of contact or interactions with the cats' primary caretaker, changes in time of day of routine husbandry, unfamiliar caretakers, and a delay of three hours

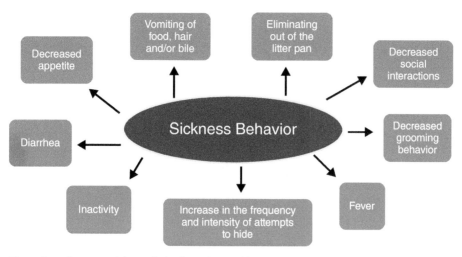

Figure 7.6   Common sickness behaviors observed in domestic cats.

in feeding time.[36] These events resulted in a 3.2-fold increased relative risk (RR) for SB compared to control weeks, and larger increases in risk for decreased food intake (RR = 9.3) and eliminations (RR = 6.4), and an increased risk for elimination of feces (RR = 9.8) and urine (RR = 1.6) outside the litter pan. Subsequently, changes in immune system function associated with stressors were found, including a decrease in circulating lymphocytes and an increase in the neutrophil to lymphocyte ratio from baseline. Additionally, gene expression for the pro-inflammatory cytokines IL-6 and TNF-α were altered.[30]

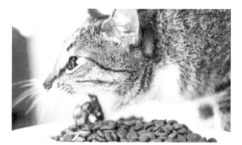

Figure 7.7   Vomiting is not a normal feline behavior; the cause should be explored.

We have consistently found that the most common SB in response to psychological stressors in confined cats include decreased appetite, increased eliminations out of the litter pan, and vomiting of food, hair, and/or bile (Figure 7.7). The most common owner reported SB include excessive appetite (34%), vomiting of hair, food or bile (25%), nervous/anxious/fearful behavior (22%), and urination or defecating out of the litter pan (11%).[82] These and other SBs also are frequently identified in pet cats brought to veterinarians for evaluation.[83] These results demonstrate that daily monitoring of cats for SB can offer a practical, non-invasive method to assess stress responses and the quality of their environment and thus, gauge overall welfare for cats confined in homes or veterinary hospitals, as well as those housed in shelters or research colonies.

Management

The housing space of confined cats is generally reduced in both quantity and quality in comparison to options available to their free-roaming counterparts. There are many aspects of the captive environment that may impact the welfare of cats. Individuals must adapt to their physical environment, which often does not match the physical environment in which their species evolved. Captive housing environments are typically built and maintained for human comfort and convenience. Cats perceive their environments very differently from how humans do, so many environmental factors may be aversive or stressful to them. Factors pertaining to the macro-environment (the room), the micro-environment (the individual cage or restricted area available to the cat), predictability and control of the environment, and the quality of the social environment (including the human–cat relationship), as well as interactions with conspecifics and other animals in the environment, such as dogs housed within auditory or olfactory proximity, all influence cats' perception of threat.[18,84–86] The impact of stress caused by human intervention(s) should be minimized to support both the psychological and physiological health of confined cats. Understanding the cats' sensorium and how they are likely to perceive stimuli will aid caretakers in monitoring and improving the housing environment. Finally, the environment should be behaviorally relevant, with the quantity and quality of space provided allowing for the development and normal expression of species-typical behavior patterns.

Perhaps the greatest stressor cats experience when confined in a home or cage is the perception or actual lack of ability to control their surroundings. Confined cats have little or no control over:[32]

- Who their social partners are.
- How much space they can put between themselves and others.
- The type, amount, or availability of food.
- The quality or quantity of environmental stimuli they experience, including
  - Lighting
  - Noise
  - Odor
  - Temperature.

Predictability, or the lack thereof, is another environmental aspect that cats may perceive to be stressful. Studies have shown that, given a choice, animals will choose predictability over unpredictability, especially in relation to aversive events.[32,87,88] Predictability refers both to temporal consistency (the time when events happen), as well as familiarity with caretakers and the environment. A consistent, predictable daily routine is essential, particularly when an animal is confined. Daily cleaning and feeding procedures conducted at the same time of day and performed by a familiar person allow cats to predict potentially aversive events.

Finally, individual personality differences have been identified in cats, indicating that personality traits may play a role in cat preferences for or use of resources. A recent study of coping styles in cats reported that cats housed in an enriched housing environment that was quiet, predictable, and enriched, to minimize stress and promote acclimation, used hiding and perching resources differently. Although hiding decreased and perching increased across days overall, cats that were identified as having a reactive coping style spent more time in the hide box, whereas cats identified as having a proactive coping style spent more time on the perch.[89] These results reinforce the importance of addressing individual differences by providing enriched caging with *both* hiding and perching opportunities to confined cats, as previously reported.[18,31,81,90,91]

Behavioral Approaches to Helping Cats Showing Chronic Pain Or Sickness Behaviors[92,93]

The Client

Owners of cats with chronic pain come to us for a diagnosis for the cause of whatever signs concern them most, and may not know that their cat suffers from chronic pain. In our experience, the most important consideration for a successful outcome for cats with chronic pain related to FIC (and apparently other chronic pain states as well)[94] is effective and empathic client communication.[92] After performing a complete evaluation of the cat and concluding that chronic pain is likely to be present, we can explain to the client that while no cure currently is available, appropriate therapeutic and palliative procedures can generally keep the cat's clinical signs to a minimum and increase the disease-free interval, and that most of their care can be provided in collaboration with a trained technician. We also demonstrate compassion by listening carefully to the client's story of the effects of having a cat with chronic pain, provide a satisfactory explanation for the sources of the signs, express care and concern for the situation, and enhance the *client's* perception of control. Effective caregiver–client interactions appear to enhance patient adherence to treatments, and quality of life outcomes of therapy.[95] We can then prescribe any therapies appropriate to the presenting manifestation(s), and (when possible) introduce the client to the technician or other staff member trained to care for cats with chronic pain, who will coach the client to implement multimodal environmental modification (MEMO) [66,96] for the patient in an attempt to minimize the effects of perception of environmental threat on the cat's signs. The formality of this introduction demonstrates that we intend to sustain the partnership with the client through our technical support staff to support their efforts to gain and maintain control of the patient's clinical signs.

The Cat

Pharmacotherapy

Choices for drug therapy, if any, depend on the individual cat's manifestation(s) of chronic pain, and are beyond the scope of this chapter. Excellent references are available elsewhere.[28,97] Medicating cats can be challenging and if forced on them will increase fear and distress, damage the cat–owner relationship, and has the potential to shorten their life if the owner is unable to provide the necessary treatment, especially for chronic conditions. Therefore, we recommend utilizing low-stress techniques and training cats to accept examination, medication, and treatments, ideally before they are necessary, to minimize fear and distress and optimize care. A full discussion of cooperative care is beyond the scope of this chapter but can found elsewhere.[98]

Diet and Feeding Management

Some diets are marketed for "stressed" cats, but the evidence for their effectiveness in management of chronic pain has yet to be evaluated, and their salutary effects, if any, seem modest.[99,100] Moreover, studies have shown that many cats with chronic visceral pain (FIC) can be effectively managed without any diet change.[36,96,101,102] In most cases we recommend that owners choose whichever (Association of American Feed Control Officials labeled) diets fit their personal preferences, and then to offer a few examples of these at mealtime so their cat can express its preferences. We recommend this to minimize the effects of their perception of diet on the activation of the SRS of both the client and the cat. A detailed discussion of the pros and cons of diet therapy for all manifestations of chronic pain is beyond the scope of this article, and unfortunately most studies of dietary management of pain have been either supported or conducted by food companies.[103] If a diet change seems appropriate, only attempt to implement it after the cat has returned home and is feeling better to reduce the risk of inducing a learned aversion to the new food.

The Environment

Environmental conditions are known to affect the behavior and health of animals,[104] particularly captive animals.[32,105] Environmental enrichment has been shown to relieve chronic pain in a variety of animal studies.[106-108] If cats with chronic pain have a sensitized SRS, then treatments that increase their perception of control *and* reduce their perception of threat are more likely to be effective than those that do not. Effective MEMO creates conditions that permit the patient to feel safe, and to have unrestricted access to species-appropriate novelty, activity, and interactions with other animals (including humans). Effective MEMO for cats means provision of all "necessary" resources, refinement of interactions with owners, a tolerable intensity of conflict, and thoughtful institution of change(s) to the cat's environment (its "territory"). It also extends the "1+1" rule traditionally applied to litter boxes (one for each cat in the home, plus one more) to all pertinent resources (particularly resting areas, and food, water, and litter containers) in the home.

Space

Each cat needs a safe "refuge"; a cozy carrier in a desirable (to the cat) location in the home and outfitted for the cat's comfort. Habituating the cat to the carrier also facilitates crating the cat for medical care and other travel. Cats also interact with the physical structures in their environment, and need opportunities to scratch (both horizontal and vertical may be necessary), climb, hide, and rest; preferably in multiple locations in the home.

A recent study reported that some cats may enjoy olfactory enrichment, including catnip, silver vine, Tatarian honeysuckle and valerian (a constituent of Feliway spray).[109,110] Another recent study reported pet cats' preferences for social interaction with the owner (50% of cats), food (37%), toys (11%), and scent (2%).[111] Significantly more cats preferred social interaction to toys and food to scent, but no differences were found between social interaction and food, food and toys, or toys and scent.

Food

Cats prefer to eat individually in a safe, quiet location where they will not be startled by other animals, sudden movement, or activity of air ducts or appliances that may begin operation unexpectedly.[112] Some cats also prefer wet foods, possibly due to differences in flavors or the potentially more natural "mouth feel," whereas other cats prefer dry foods. When a diet change is appropriate (and agreed to by the owner), offering the new diet in a separate, adjacent container at mealtime rather than removing the usual food and replacing it with the new food or mixing foods permits cats to express their preferences. Natural cat-feeding behavior also includes predatory activities such as stalking and pouncing. These may be simulated by hiding small amounts of food around the house, or by putting food into food puzzles.[113]

Litter Boxes

Litter box issues may be present even when LUTS are not observed. A detailed discussion of litter-box location (safe), size (big), litter type (ask the cat) and management is beyond the scope of this article; excellent recommendations are available elsewhere.[92,93,114]

Play

Cats may enjoy play interactions with owners, and many can be trained to perform behaviors ("tricks") to the extent that their condition permits.[115] Owners need to understand that while cats readily respond to positive reinforcement (food), they cannot respond to punishment like more group-living social species, because this form of "teaching" apparently never entered their behavioral repertoire.[116] Cats also seem to be more amenable to learning if the behavior is shaped *before* feeding. Many cats appear to like novelty, so providing a variety of toys, rotated or replaced regularly, can sustain their interest. Some cats also seem to have preferences for specific prey. For example, some cats prefer to chase birds, whereas others may prefer to chase mice, lizards, or bugs. Identifying a cat's "prey preferences" allows owners to provide toys that the cat will be most likely to play with.

Not all cats enjoy play; some seem to prefer to be petted and groomed.

Conflict

Like the rest of us, when a cat feels threatened, it often responds by attempting to restore its perception of control. During such responses, some cats become aggressive, some become withdrawn, and some become ill. Inter-cat conflict may be present when multiple cats are housed indoors together.[117] Conflict among cats can develop because of perceived threats to their status in the home, over access to valued (or scarce) resources (food, resting areas, litter boxes, owner attention, etc.), from other animals in the home, or from outside cats. Providing a "house of plenty," one with more resources than all the cats can use at once, may minimize these risks.

Follow-up

All the information clients sometimes need can overwhelm them.[92] One can help support the client by focusing conversations on those changes the client perceives to be most important, and is willing to make, by providing written instructions for implementing the desired changes, and then following up with the client in a few days to see what questions have come to their mind, and what they have managed to do in the interim. We always ask *both*, "How is your cat doing?" and "How are *you* doing?" We then re-contact them in a week or two to learn how things are going and to provide support. If implementation of the changes has been successful, one can move on to additional changes. In our experience, a time usually comes (and often quite quickly) when the client "gets it" and can continue on without additional coaching.

Prevention

Vulnerability for a chronic pain condition can develop after significant adverse experiences, particularly early in life.[118] This vulnerability may be unmasked by chronic and or overwhelming perception of threat later in life, and also may be mitigated by effective MEMO.[119,120] The husbandry implications of this information is clear; to the extent that we can convince ourselves and our clients of the value of effective environmental enrichment for all cats, and then find and implement ways to provide it, we all – cats, clients, and caregivers – are likely to enjoy better health and wellbeing, and may minimize the risk of chronic pain.

Conclusions

Many confined cats appear to cope with less-than-optimal environments. The underlying, early adverse event-mediated, differences in neuro-endocrine-immune responses identified in some cats with chronic pain, however, may limit their adaptive capacity, so these cats may represent a separate population of individuals with increased vulnerability to provocative environments. Moreover, we are concerned more with optimizing the environments of cats than with identifying and implementing minimum requirements for their survival.

Providing an environment that is compatible with cats' behavioral needs often seems to mitigate the effects of at least some manifestations of chronic pain in addition to promoting their general health and welfare. This is not to say that the absence of environmental enrichment causes chronic pain in cats, only that it may unmask an underlying vulnerability in some cats.[121]

Resources for Practices

The science of Feline OA Pain https://www.zoetisus.com/oa-pain/feline-oa-pain.aspx

Degenerative Joint Disease in Cats https://catvets.com/public/PDFs/ClientBrochures/DJD-Webview.pdf

WSAVA Global Pain Council https://wsava.org/committees/global-pain-council

WSAVA Assessment, recognition and treatment of pain, 2022 AAFP/AAHA Pain Management Guidelines Dogs and Cats https://www.aaha.org/aaha-guidelines/2022-aaha-pain-management-guidelines-for-dogs-and-cats/home https://www.wsava.org/WSAVA/media/Documents/CommitteeResources/GlobalPainCouncil/Chronic-Pain_Cats.pdf

Resources for Clients

How do I know if my cat is in pain? https://catfriendly.com/keep-your-cat-healthy/know-cat-pain

How to tell if your cat is in pain https://www.aaha.org/globalassets/02-guidelines/pain-management/painmanagement_cats_web.pdf

Chronic pain in cats Owner webinar – www.youtube.com/watch?v=_f18kjTbuCc

Degenerative Joint Disease (Arthritis) in cats https://catfriendly.com/feline-diseases/degenerative-joint-disease-arthritis

Joint pain in cats – http://painfreecats.org/for-owners/#diagnosing

References

1 Aydede M. Does the IASP definition of pain need updating? *Pain Rep.* 2019;4(5):e777.
2 Merola I, Mills DS. Behavioural signs of pain in cats: An expert consensus. *PLoS One.* 2016;11(2):e0150040.
3 Merola I, Mills DS. Systematic review of the behavioural assessment of pain in cats. *J Feline Med Surg.* 2016;18(2):60–76.
4 Steagall P, Robertson SA, Taylor P. *Feline anesthesia and pain management.* Hoboken, NJ: John Wiley & Sons; 2017.

5   Lascelles B, Cripps P, Mirchandani S, Waterman A. Carprofen as an analgesic for postoperative pain in cats: Dose titration and assessment of efficacy in comparison to pethidine hydrochloride. *J Small Anim Pract*. 1995;36(12):535–541.

6   Demaline B. Fear in the veterinary clinic: History and development of the fear free℠ initiative. *Conspectus Borealis*. 2018;4(1):2.

7   Steagall PV, Monteiro BP. Acute pain in cats: Recent advances in clinical assessment. *J Feline Med Surg*. 2018;21(1):25–34.

8   Robertson S. How do we know they hurt? Assessing acute pain in cats. *In Practice*. 2018;40(10):440–448.

9   Mathews K, Kronen PW, Lascelles D, et al. Guidelines for recognition, assessment and treatment of pain: WSAVA Global Pain Council members and co-authors of this document. *J Small Anim Pract*. 2014;55(6):E10–E68.

10 Waran N, Best L, Williams V, Salinsky J, Dale A, Clarke N. A preliminary study of behaviour-based indicators of pain in cats. *Anim Welfare*. 2007;16(S):105–108.

11 Robertson S. Assessment and recognition of acute (adaptive) pain. In: Steagall P, Robertson S, Taylor P, eds. *Feline anesthesia and pain management*. Hoboken, New Jersey; 2017:199–220.

12 Corletto F. *Using acute pain scales for cats*. British Medical Journal Publishing Group; 2017.

13 Brondani JT, Mama KR, Luna SP, et al. Validation of the English version of the UNESP-Botucatu multidimensional composite pain scale for assessing postoperative pain in cats. *BMC Vet Res*. 2013;9(1):143.

14 Benito J, Monteiro BP, Beauchamp G, Lascelles BDX, Steagall PV. Evaluation of interobserver agreement for postoperative pain and sedation assessment in cats. *J Am Vet Med Assoc*. 2017;251(5):544–551.

15 Doodnaught GM, Benito J, Monteiro BP, Beauchamp G, Grasso SC, Steagall PV. Agreement among undergraduate and graduate veterinary students and veterinary anesthesiologists on pain assessment in cats and dogs: A preliminary study. *Can Vet J*. 2017;58(8):805.

16 Reid J, Scott E, Calvo G, Nolan A. Definitive Glasgow acute pain scale for cats: Validation and intervention level. *Vet Rec*. 2017;108(18):449.

17 Zeiler GE, Fosgate GT, Van Vollenhoven E, Rioja E. Assessment of behavioural changes in domestic cats during short-term hospitalisation. *J Feline Med Surg*. 2014;16(6):499–503.

18 Stella J, Croney C, Buffington T. Environmental factors that affect the behavior and welfare of domestic cats (Felis silvestris catus) housed in cages. *App Anim Behav Sci*. 2014;160:94–105.

19 Buisman M, Hasiuk MM, Gunn M, Pang DS. The influence of demeanor on scores from two validated feline pain assessment scales during the perioperative period. *Vet Anaesth Analg*. 2017;44(3):646–655.

20 Evangelista MC, Watanabe R, Leung VS, et al. Facial expressions of pain in cats: The development and validation of a Feline Grimace Scale. *Sci Rep*. 2019;9(1):1–11.

21 Calvo G, Holden E, Reid J, et al. Development of a behaviour-based measurement tool with defined intervention level for assessing acute pain in cats. *J Small Anim Pract*. 2014;55(12):622–629.

22 Shipley H, Guedes A, Graham L, Goudie-deangelis E, Wendt-Hornickle E. Preliminary appraisal of the reliability and validity of the Colorado State University Feline Acute Pain Scale. *J Feline Med Surg*. 2019;21(4):335–339.

23 McLennan KM., Miller AL, Dalla Costa E, et al. Conceptual and methodological issues relating to pain assessment in mammals: The development and utilisation of pain facial expression scales. *App Anim Behav Sci*. 2019;217:1–5.

24 Carney HC, Little S, Brownlee-Tomasso D, et al. AAFP and ISFM feline-friendly nursing care guidelines. *J Feline Med Surg*. 2012;14(5):337–349. doi:10.1177/1098612X12445002.

25 Lefman SH, Prittie JE. Psychogenic stress in hospitalized veterinary patients: Causation, implications, and therapies. *J Vet Emerg Crit Care*. 2019;29(2):107–120.

26 Grubb T, Sager J, Gaynor JS, et al. AAHA anesthesia and monitoring guidelines for dogs and cats. *J Am Anim Hosp Assoc*. 2020;56(2):59–82.

27 Steagall PV. Analgesia: What makes cats different/challenging and what is critical for cats? *Vet Clin Small Anim Pract*. 2020;50(4):749–767.

28 Self I. *BSAVA guide to pain management in small animal practice*, 1st ed. Gloucester, UK: British Small Animal Veterinary Association; 2019.

29 Epstein ME, Rodan I, Griffenhagen G, et al. AAHA/AAFP pain management guidelines for dogs and cats. *J Feline Med Surg*. 2015;17(3):251–272.

30 Stella J, Croney C, Buffington T. Effects of stressors on the behavior and physiology of domestic cats. *App Anim Behav Sci*. 2013;143(2):157–163. doi:10.1016/j.applanim.2012.10.014.

31 Gourkow N, Fraser D. The effects of housing and handling practices on the welfare, behaviour and selection of domestic cats (Felis sylvestris catus) by adopters in an animal shelter. *Anim Welfare*. 2006;15:371–377.

32 Morgan KN, Tromborg CT. Sources of stress in captivity. *App Anim Behav Sci*. 2007;102(3–4):262–302. doi:10.1016/j.applanim.2006.05.032.

33 Snowdon CT, Teie D, Savage M. Cats prefer species-appropriate music. *App Anim Behav Sci*. 2015;166:106–111. doi:10.1016/j.applanim.2015.02.012.

34 NRC. Thermoregulation in Cats. In: *Nutrient requirements of dogs and cats*. Washington, DC: The National Academies Press; 2006:270–271. https://doi.org/10.17226/10668.

35 Herron ME, Shreyer T. The pet-friendly veterinary practice: A guide for practitioners. *Vet Clin North Am Small Anim Pract*. 2014;44(3):451–481.

36 Stella JL, Lord LK, Buffington CA. Sickness behaviors in response to unusual external events in healthy cats and cats with feline interstitial cystitis. *J Am Vet Med Assoc*. 2011;238(1):67–73. doi:10.2460/javma.238.1.67.

37 Gruen ME, Lascelles BDX, Colleran E, et al. AAHA pain management guidelines for dogs and cats. *J Am Anim Hosp Assoc*. 2022;58(2):55–76.

38 Burns K. Cat friendly practice program takes off: American Association of Feline Practitioners growing with program. *J Am Vet Med Assoc*. 2012;241(10):1264.

39 Duncan G. Mind-body dualism and the biopsychosocial model of pain: What did Descartes really say? *J Med Philos*.

40 Wall PD. On the relation of injury to pain the John J. Bonica Lecture. *Pain*. 1979;6(3):253–264.

41 Melzack R, Wall PD. *Pain mechanisms: A new theory*. 1965.

42 Westropp JL, Kass PH, Buffington CA. Evaluation of the effects of stress in cats with idiopathic cystitis. *Am J Vet Res*. 2006;67(4):731–736.

43 Harte SE, Harris RE, Clauw DJ. The neurobiology of central sensitization. *J Appl Biobehav Res*. 2018;23(2):e12137.

44 Vachon-Presseau E. Effects of stress on the corticolimbic system: Implications for chronic pain. *Prog Neuro-Psychopharmacol Biol Psychiatry*. 2018;87:216–223.

45 Timmers I, Quaedflieg CW, Hsu C, Heathcote LC, Rovnaghi CR, Simons LE. The interaction between stress and chronic pain through the lens of threat learning. *Neurosci Biobehav Rev*. 2019;107:641–655.

46 Treede R-D, Rief W, Barke A, et al. Chronic pain as a symptom or a disease: The IASP classification of chronic pain for the: International classification of diseases:(: ICD-11:). *Pain* 2019;160(1):19–27.

47 Bravo L, Llorca-Torralba M, Suárez-Pereira I, Berrocoso E. Pain in neuropsychiatry: Insights from animal models. *Neurosci Biobehav Rev*. 2020;115:96–115.

48 Larauche M, Moussaoui N, Biraud M, et al. Brain corticotropin-releasing factor signaling: Involvement in acute stress-induced visceral analgesia in male rats. *Neurogastroenterol Motil.* 2019;31(2):e13489.

49 Bonica JJ. *The management of pain*. Philadelphia: Lea and Febiger; 1953:1243–1244.

50 Treede R-D, Rief W, Barke A, et al. A classification of chronic pain for ICD-11. *Pain.* 2015;156(6):1003.

51 Kosek E, Cohen M, Baron R, et al. Do we need a third mechanistic descriptor for chronic pain states? *Pain.* 2016;157(7):1382–1386.

52 Buffington CAT. Bladder pain syndrome/interstitial cystitis – Etiology and animal research. In: Baranowski A, Abrams P, Fall M eds. *Urogenital pain in clinical practice*. New York: Informa; 2007:169–183:chap19.

53 Monteiro BP, Steagall PV. Chronic pain in cats: Recent advances in clinical assessment. *J Feline Med Surg.* 2019;21(7):601–614.

54 Scholz J, Finnerup NB, Attal N, et al. The IASP classification of chronic pain for ICD-11: Chronic neuropathic pain. *Pain.* 2019;160(1):53.

55 Epstein ME. Feline neuropathic pain. *Vet Clin North Am Small Anim Pract.* 2020;50(4):789–809.

56 Monteiro B, Lascelles B. Assessment and recognition of chronic (maladaptive) pain. In: Steagall PVM, Robertson SA, Taylor PM, eds, *Feline anesthesia and pain management*. Hoboken, NJ: Wiley/Blackwell; 2017:241–256.

57 Monteiro BP. Feline chronic pain and osteoarthritis. *Vet Clin North Am Small Anim Pract.* 2020;50(4):769–788.

58 Kean J, Monahan P, Kroenke K, et al. Comparative responsiveness of the PROMIS pain interference short forms, brief pain inventory, PEG, and SF-36 bodily pain subscale. *Med Care.* 2016;54(4):414.

59 Reid J, Nolan A, Scott E. Measuring pain in dogs and cats using structured behavioural observation. *Vet J.* 2018;236:72–79.

60 Noble CE, Wiseman-Orr LM, Scott ME, Nolan AM, Reid J. Development, initial validation and reliability testing of a web-based, generic feline health-related quality-of-life instrument. *J Feline Med Surg.* 2019;21(2):84–94.

61 Tatlock S, Gober M, Williamson N, Arbuckle R. Development and preliminary psychometric evaluation of an owner-completed measure of feline quality of life. *Vet J.* 2017;228:22–32. doi:10.1016/j.tvjl.2017.10.005.

62 Niessen S, Powney S, Guitian J, et al. Evaluation of a quality-of-life tool for cats with diabetes mellitus. *J Vet Int Med.* 2010;24(5):1098–1105.

63 Noli C, Borio S, Varina A, Schievano C. Development and validation of a questionnaire to evaluate the Quality of Life of cats with skin disease and their owners, and its use in 185 cats with skin disease. *Vet Dermatol.* 2016;27(4):247.

64 Scott EM, Davies V, Nolan AM, et al. Validity and responsiveness of the generic health-related quality of life instrument (VetMetrica™) in cats with osteoarthritis. Comparison of vet and owner impressions of quality of life impact. *Front Vet Sci.* 2021;8:1124.

65 Freeman LM, Rodenberg C, Narayanan A, Olding J, Gooding MA, Koochaki PE. Development and initial validation of the Cat HEalth and Wellbeing (CHEW) Questionnaire: A generic health-related quality of life instrument for cats. *J Feline Med Surg.* 2016;18(9):689–701.

66 Westropp JL, Delgado M, Buffington C. Chronic lower urinary tract signs in cats: Current understanding of pathophysiology and management. *Vet Clin Small Anim Pract.* 2019;49(2):187–209. doi:10.1016/j.cvsm.2018.11.001.

67 Hart BL. Biological basis of the behavior of sick animals. *Neurosci Biobehav Rev.* 1988;12(2):123–137. doi:10.1016/S0149-7634(88)80004-6.

68 Kirsten K, Soares SM, Koakoski G, Kreutz LC, Barcellos LJG. Characterization of sickness behavior in zebrafish. *Brain Behav Immun.* 2018;73:596–602.

69 Broom DM. Behaviour and welfare in relation to pathology. *App Anim Behav Sci.* 2006;97(1):73–83. doi:10.1016/j.applanim.2005.11.019.

70 Fogsgaard KK, Røntved CM, Sørensen P, Herskin MS. Sickness behavior in dairy cows during Escherichia coli mastitis. *J Dairy Sci.* 2012;95(2):630–638.

71 Shattuck EC, Muehlenbein MP. Towards an integrative picture of human sickness behavior. *Brain Behav Immun.* 2016;57:255–262.

72 Marques-Deak A, Cizza G, Sternberg E. Brain-immune interactions and disease susceptibility. *Mol Psychiatry.* 2005;10(3):239–250.

73 Dantzer R. Neuroimmune interactions: From the brain to the immune system and vice versa. *Physiol Rev.* 2018;98(1):477–504.

74 Danese A, McEwen BS. Adverse childhood experiences, allostasis, allostatic load, and age-related disease. *Physiol Behav.* 2012;106(1):29–39. doi:10.1016/j.physbeh.2011.08.019.

75 Raison CL, Miller AH. When not enough is too much: The role of insufficient glucocorticoid signaling in the pathophysiology of stress-related disorders. *Am J Psychiatry.* 2003;160(9):1554–1565. doi:10.1176/appi.ajp.160.9.1554.

76 Dantzer R, O'Connor JC, Freund GG, Johnson RW, Kelley KW. From inflammation to sickness and depression: When the immune system subjugates the brain. *Nat Rev Neurosci.* 2008;9(1):46–56. doi:10.1038/nrn2297.

77 Sapolsky RM. *Why zebras don't get ulcers*, 3rd ed. New York, NY: Holt paperbacks; 2004.

78 Marques-Deak A, Cizza G, Sternberg E. Brain-immune interactions and disease susceptibility. *Mol Psychiatry.* 2005;10(3):239–250. doi:10.1038/sj.mp.4001643.

79 Dantzer R, Kelley KW. Twenty years of research on cytokine-induced sickness behavior. *Brain Behav Immun.* 2007;21(2):153–160.

80 Bain MJ, Buffington CT. The relationship between mental and physical health. In: McMillan FD ed. *Mental health and well-being in animals*, 2nd ed. Oxfordshire, UK: CABI; 2019:33–49.

81 Stella JL, Croney CC, Buffington CT. Behavior and welfare of domestic cats housed in cages larger than US norm. *J Appl Anim Welfare Sci.* 2017;20(3):296–312.

82 Stella JL, Croney CC. Management practices of cats owned by faculty, staff, and students at two Midwest veterinary schools. *Sci World J.* 2016;2016.

83 Buffington CA, Westropp JL, Chew DJ, Bolus RR. Risk factors associated with clinical signs of lower urinary tract disease in indoor-housed cats. Research Support, N.I.H., Extramural Research Support, Non-U.S. Gov't. *J Am Vet Med Assoc.* 2006;228(5):722–725. doi:10.2460/javma.228.5.722.

84 Amat M, Camps T, Manteca X. Stress in owned cats: Behavioural changes and welfare implications. *J Feline Med Surg.* 2016;18(8):577–586. doi:10.1177/1098612X15590867.

85 Stella JL, Croney CC. Environmental aspects of domestic cat care and management: Implications for cat welfare. *Sci World J.* 2016;ArticleID: 6296315. doi:10.1155/2016/6296315.

86 Vinke C, Godijn L, Van der Leij W. Will a hiding box provide stress reduction for shelter cats? *App Anim Behav Sci.* 2014;160:86–93.

87 Weiss JM. Psychological factors in stress and disease. *Sci Am.* 1972;226(6):104–113.

88 Weiss JM. Effects of coping behavior in different warning signal conditions on stress pathology in rats. *J Comp Physiol Psychol.* 1971;77(1):1–13. doi:10.1037/h0031583.

89 Stella J, Croney C. Coping styles in the domestic cat (Felis silvestris catus) and implications for cat welfare. *Animals.* 2019;9(6):370.

90 Kry K, Casey R. The effect of hiding enrichment on stress levels and behaviour of domestic cats (Felis sylvestris catus) in a shelter setting and the implications for adoption potential. *Anim Welfare.* 2007;16(3):375–383.

91 Rochlitz I. Feline welfare issues. In: Turner DC, Bateson P, eds. *The domestic cat – The biology of its* behavior. Cambridge, UK: Cambridge University Press; 2000:208–226.

92 Herron ME, Buffington CA. Environmental enrichment for indoor cats: Implementing enrichment. *Compend Contin Educ Vet*. 2012;34(1):E1–E5.

93 Ellis SL, Rodan I, Carney HC, et al. AAFP and ISFM feline environmental needs guidelines. *J Feline Med Surg*. 2013;15(3):219–230. doi:10.1177/1098612X13477537.

94 Monteiro B, Troncy E. Treatment of chronic (Maladaptive) pain. In: Steagall PV, Robertson SA, Taylor P eds. *Feline anesthesia and pain management*. Hoboken, NJ: John Wiley & Sons; 2018:257–280:chap 15.

95 Frankel RM. Pets, vets, and frets: What relationship-centered care research has to offer veterinary medicine. *J Vet Med Educ*. Spring 2006;33(1):20–27.

96 Buffington CAT, Westropp JL, Chew DJ, Bolus RR. Clinical evaluation of multimodal environmental modification in the management of cats with lower urinary tract signs. *J Feline Med Surg*. 2006;8:261–268.

97 Steagall PV, Robertson SA, Taylor P. *Feline anesthesia and pain management*. Hoboken, NJ: John Wiley & Sons; 2018:301.

98 Howell A, Feyrecilde M. *Cooperative veterinary care*. Hoboken, NJ: John Wiley & Sons; 2018.

99 Kruger JM, Lulich JP, MacLeay J, et al. Comparison of foods with differing nutritional profiles for long-term management of acute nonobstructive idiopathic cystitis in cats. *J Am Vet Med Assoc*. 2015;247(5):508–517. doi:10.2460/javma.247.5.508.

100 Landsberg G, Milgram B, Mougeot I, Kelly S, de Rivera C. Therapeutic effects of an alpha-casozepine and L-tryptophan supplemented diet on fear and anxiety in the cat. *J Feline Med Surg*. 2017;19(6):594–602. 1098612X16669399.

101 Seawright A. A case of recurrent feline idiopathic cystitis: The control of clinical signs with behavior therapy. *J Vet Behav Clin Appl Res*. 2008;3(1):32–38. doi:10.1016/j.jveb.2007.09.008.

102 Chew DJ, Bartges JW, Adams LG, Kruger JM, Buffington CAT. *Randomized, placebo-controlled clinical trial of pentosan polysulfate sodium for treatment of feline interstitial (idiopathic) cystitis presented at: 2009 ACVIM Forum*; June 4, 2009; Montreal, Quebec.

103 Mozaffarian D. Conflict of interest and the role of the food industry in nutrition research. *JAMA* 2017;317(17):1755–1756.

104 Hannan AJ. Review: Environmental enrichment and brain repair: Harnessing the therapeutic effects of cognitive stimulation and physical activity to enhance experience-dependent plasticity. *Neuropathol Appl Neurobiol*. 2014;40(1):13–25. doi:10.1111/nan.12102.

105 Hoy JM, Murray PJ, Tribe A. Thirty years later: Enrichment practices for captive mammals. *Zoo Biol*. 2010;29(3):303–316. doi:10.1002/zoo.20254.

106 Vachon P, Millecamps M, Low L, et al. Alleviation of chronic neuropathic pain by environmental enrichment in mice well after the establishment of chronic pain. *Behav Brain Funct*. 2013;9:22. doi:10.1186/1744-9081-9-22.

107 Bushnell MC, Case LK, Ceko M, et al. Effect of environment on the long-term consequences of chronic pain. *Pain* 2015;156(4):S42–S49. doi:10.1097/01.j.pain.0000460347.77341.bd.

108 Tai LW, Yeung SC, Cheung CW. Enriched environment and effects on neuropathic pain: Experimental findings and mechanisms. *Pain Pract*. 2018(8):1068–1082. doi:10.1111/papr.12706.

109 Pageat P. Properties of cats' facial pheromones. *Google Patents*; 1998.

110 Bol S, Caspers J, Buckingham L, et al. Behavioral responsiveness of cats (Felidae) to silver vine (Actinidia polygama), Tatarian honeysuckle (Lonicera tatarica), valerian (Valeriana officinalis) and catnip (Nepeta cataria). *BMC Vet Res*. 2017;13(70):1–15.

111 Shreve KRV, Mehrkam LR, Udell MA. Social interaction, food, scent or toys? A formal assessment of domestic pet and shelter cat (Felis silvestris catus) preferences. *Behav Processes* 2017;141:322–328.

112 Masserman JH. Experimental neuroses. *Sci Am.* 1950;182:38–43.

113 Dantas LM, Delgado MM, Johnson I, Buffington CT. Food puzzles for cats: Feeding for physical and emotional wellbeing. *J Feline Med Surg.* 2016;18(9):723–732. doi:10.1177/1098612X16643753.

114 de Souza Dantas LM. Vertical or horizontal? Diagnosing and treating cats who urinate outside the box. *Vet Clin North Am Small Anim Pract.* 2018;48(3):403–417.

115 Bradshaw J, Ellis S. *The trainable cat: A practical guide to making life happier for you and your cat.* New York, NY: Basic Books; 2016.

116 Barnett S. The "instinct to teach". *Nature.* 1968;220(5169):747–749.

117 Elzerman AL, DePorter TL, Beck A, Collin J-F. Conflict and affiliative behavior frequency between cats in multi-cat households: A survey-based study. *J Feline Med Surg.* 2019;22(8):705–717. 1098612X19877988.

118 Williams MD, Lascelles BDX. Early neonatal pain-A review of clinical and experimental implications on painful conditions later in life. *Front Pediatr.* 2020;8:30. doi:10.3389/fped.2020.00030.

119 Buffington CA. Idiopathic cystitis in domestic cats – beyond the lower urinary tract. *J Vet Int Med.* 2011;25(4):784–796. doi:10.1111/j.1939-1676.2011.0732.x.

120 Withey SL, Maguire DR, Kangas BD. Developing improved translational models of pain: A role for the behavioral scientist. *Perspect Behav Sci.* 2020;43(1):39–55.

121 Buffington CA. Developmental influences on medically unexplained symptoms. *Psychother Psychosom.* 2009;78(3):139–144. doi:10.1159/000206866.

8

Fear, Anxiety, Stress Behaviors in Cats

Amanda Rigterink

Introduction

Among the most common behavior problems in cats – weakening the human–animal bond and resulting in relinquishment – are house soiling, aggression (inter-cat and human-directed), and social avoidance.[1] Fear, anxiety, and stress tend to underlie these problems, but it can be difficult for owners to recognize subtle signs of emotional distress in their cats (Figure 8.1). When fear and anxiety evolve into a state of chronic stress, cats may begin to show such abnormal behaviors as appetite changes, poor grooming, and eliminating outside the litter box. Veterinarians often have difficulty sorting out how emotional disturbances and physical factors may be contributing to behavioral diagnoses.[2]

What is normal?

Like humans, cats are sentient beings with the ability to experience and respond to both positive and negative emotions. Fear in cats can be a normal adaptive response to a direct trigger or threat; for example, a cat experiences fear when confronted by a hostile dog. The "flight or fight" response kicks in so that the cat can neutralize the threat by fleeing or fighting in order to remain safe (and alive). To a lesser extent, anxiety also can be a normal self-preserving response in cats. A cat sees a dog across the street and anticipates that the dog may be a threat. The anxiety (anticipation of danger) experienced by the cat is an adaptive response that motivates the cat to distance itself from the dog.

What is normal but unacceptable?

First, aggression can be a normal response to fear – but many cat owners find it unacceptable, particularly if it is directed at a person or pet in the home. For instance, a child trying to pet and pick up the cat may trigger fear in the cat, who then growls or swats at the child.

Second, a cat might respond to the child by retreating or hiding; although this is a generally more "acceptable" response than growling and swatting, some owners may struggle to understand why the cat does not want to be interact with the child and deem the behavior "abnormal."

(Continued)

Clinical Handbook of Feline Behavior Medicine, First Edition. Edited by Elizabeth Stelow.
© 2023 John Wiley & Sons, Inc. Published 2023 by John Wiley & Sons, Inc.
Companion Website: www.wiley.com/go/stelow/behavior

(Continued)

> **What is abnormal but acceptable?**
> Due to anxiety, a cat may perceive a completely innocuous stimulus as threatening and retreat or hide. If the owner cannot interpret the cat's behavior as retreating in response to the innocuous stimulus, the owner will not likely feel this behavior is problematic (or realize that it is abnormal).
>
> **What is abnormal and generally unacceptable?**
> Owners of very fearful or anxious cats – or savvy owners of slightly fearful or anxious cats – will understand that their cats' responses are abnormal and will seek help. This is particularly true when the fear and anxiety lead to unwanted behaviors like aggression and house soiling.

Unfortunately, animal welfare research regarding assessment and treatment of behavioral disorders in domestic cats largely has been neglected. Reasons for this include lack of funding opportunities, societal expectations regarding feline behavior, and limited recognition of fear/anxiety in cats as compared to dogs. For example, owners may expect cats to be "low-maintenance" pets as compared to dogs, viewing the cat as more independent, more stoic, and having less need for human interaction.[3,4] Owners also may overlook cues regarding feline fear or misinterpret such feline behaviors as passivity (hiding, decreased motion) and increased self-maintenance behaviors (displacement over-grooming) as indicative of lack of fear or less severe fear when encountering fearful stimuli.[5] In the veterinary office setting, veterinary staff also may fail to recognize the feline body language and vocalizations (or lack of) that communicate fear and stress.[6,7]

Data from an online cross-sectional survey of 547 US cat owners showed that greater owner knowledge about cats, owner-pet interactions, and perceptions of affordability of cat ownership were significant predictors of a lower number of reported behavior problems. In addition, greater owner knowledge about cats correlated with less use of positive-punishment-based responses to misbehavior and increased tolerance of potential behavior problems when present.[8] A study from Italy examined whether and how owners recognize when the welfare of their cats is impaired. Out of 194 cat owners surveyed, most (71%) correctly included both physical and psychological components when defining stress; however, approximately 10% of owners believed that the presence of stress

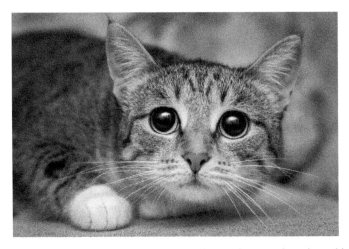

Figure 8.1 Cats can experience fear, anxiety, and stress – how do we identify it and what do we do about it? Courtesy of Елена Беляева / Adobe Stock

would not impact the welfare of their cats. The study also found that owners tended to miss signs of stress in their cats, and perception of stress often depended on faulty preconceived ideas about normal cat behavior in terms of play, social interactions, and aggression. Thus, distorted perceptions of what constitutes stress in cats can prevent owners from intervening to correct harmful situations.[9]

Veterinary professionals can aid owners in recognizing when cats fail to cope with fear and anxiety and help owners facilitate changes in the cat's physical and social home environment.[10] Both "well" and "sick" visits should include routine discussions about the emotional well-being of the cat. Moreover, veterinary hospitals must strive to minimize even short-term aversive emotional experiences that may have long-term effects.[11,12] Please see Chapter 15: Cats in the Clinic for more information.

This chapter explores:

- Working definitions for fear, anxiety, and stress
- How these occur physiologically
- How they present in our feline patients
- Behavioral disorders that may result
- How to uncover them during history taking
- How to treat them once they are diagnosed

Fear and Anxiety

Fear and anxiety are stress responses that require compensatory mechanisms to maintain a state of homeostasis.[13] While fear and anxiety are overlapping aversive emotional states that seem similar, they are very different. Fear is an adaptive response to a readily identifiable stimulus/trigger that impels the animal to save itself from a perceived *direct* threat. On the other hand, anxiety is the *anticipation* of a future threat or danger that may be actual, imagined, or unknown. Some consider the development of anxious behaviors to be a failure of coping with fear.[6] It should be noted that *perception* is a key concept common to both fear and anxiety; the threat or danger *perceived* by the fearful or anxious cat is its reality.[1,14] This likely relates to why stress is overlooked: owners don't understand how their cats can perceive an "innocuous" stimulus as stressful.

Responses to a stressor involve physiologic pathways mediated by the autonomic nervous system and hypothalamic-pituitary-adrenal axis (HPA). Fear triggers the sudden increase in autonomic arousal needed to facilitate the classic "fight or flight" response for escaping immediate danger. Anxiety tends to be associated more with increased muscle contraction, hypervigilance, and avoidance.[6,15] Both fearful and anxious cats may experience increase in blood pressure, heart rate, and respiratory rate, as well as pupillary dilatation, trembling, salivation, pacing, aggression, and avoidance.[16]

When evaluating the consequences of a potential aversive trigger (such as an unfamiliar person approaching the cat), behavioral, physical, and physiological changes must be considered. It is vital to understand how the cat perceives the specific trigger, and how a cat reacts can vary considerably due to its current living circumstances, past experiences, and genetic background. Appropriate treatment plans can be developed only when the underlying emotions motivating problem behaviors are identified and addressed. As a result, it is critical that behavioral assessment questions be part of every feline veterinary visit.[17] In addition, an understanding of the neurophysiologic pathways involved in fear and anxiety is critical when the behavior treatment plan includes the use of targeted behavioral medications.[14,18]

Although cats are not limited in the stimuli they find fear-inducing, anxiety diagnosed in cats commonly is associated with "historical" fear-inducing stimuli. Past aversive triggers that can result in feline anxiety commonly are related to animate stimuli (e.g., other animals, familiar and unfamiliar people) and inanimate stimuli (e.g., certain noises). In addition, many cats experience anxiety associated with certain situations and places; a change in environment like moving to a new home can trigger anxiety, and certain situations such as riding in the car or visiting the veterinary hospital also can be anxiety-provoking. Separation anxiety also is diagnosed in cats; like dogs, cats are social creatures and can experience anxiety when separated from their owners and house mates. Last, painful conditions such as arthritis and illness/disease can underlie feline anxiety.[6,12]

Stress and Stressors

Stress, acute and chronic, develops when fear and anxiety cease to act as adaptive mechanisms for self-preservation, and the fearful or anxious cat finds itself in an environment that is neither predictable nor controllable.[16] Frequent and recurrent episodes of fear and anxiety result in over-stimulation of the autonomic nervous system and HPA; such stress hormones as epinephrine, norepinephrine, and cortisol rise and physical homeostasis is disrupted.[13,16,19] The ensuing state of chronic stress impacts both the emotional and the physical welfare of the cat.

Some of the most common stressors experienced by domestic cats include changes in environment, inter-cat conflict, poor human–animal bonding, and the inability to carry out normal species-specific motivated behaviors. Stress may result in such behavioral disorders as inter-cat aggression, redirected aggression, urine marking, and compulsive disorders.[20] Like stress caused by physical factors, chronic emotional stress can lead to physical disorders such as Feline Interstitial Cystitis (FIC), immunosuppressive disorders such as Feline Herpes Virus-1 (FHV-1), and skin disease due to overgrooming.[2,16,18] It has been shown that FIC is associated directly with increased catecholamine levels resulting from stress-induced increase in the activity of tyrosine hydroxylase which catalyzes the rate-limiting step in catecholamine synthesis.[21] Unlike episodic fear and anxiety, chronic stress may be harder to recognize in cats, since it so often manifests as something else. Addressing stress that underlies medical and behavioral disorders is of critical importance to the physical, emotional, and social welfare of the cat.

Physiology of Fear, Anxiety, Stress

Fear, anxiety, and stress share certain neuroanatomic pathways that involve the amygdala, autonomic nervous system, and the HPA. When the cat encounters an aversive stimulus, detection of the threat by the "defense" circuits of the central amygdala activates neuromodulatory peripheral hormonal systems that stimulate neuronal release of norepinephrine, dopamine, serotonin, and ace-tylcholine into various areas of the brain. The central amygdala also targets neurons that act upon the sympathetic division of the autonomic nervous system to trigger the release of epinephrine and norepinephrine from the adrenal medulla.[14,22,23] In addition, fear and anxiety stimulate the anterior pituitary gland to release corticotropin releasing factor (CRF) which in turn acts upon the adrenal cortex to release cortisol into the bloodstream. Thus, fear and anxiety not only trigger the immediate self-survival defensive fight/flight responses but also result in a state of generalized arousal.[23]

While high levels of cortisol are found in stressed cats, this biomarker only indicates a state of arousal in response to changes in the environment that can be positive or negative.[18] Dysregulation of the stress neurophysiologic system occurs when aversive conditions become more permanent or chronic. The anabolic and immunosuppressive actions of cortisol can lead to disruption of physiologic homeostasis and to a variety of behavioral and multi-system physical disorders that threaten the emotional and physical welfare of the cat.[6,14,24] Due to these sequelae, corticosteroids should be prescribed judiciously; in particular, long-term corticosteroid use can result in the emergence of new behavior problems and exacerbate pre-existing behavior disorders.[18]

Neurotransmitters such as serotonin and ᴕ-aminobutyric acid also may be associated with how animals respond to aversive stimuli, resulting in increased passive avoidance responses and enhanced sensitivity to negative associations.[19,25]

What Do Fear and Anxiety Look Like?

Fear, a normal emotional response to actual and perceived threats, increases when the cat is in an unfamiliar environment or situation. For example, a veterinary clinic visit, the presence of other cats, unfamiliar people, and unwanted interactions with familiar people can be fear-evoking threats. How a cat responds in a given situation depends on multiple factors including its genetic predisposition, previous experiences, and environment.[6] Under identical fear-inducing conditions, some cats may attempt to run away while others freeze, use displacement behaviors, or become aggressive.[26]

Fear responses also differ between dogs and cats. Fearful or anxious dogs tend to pant, tremble, cower, vocalize, and eliminate. Cats are more likely to hide, withdraw, or practice displacement behaviors such as grooming. The passivity of cats when exposed to aversive stimuli often is misinterpreted by owners, who may assume that the cat's lack of an active response represents the absence of fear. Moreover, even when cat owners recognize that certain passive responses such as hiding and displacement behaviors are due to fear, they may be less likely to consider the fear to be severe.[5]

Cats communicate fear and other emotions though a variety of subtle body postures, tail positions, facial expressions, and release of fear pheromones from skin glands and emptying of anal sacs.[11] Cats also may exhibit fearful/anxious responses by such behaviors as yawning, lip licking, and circling. In some instances, fear actually may result in suppression of distress vocalization.[2,27.] On the other hand, anxiety is related more to anticipation and uncertainty, and the anxious cat may exhibit hypervigilance, restlessness, and distress vocalization, as well as avoidance and displacement behaviors.[1]

These various modes of communication enable cats to avoid direct confrontations with other cats, familiar and unfamiliar. Recognition of feline fear and anxiety by owners, animal handling staff, and veterinarians can prevent or de-escalate arousal that may lead to aggression.[11,28] Additionally, identifying and alleviating stress in the cat's home environment and in the veterinary hospital are of critical importance, since a state of chronic arousal associated with long-term stress may result in a variety of behavioral disorders and physical health problems.[29,30]

Common indicators of feline fear, anxiety, and stress include decreased grooming, decreased social interaction, decreased play and exploration, hypervigilance during the day instead of sleeping, increased hiding attempts, decreased mating behaviors, and changes in appetite (inappetence or overeating).[31] Even experienced cat owners tend to miss the signs and symptoms of fear, anxiety, and stress in their cats.

Dawson et al. studied the ability of people to identify cats' affective states from subtle facial expressions as shown on video clips. Approximately 6,300 individuals each viewed 20 video clips of cats in "carefully operationalized" positive or negative states. Interestingly, although women and younger individuals were the most successful at correctly identifying positive versus negative feline facial expressions, cat owners in general did no better than non-owners. The study, however, showed that it is possible to interpret the emotional state of cats from subtle facial expressions.[10]

Body Posture and Facial Expressions

Body posture, overt and subtle, usually can identify a fearful cat from a distance. The cat may be frozen in position, hiding, or crouching (Figure 8.2). It may flee to safety, fight, or "fiddle" (exhibiting displacement behaviors like grooming) (Figure 8.3).[11] When defensive, the tense fearful cat

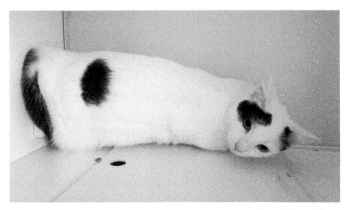

Figure 8.2   This cat is crouched and trying to make himself "small" at the back of a cage.

may attempt to make itself appear smaller by lowering its head and leaning away. Conversely, fearful cats also may "bluff" their way out of danger; the sympathetic nervous system triggered by fear can cause involuntary piloerection that makes the body appear fluffier and larger. Along with piloerection, the cat also may assume the classic "Halloween Cat" pose by standing tip-toed with arched back and tail straight up or down.[26]

Tail position is another expressive feline feature. For example, a tail held straight up vertically or wrapped around the body when seated indicates a friendly demeanor, while a tail held straight down or perpendicular to the ground is associated with an offensive attitude. A whipping tail is shown by an agitated, aroused cat and serves as a possible prelude to aggression.[11] Of note, an acutely stressed cat may appear either drowsy or hypervigilant, and the cat that rolls onto its side in the veterinary hospital setting is more likely preparing to defend itself than requesting a belly rub.[26]

While body posture changes provide easily visible indications of feline fear and anxiety, facial expressions are more subtle, change more quickly, and provide a better indication of in-the-moment fear, anxiety, or impending aggression. Of all feline facial characteristics, the pupils are most informative. Slit-like pupils indicate calmness, dilated pupils reflect the acute fear responses of fight or flight (the more dilated, the higher the level of arousal), and oblong pupils are associated

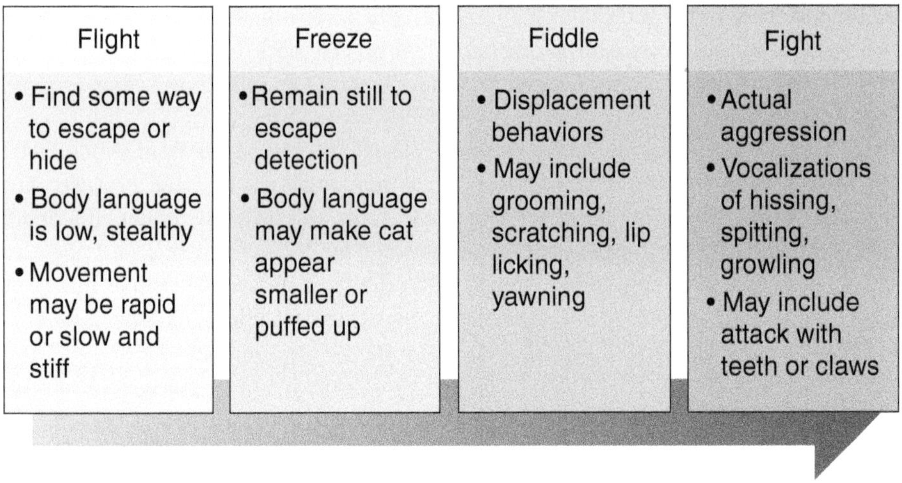

Flight	Freeze	Fiddle	Fight
• Find some way to escape or hide • Body language is low, stealthy • Movement may be rapid or slow and stiff	• Remain still to escape detection • Body language may make cat appear smaller or puffed up	• Displacement behaviors • May include grooming, scratching, lip licking, yawning	• Actual aggression • Vocalizations of hissing, spitting, growling • May include attack with teeth or claws

Figure 8.3   The "fight-flight-freeze-fiddle" response to fear. *When frightened, cats may proceed from an attempt to escape through outright aggression, should escape not be possible. Figure created by Liz Stelow.*

with aggression (Image 8.4). It may be difficult for humans to identify pupillary shape and size at a distance, but cats depend on these cues to avoid fights with other cats.[11,32]

Ears also can speak volumes about feline fear and anxiety. Ears held in an erect position indicate that the cat is focusing on a stimulus of some sort; this attention can represent benign curiosity or the beginnings of concern (Figure 8.5). When the ears are pointing downwards and sidewards, the cat is in defensive mode, while ears swiveled to display the inner pinnae indicate an aggressive stance (Figure 8.6).[11,32]

Behavioral and Physical Disorders Related to Fear, Anxiety, and Stress

The Behavior Manifestations of Fears and Anxieties

Among behavioral diagnoses in cats associated with fear and anxiety are:

- Generalized anxiety; this reflects concern about many stimuli in the environment.
- Separation anxiety; this reflects concerns about being left alone or separated from key individuals.
- Situational fear; as the name implies, this reflects fears of certain situation, like veterinary visits.
- Fear of unfamiliar and familiar people.
- Inanimate fear; this reflects fear of objects, noises, odors, and other non-living stimuli.

Domestic house cats generally have restricted exposure to things outside their immediate home environment. As a result, perception of unfamiliar animate and inanimate objects may trigger fear and anxiety.

Situational fear and anxiety related to veterinary visits are of major concern as they significantly impact feline health and welfare.[6] One study reported that approximately half of cat owners state that their cats "hate" going for veterinary visits, and over a third of owners relate that just the thought of taking their cat to

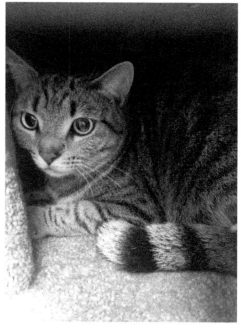

Figure 8.4 This cat's dilated pupils, curled posture, and focus away from the camera suggest that the cat is fearful.

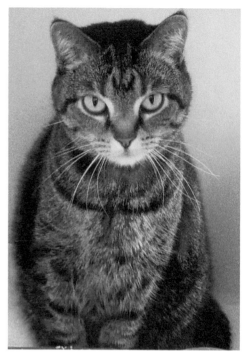

Figure 8.5 This cat is focused intently on the camera, either out of curiosity or the beginnings of concern.

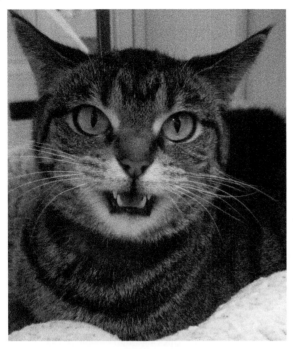

Figure 8.6 This cat's sideways-swiveled ears indicate a defensive aggressive stance.

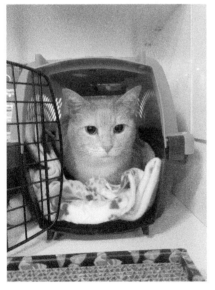

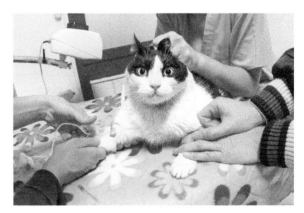

Figures 8.7 and 8.8 These cats' dilated pupils suggest that they are finding their veterinary visits frightening. Courtesy of bennymarty / Adobe Stock

the veterinarian is stressful.[30] Difficulty getting the cat into the carrier to go to a veterinary visit, the stress experienced by cat and owner at the clinic, and residual stress for the cat at home post-visit likely result in fewer veterinary visits (Figures 8.7 and 8.8).[6]

The Behavior Manifestations of Stress

Stress-related behavioral problems include inter-cat aggression, elimination outside the litter box, urine spraying, separation anxiety, pica/wool sucking, and compulsive disorders (e.g., psychogenic alopecia from excessive grooming).[6,14,20]

The Medical Manifestations of Stress

When fear and anxiety become overwhelming, the resulting state of chronic stress may be expressed through physical disorders. As in humans, multi-system diseases in cats can be associated with chronic stress. Some examples are feline idiopathic cystitis (FIC) and such immunosuppression disorders as feline herpesvirus-1 (FHV-1), feline infectious peritonitis (FIP), feline leukemia virus (FeLV), and feline immunodeficiency virus (FIV).[21]

Other conditions may be exacerbated by chronic stress such as feline orofacial pain syndrome (FOPS) and gastrointestinal disease manifested by vomiting, diarrhea, stress colitis, and repeated hairballs due to stress-induced overgrooming.[2,20] Stress also can impact cognition particularly in senior cats; increased levels of endogenous steroids associated with chronic stress can impair cognitive processing and result in greater sensitivity to negative stimuli in the cat's environment.[18]

Veterinary Behavior Assessment through History Taking

Recognition of changes in behavior can provide invaluable information regarding the presence of pain and disease. Owners should be made aware that the presence of fear, anxiety, stress, and behavioral changes are just as important to report as physical symptoms. Thus, a thorough veterinary wellness or illness assessment should include questions aimed at determining the presence of any behavioral changes that may be impacting or reflecting the emotional or physical health and well-being of the cat.[31] The sooner the identification of fear, anxiety, and stress, the better the chances of preventing these aversive responses from evolving into full-blown behavioral disorders.

As part of history-taking during every veterinary visit, behavior-oriented questions should aim to assess any changes in the cat's activity, appetite, water consumption, sleep, elimination pattern, grooming, and vocalization.[2] Specific questions should include:[31]

- Any elimination outside the litter box or urine spraying on vertical surfaces?
- Aggression (hiss, scratch, bite) towards unfamiliar or familiar people?
- Frequent fearful behaviors?
- Destruction of things in the home?
- Any problematic interactions with other cats or pets in the household?
- Any changes in disposition or activity?

A more standardized way to obtain behavioral history during veterinary visits is the Feline Behavioral Assessment & Research Questionnaire (FeBARQ). Similar to the C-BARQ for dogs, FeBARQ is a questionnaire instrument developed and validated for the quantitative assessment of cat behavior and behavioral problems by cat owners.[33]

It is important, during history taking, to identify any triggers for the fears, anxieties, or stress being manifested by the cat. These specific stimuli will become very important to the tailoring of an effective treatment plan. Triggers are typically very apparent, as behavior evidence of the cat's concern usually relates to triggers in a cause-and-effect manner. But, if triggers are not readily identifiable by the owner, ask them to keep a journal to try to narrow down the possibilities.

Treatment of Fear, Anxiety, Stress

Once identified, fears, anxieties, and stress in feline patients should be treated. The goal of treatment is the relief from fear, anxiety, or chronic stress – but attention may also need to be paid to any medical sequelae that may have resulted.

As for all diagnoses, especially those of a behavioral or emotional nature, a multipronged approach is often necessary. In the treatment of fears, anxieties, and stress, a good first step is to plan for the management of the cat's home environment, including avoidance of all triggering stimuli that have been identified. Then, the cat can be conditioned to feel more calm or positive about fearful stimuli using behavior modification in the form of desensitization and counterconditioning. Finally, the cat's improvement may be enhanced through the use of pheromones or pharmaceuticals designed to reduce fears or anxiety. Following is information on the use of management, environmental enrichment, behavior modification, pheromones, and medications in a treatment plan for feline fears, anxieties, and stress.

Management

Home environments of domestic cats contain multiple potential sources of stress that may be avoidable or not. Some cats may not be able to cope with environmental stressors, and supportive care on a personal level is key in helping those cats and their owners. With the owner's input, veterinary personnel should strive to help identify the triggers of fear and anxiety in the home environment so that owners can remove or avoid them as much as possible. Clinicians (and owners) also should assess the presence of chronic or background stress. Management is the first and most important step in addressing feline fear, anxiety, and stress. Successful management, whereby triggers can be eliminated or avoided, is dependent on interventions that are individualized to the cat and its environment.[20] Veterinarians should seek to recognize those cats that are unable to cope and guide owners in providing reasonable environmental changes and social approaches that will aid in reducing the stress.[12] Decreasing the cat's exposure to perceived aversive stimuli will help reduce overall stress, and managing fear-evoking triggers can help reduce emotional arousal that may motivate aggression and other fear-related behaviors.[18]

The cat should have options available to enable "control" in its environment. For example, a "safe place" that is a haven should be set up for hiding/resting to avoid or neutralize environmental stressors. A cat that is fearful of unfamiliar people should be able to go to its "safe place" while visitors are in the home; playing calming music or white noise to reduce fear-eliciting noises and using pheromonatherapy near the "safe place" also are helpful.[6,20] Finally, reducing exposure to a specific trigger will prevent the cat from practicing undesirable behaviors that, from its perspective, are responsible for causing the feared stimulus to go away. Owners should be reminded that punishment for undesirable behaviors triggered by fear and anxiety only will increase the cat's distress and exacerbate behavior issues over time.[12] In the veterinary office/hospital setting, minimizing stress for patients should be a priority. While a "no stress" environment is not possible, understanding how to create a "low stress" environment and how to handle animals in a less stressful manner benefits patients, owners, and veterinary staff.[26,34]

Environmental Enrichment

Environmental enrichment is another important component of a behavior treatment plan since it also can help reduce chronic stress resulting from fear and anxiety. Provide places for climbing, hiding, and resting (such as cat trees and shelving) where the cat will not be disturbed by other cats, pets, or people. Hide food/treats for "foraging" and provide puzzle feeders. Toys that move and bounce (simulating prey) particularly are mentally and physically stimulating and should be rotated to keep the cat's interest. Some cats have the need to scratch and engage in facial rubbing so that provision of scratching materials is another good enrichment tool.[20]

Behavior Modification (Desensitization and Counter Conditioning)

Just as in the treatment of canine behavior disorders, behavior modification techniques can be used in cats to change the perception of and response to certain aversive triggers in a carefully controlled stepwise manner. For example, in inter-cat aggression, the cats are kept separated for a period of time to lessen daily fear and anxiety and then slowly are exposed to one another in a limited and controlled manner (desensitization). Reading the cats' body language is crucial in determining when to proceed with the next step in the procedure. Then, the cats' perceptions of one another gradually are changed by associating the other cat's presence with positive things such as food rewards (counter conditioning).[12]

Pheromonatherapy

Pheromonatherapy is another modality used as a behavioral intervention. Pheromones, naturally produced and used by cats as a means of communication, can aid in altering the cat's emotional response to a stressor. Thus, pheromonatherapy can act to improve the cat's feeling of safety and well-being when used correctly and effectively. Cats apply their own pheromones by rubbing, rolling, scratching, and bunting against surfaces and humans. Synthetic pheromones are available in various fractionated forms (facial F1-F5) and physical forms (sprays, plug-in diffusers, towelettes); the fraction and form used are determined by the particular need. For example, the Feliway diffuser contains a facial pheromone analogue that can be plugged in near the cat's safe haven or resting location to decrease anxiety during stressful events such as thunderstorms, fireworks, and household visitors. The spray form can be used to reduce the impact of urine markings when sprayed on previously marked areas and to reduce the anxiety of travel when sprayed inside the cat carrier.[35–37]

Medications and Supplements

Several psychopharmaceuticals are used to treat veterinary behavior disorders. The use of psychotropic agents never should be the first or only part of a behavior treatment plan; they can serve as an important part of a multi-faceted behavior modification program that includes management and behavior modification. Psychopharmaceutical medications act by reducing fear, anxiety, and arousal that often motivate aggressive behavior. Moreover, the medications can aid in reducing impulsivity, thereby increasing responsiveness to behavior. While medication treatments are based on the presumed neurochemistry of the underlying stress response, individuals with the same behavioral diagnoses may respond differently to the same medication.[38]

Conclusion

Fear, anxiety, and stress underlie common feline behavior problems that often result in relinquishment. Recognizing when a cat is fearful or anxious can be difficult due to passive feline coping mechanisms that include hiding and withdrawing. In addition, what appears harmless to owners may be perceived as fear-inducing to their cats. As a result, chronic emotional stress in cats may not be addressed in a timely manner, leading to both behavioral and physical disorders.

With appropriate education and guidance, owners can learn how cats communicate their emotions and that changes in behavior are just as important as physical changes. Every veterinary visit presents an opportunity to ask owners behavior-oriented questions that may reveal the presence of emotional distress in their cats. Then, veterinary professionals can guide owners in taking steps to reduce their cat's chronic stress through environmental management and enrichment opportunities. Behavior modification techniques, pheromonatherapy, and pharmacologic treatment also may be utilized to reduce fear, anxiety, and stress that motivate feline behavioral disorders.

Last, the concept of low-stress handling should be adopted by all veterinary practices. A major source of stress to veterinary patients and their owners is the veterinary environment itself. Adverse veterinary experiences can cause harm to feline patients, owners, and veterinary staff. Minimizing stress in the veterinary setting is a win-win situation for all.

References

1 Landsberg G, Milgram B, Mougeot I, et al. Therapeutic effects of an alpha-casozepine and L-tryptophan diet on fear and anxiety in the cat. *J Feline Med Surg.* 2017;19(6):594–602.
2 Horwitz DF, Rodan I. Behavioral awareness in the feline consultation: Understanding physical and emotional health. *J Feline Med Surg.* 2018;20:423–436.
3 Baillie KU. Demystifying feline behavior: Q & A with James Serpell and Carlos Siracusa. *Penn Today.* February 19, 2020. https://penntoday.upenn.edu/news/demystifying-feline-behavior.
4 Schwartz S. Separation anxiety syndrome in cats: 136 cases (1991–2000). *JAVMA.* 2002;220(7):1028–1033.
5 Dale AR, Walker JK, Farnworth MJ, et al. A survey of owners' perceptions of fear of fireworks in a sample of dogs and cats in New Zealand. *NZ Vet J.* 2010;58(6):286–291.
6 Stepita M. Feline anxiety and fear-related disorders. In: Little SE, ed. *August's consultations in feline internal medicine*, Vol. 7. Chapter 90. Elsevier E-books; 2016:900–910.
7 Bennett V, Gourkow N, Mills DS. Facial correlates of emotional behaviour in the domestic cat (Felis catus). *Behav Processes.* 2017;141(3):342–350.
8 Grigg EK, Kogan LR. Owners' attitudes, knowledge, and care practices: Exploring the implications of domestic cat behavior and welfare in the home. *Animals.* 2019;9:1–22.
9 Mariti C, Guerrini F, Vallini V, et al. The perception of cat stress by Italian owners. *J Vet Behav.* 2017;20:74–81.
10 Dawson LC, Cheal J, Niel L, Mason G. Humans can identify cats' affective states from subtle facial expressions. *Anim Welf.* 2019;28:519–531.
11 Rodan I. Understanding feline behavior and application for appropriate handling and management. *Top Companion Anim Med.* 2010;25(4):178–188.
12 Hargrave C. Let's talk about stress. *UK-Vet: The Vet Nurse.* March 2, 2017.
13 Radley JJ, Morrison JH. Repeated stress and structural plasticity in the brain. *Ageing Res Rev.* 2005;4:271–287.
14 Levine ED. Feline fear and anxiety. *Vet Clin Small Anim.* 2008;38:1065–1079.

15 Muskin PR (physician rev). What are anxiety disorders? *Am Psych Assoc.* 2021. https://www.psychiatry.org/patients-families/anxiety-disorders/what-are-anxiety-disorders.

16 Tynes VV. The physiologic effects of fear. *DVM 360.* 2014. https://www.dvm360.com/view/physiologic-effects-fear.

17 Incorporating behavioral assessments into every examination. In: Hammerle M, Horst C, Levine E, Overall K, Radosta L, Rafter-Richie M, Yin S (Task Force). 2015 AAHA canine and feline behavior management guidelines. *J Am Anim Hosp Assoc.* Jul-Aug 2015;51(4):205–221.

18 Mills D, Karagiannis C, Zulch H. Stress- it's effect on health and behavior: A guide for practitioners. *Vet Clinic Sm Anim.* 2014;44:525–541.

19 Koolhaas JM, Bartolomucci A, Buwalda B, et al. Stress revisited: A critical evaluation of the stress concept. *Neurosci Biobehav Rev.* 2011;35(5):1291–1301.

20 Amat M, Camps T, Manteca X. Stress in owned cats: Behavioural changes and welfare implications. *J Feline Med Surg.* 2016;18(8):577–586.

21 Westropp JL, Kass PH, Buffington CAT. Evaluation of the effects of stress in cats with idiopathic cystitis. *Am J Vet Res.* 2006;67(4):731–736.

22 Johnson LR. How fear and stress shape the mind. *Frontiers in Behav Neurosci.* 2016;10(24):1–3.

23 LeDoux J. Rethinking the emotional brain. *Neuron.* 2012;73(4):653–676.

24 Tsigos C, Kyrou I, Kassi E, Chrousos GP. Stress: Endocrine physiology and pathophysiology. *Endotext (Internet).* Oct 17, 2020. https://www.ncbi.nlm.nih.gov/books/NBK278995.

25 Steimer T. The biology of fear- and anxiety-related behaviors. *Dialogues in Clin Neurosci.* 2002;4(3):231–244.

26 Lloyd JKF. Minimizing stress for patients in the veterinary hospital: Why it is important and what can be done about it. *Vet Sci.* 2017;4(22):1–19.

27 deRivera C, Ley J, Milgram B, Landsberg G. Development of a laboratory model to assess fear and anxiety in cats. *J Feline Med Surg.* 2017;19(6):586–593.

28 Overall K. How to deal with anxiety and distress responses: Cats and elimination, and cats and aggression. *Atlantic Coast Veterinary Conference* 2001. https://www.vin.com/apputil/content/defaultadv1.aspx?id=3844025&pid=11131&print=1.

29 Tateo A, Zappaterra M, Covella A, Padalino B. Factors influencing stress and fear-related behaviour of cats during veterinary examinations. *Ital J Anim Sci.* 2021;20(1):46–58.

30 Spinks I. *Bayer Veterinary Care Usage Study III: Feline findings.* 2013. https://www.brakkeconsulting.com/wp-content/uploads/2018/01/BayerBCI_BVCUS_III_Feline_Findings_2013.pdf.

31 Overall K, Rodan I, Beaver BV, Carney H, Crowell-Davis S, Hird N, Kudrak S, Wexler-Mitchell E. *Feline Behavior Management Guidelines AAFP 2005.*

32 Overall K. *Clinical behavioral medicine for small animals.* St. Louis: Elsevier Mosby; 2013.

33 Duffy DL, Diniz demoura RT, Serpell JT. Development and evaluation of Fe-BARQ: A new survey instrument for measuring behavior in domestic cats (Felis s. catus). *Behav Processes.* 2017;141:329–341.

34 Yin S. *Low stress handling restraint and behavior modification of dogs & cats.* Davis, CA: Cattle Dog Publishing; 2009.

35 Pereira JS, Fragoso S, Beck A, et al. Improving the feline veterinary consultation: The usefulness of Feliway spray in reducing cats' stress. *J Feline Med Surg.* 2015;18(12):1–6.

36 Mills DS, Redgate SE, Landsberg GM. A meta-analysis of studies of treatments for feline urine spraying. *PloS ONE.* 2011;6(4). https://pubmed.ncbi.nlm.nih.gov/21525994.

37 DePorter TL. Use of pheromones in feline practice. In: Rodan I, Heath S, eds. *Feline behavioral health and welfare*, 1st ed. Elsevier E-books; 2015 Chapter 18. Kindle Edition.

38 Medications for fearful dogs and cats. In: Hammerle M, Horst C, Levine E, Overall K, Radosta L, Rafter-Richie M, Yin S (Task Force). 2015 AAHA canine and feline behavior management guidelines. *J Am Anim Hosp Assoc.* Jul-Aug 2015;51(4):205–221.

9

Compulsive and Displacement Behaviors

Melissa Bain

Introduction

Repetitive behaviors can be due to a number of underlying psychological and physiological reasons, ranging from compulsive, displacement, and stereotypic behaviors to those due to an underlying medical condition arising from numerous etiologies. They can be classified as a sequence of movements usually derived from normal maintenance behaviors (grooming, walking, eating) that are performed out of context in a repetitive, exaggerated, ritualistic, and/or sustained manner. In two studies of cats visiting a veterinary behaviorist, approximately 5% were diagnosed with a compulsive behavior.[1,2]

When evaluating any problem behavior, it can be helpful to separate it into normal or abnormal, and acceptable or unacceptable (Table 9.1).

How to Diagnose

The History/Background of the Problem

History-taking, while somewhat different for helping identify behavior problems, is not much different than what is used in a more general sense.[3,4] It takes time for veterinarians and staff to become fluent in order to most effectively gather information, as well as be comfortable asking open-ended questions to more efficiently gather information. Veterinarians may be less comfortable in gathering information from owners regarding problem behaviors; however, despite their discomfort, they believe that it is still very important.[5,6] Training in successful communication has received more attention in veterinary schools as of late, and is listed as highly sought after by veterinary employers.[7,8] Table 9.2 provides some highlights on information to collect from owners to help determine the diagnosis. It should be noted, however, that owner-reports and video-recorded evidence are more central for behavioral diagnoses than for physiological diagnoses.[9,10]

An important technique to help differentiate between the differential diagnoses is to ask for a video recording of the cat when people are present, when they are completely away from the home, and a walkthrough of the environment in which the cat resides. If a cat has a true compulsive disorder, it likely will still perform the behavior if no one is present.

Videos can also help the veterinarian identify environmental factors that could play a role in the cat's behavior, especially if the appointment is in-clinic compared as opposed to being a house call.

Clinical Handbook of Feline Behavior Medicine, First Edition. Edited by Elizabeth Stelow.
© 2023 John Wiley & Sons, Inc. Published 2023 by John Wiley & Sons, Inc.
Companion Website: www.wiley.com/go/stelow/behavior

Table 9.1 Repetitive behaviors differentiated into normal vs. abnormal and acceptable vs. unacceptable.

What is Normal?

Many cats perform what could be considered "quirky" behaviors. Often we are unable to come up with a reason for these one-off behaviors that don't interfere with a cat's quality of life, nor signal an underlying pathological state.

What is normal but often unacceptable?

Repetitive behaviors can be disturbing for an owner to observe. If a cat chases its tail, even if this behavior doesn't interfere with its welfare or indicative of an underlying medical condition, and trips an owner, it is unacceptable.

What is abnormal but often acceptable?

Owners may be tolerant of a cat performing repetitive behaviors that signal underlying anxiety or a medical condition, and sometimes even write it off as "cute." They may also encourage these behaviors by rewarding the cat, sometimes inadvertently, when it is performing this behavior. They may also not seek veterinary care for a potential underlying medical condition if they don't perceive the behavior as abnormal or disruptive to their lives.

What is abnormal and typically unacceptable?

If a cat engages in repetitive behaviors that are either interfering with the owner's quality of life, such as performing these behaviors in the middle of the night, interfering with the cat's welfare, or overtly appearing to be due to an underlying physical condition, owners may be more likely to seek veterinary care.

Such factors that can be investigated are particular locations in which the cat performs the behavior (i.e. by the door in the kitchen), potential stressors (i.e. too few litterboxes and inappropriate locations, feeding locations), and perhaps owner engagement with the cat. There could be subtle signs that the veterinarian may notice, especially if the behavior is caught on video. A subtle body movement, a specific direction in which the cat moves, and/or other physiological signs may be more apparent in a video compared to in-clinic.

Some veterinarians prefer doing house calls for behavioral cases. It should be noted, however, that some cats will hide for the entire visit, and may not perform the behavior in front of unfamiliar people. Additionally, there may be other distractions in a home environment that play a role in how efficient an appointment can be handled. It may be necessary for the cat to eventually come to the veterinary clinic to have diagnostic tests performed.

Basic Information

As with any patient, it is imperative to gather information on the cat's previous and current medical history, including current and prior medications and medical conditions. Especially important is the use of flea and tick preventatives if a cat is presenting for repetitive behaviors with a possible underlying dermatological condition. It is also important to perform a physical examination and applicable medical workup as indicated.

If available, one should gather information on the source of the cat, and whether there is any information on relatives, as there is a potential heritable factor for some repetitive behaviors.

Environmental Information

Since there are multiple causes of repetitive behaviors, some resulting from environmental stressors, one should gather information on the cat's daily routine, as well as interactions with people and other pets in the household. While not a direct cause of repetitive behaviors, household cat aggression can be enough of a stressor to cause a cat to perform displacement behaviors. Evaluation of the environment, through videos, drawings, and/or in-home visits, can provide information that may otherwise seem unimportant to the owner.

Table 9.2 Gathering a behavioral history for a cat displaying repetitive behaviors.

Basic information	Medical history, including medications and medical conditions
	Age, source of the cat/lineage, if known
	⊚ May help identify a genetic predisposition
	Incidence of behavior in affected relatives
	⊚ Heritable factor of compulsive disorders support likelihood of compulsive behavioral patterns in relatives
Environmental information	Household composition and interactions, including people and other pets
	⊚ May help identify sources of conflict for the cat
	Typical daily routine
	⊚ This can help identify specific areas of conflict, stress, or frustration; specifically look for adequate social, physical, and mental stimulation.
Incident information	Approximate or specific date of onset of behavior
	⊚ Correlation of onset with any environmental or physical changes
	Description of the condition and its progression including historical and current
	⊚ Behaviors observed during a bout including any postural changes, vocalizations, etc.
	⊚ Will help to determine if the behavior in question meets the criteria of a compulsive disorder
	Triggers for behavior including time of day, presence of others, situations, events, locations, etc.
	Frequency and duration of bouts
	⊚ Compulsive behaviors tend to appreciate an escalation over time
	Ease of distraction
	⊚ Will help to rule out seizure-related condition
	Evidence that the behavior occurs when the cat is alone
	⊚ Videos helpful to answer this question.
	Have owners recount the two most recent bouts of the behavior in question with specific details
	⊚ Time of day
	⊚ Location
	⊚ Others present (pets and people)
	⊚ Cat's behavior before, during, and after bout
	⊚ Owner's behavior before, during, and after bout
	⊚ Cat's response to any owner interventions
Response to previous treatments	Owner response
	⊚ This may help to identify inappropriate interventions
	⊚ If there is a medical component, this could provide information

Human and Non-Human Household Members and Visitors

People and other pets may play a significant role in a cat's problem behavior. Their role can be directly related to the problem, such as owners giving attention for unwanted behaviors or playing with something like a laser pointer that encourages repetitive behaviors. It can also be indirectly related to the problem, such as by the owner punishing the cat or stressful interactions with other household cats. These can cause increased anxiety or a decreased threshold for performing a behavior, leading to a displacement repetitive behavior.

Incident Information

In addition to the background information, the information on the incidents in question is the core for diagnoses, including what the behavior looks like. This is where video examples or direct observation is beneficial for diagnosis.

It is useful to focus on the "ABCs" of the behavior, which are the Antecedents, Behaviors, and Consequences, focusing on the environment, the animal, and the owner's behaviors. Antecedents may be triggers identified in the environment or owner behaviors. Was there a sudden, loud noise? Is the behavior more likely to happen at a particular time of day? Did the owner squirt the cat with a water bottle right before the behavior started? It is important to also identify antecedent behaviors of the animal. Was it resting or pacing? Was it vocalizing? Did it engage in a fight with another cat?

Information on the cat's behavior during the incident include the duration and description of the behavior, ease of distraction, and the frequency of such incidents. The owner's behavior during the incident should be noted as well. Did they yell at the cat, or try to distract with a treat? It is also important to identify whether the behavior occurs when the cat is completely alone, information that can be gathered via video recording. Once the incident has ended, how long did it take for the cat to return to its typical behavior? If other animals or people were involved, how did they respond after the fact?

Medical Workup

Underlying pathologies must be considered when presented with a cat displaying repetitive behaviors, as there could be a component of a medical problem playing a role. An appropriate medical workup is suggested for these patients, starting with a minimum database of a completely blood count, serum chemistry panel, fecal examination, and urinalysis. A complete dermatological workup should be performed for cats displaying overgrooming or abnormal grooming. This would include evaluation of skin scrapings, Wood's lamp evaluation, fungal culture of hairs, and assessment of response to parasiticides. Further testing can include skin biopsies, response to a diet trial for food allergies, intradermal allergy tests, and assessment for endocrinopathies. Medical causes of pruritis were found for 90% of cats presenting for presumptive "psychogenic alopecia."[11] Similarly, medical differentials should be considered for dogs with acral lick dermatitis, which is a self-injurious behavior usually directed toward a limb.[12,13]

Medical Differentials

Many medical differentials should be considered based on the presenting complaint. While one frequently thinks of determining an animal has a medical OR behavioral problem, they should be considered synergistically. If you diagnose an underlying medical problem seemingly the cause of the repetitive behavior, you must still investigate the role, if any, behavior plays in the problem. Common differentials are listed in Table 9.3.

Neurological Disease

Seizures due to any of a number of underlying conditions, including neoplastic, should be considered if the behavior cannot be interrupted. There generally is a postictal phase, and other neurological deficits are usually present on physical exam. Sensory neuropathies or cauda equina should be

Table 9.3   Physiological differential diagnoses for repetitive behaviors.

Repetitive behavior	Possible medical causes
Psychogenic alopecia/ overgrooming	Infection, allergies, abnormal nerve sensation, orthopedic problem, or pain
Pica	Gastrointestinal problem, toxin
Light chasing	Ophthalmological problem, neurological problem (seizures, tumor)
Tail chasing	Neurological problem (spinal nerve problem), inflamed anal sacs, allergies, injury to tail
Excessive licking of objects or air	Gastrointestinal problem
Circling (walking in circles)	Neurologic problem, ophthalmological problem
Pacing	Pain or discomfort that decreases time spent lying down

considered for those conditions that present as self-directed repetitive behaviors, such as tail-chasing. Developmental neurological diseases can include hydrocephalus, syringomyelia, and lissencephaly.

Dermatological Disease
As cited above, medical causes of pruritis were found for 90% of cats presenting for presumptive "psychogenic alopecia."[11] Such causes include ectoparasites, food allergies, atopy, bacterial or fungal disease, such as dermatophytosis. See Figures 9.1, 9.2 and 9.3.

Infectious, Inflammatory, and Traumatic Causes
Infectious diseases or inflammatory processes, including those causing pain, that affect any of a number of organ systems should also be considered if appropriate. Referred pain can present as a self-directed behavior. An example are painful nephroliths causing the cat to self-direct licking to the dorsal aspect over the kidneys. Infectious diseases can include rabies, feline infectious peritonitis (FIP), and feline immunodeficiency virus (FIV), and inflammatory diseases can include granulomatous meningoencephalitis.

Nutritional or Toxin
A nutritional cause of repetitive behaviors is unlikely to be seen, unless there is an absorption or storage disease. Animals on an excessively low-protein diet may display unusual behaviors, as can animals with a thiamine deficiency. While not a nutritional disease per se, a cat with a liver shunt presenting with hepatic encephalopathy and head pressing may be misinterpreted as having a repetitive behavior.

Behavioral Differentials

Once a medical problem has been either ruled out, treated, or managed, behavioral reasons for the behavior should be investigated (Table 9.4). It is often difficult to come up with a definitive diagnosis for repetitive behaviors, even for dogs for which there are more standard criteria.[14] It is a false dichotomy to state it's "either" medical or behavioral, as frequently they occur concurrently, and sometimes are difficult to determine which one came first. One must also determine comorbidity with other problem behaviors, as has been reported in roughly half of cats diagnosed with a compulsive disorder.[15]

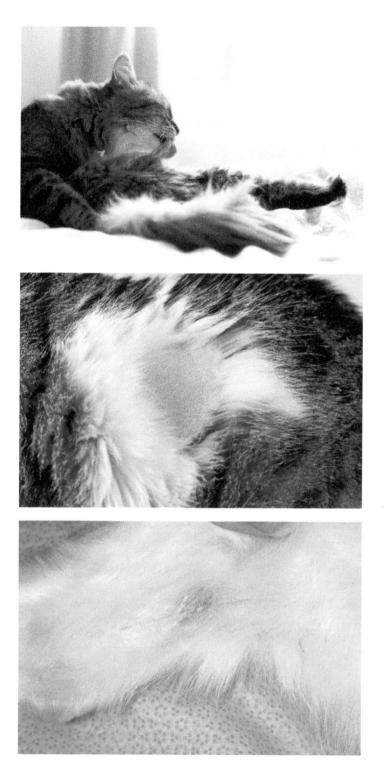

Figures 9.1, 9.2, and 9.3   For a cat that is grooming to the point of hair loss, medical causes should be ruled out before treating the problem as behavioral in nature. Image provided by Melissa Bain. sonyachny / Adobe Stock and Firn / Adobe Stock

Table 9.4 Behavioral differential diagnoses for repetitive behaviors.

Diagnosis	Definition	When it is displayed
Compulsive behavior	A behavior that is constantly repeated without an apparent purpose, often without a specific context. The cat can potentially have an underlying anxiety disorder.	In many different contexts, scenarios, and locations. Can be very difficult to interrupt. Usually interferes with normal daily functioning.
Displacement behavior	A normal behavior performed out of context for the situation, often repeated. Often starts when an external stressful event occurs. When performed excessively and out of context, it may become a compulsive disorder.	In response to a stressful event, such as with fear of unfamiliar people, other cats, or specific triggers.
Attention-seeking behavior	A behavior that cats perform for owner attention. Attention could be something positive (petting, getting a treat). It can also be something aversive (yelling, chasing) – at least it got the owner's attention.	Only when someone is present or might come into the area where the cat is. These types of behaviors are maintained by the owner paying attention to the cat in response.
Stereotypic behavior	A behavior that is constantly repeated with a possible purpose of relieving stress related to housing or feeding conditions. These are quite similar to compulsive disorders and may even be the same.	Generally, when a confined animal (zoo, laboratory animal and perhaps even a pet) is not able to perform the full range of species-typical behaviors due to the environment.

Compulsive Behaviors

To be considered compulsive, the behavioral pattern under consideration must be sufficiently pronounced to exceed that necessary to meet its apparent goal or such that it interferes with the cat's normal functioning. Compulsive behaviors are those in which the cat engages in a repetitive, relatively unvaried sequence of movements, usually derived from contextually normal maintenance behaviors (i.e. grooming, hunting). Obsessive-compulsive and related disorders (OCD) in humans are characterized by obsessions, thoughts, or urges, leading to compulsions, which are repetitive psychological or physical actions that are performed to alleviate the anxiety related to the obsessions one has.[16] It is uncertain whether animals "obsess" and have thoughts or urges to perform these behaviors.

Compulsive behaviors often interfere with normal daily activities and functioning. They generally worsen over time, and the behaviors can start to occur in more contexts and with less provocation. While not displacement behaviors, they can arise from them if practiced and/or reinforced enough. Often an owner can identify a specific stressful event (physical trauma or social upheaval) that coincided with onset of a compulsive behavior. There are links to genetic predispositions, as Oriental-type breed cats are overrepresented.[17] See Figures 9.4 and 9.5.

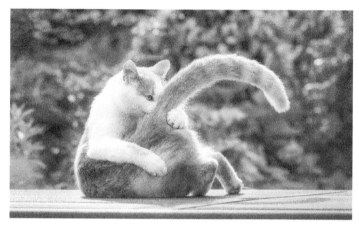

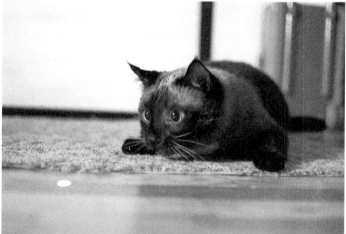

Figures 9.4 and 9.5   Although cats are less prone to tail chasing/mutilation and light/shadow chasing than dogs, these are possible diagnoses for them. Courtesy of kathomenden / Adobe Stock and Lema-lisa / Adobe Stock

Ingestive Behaviors (Pica, Fabric Chewing/Sucking)

Pica is described as the ingestion of nonfood items. It is unclear about which sex is over-represented; however, Oriental-type breeds, such as Siamese, and American Domestic Shorthair cats are over-represented in those displaying abnormal ingestive behaviors.[2,15,18] Normal exploratory behavior should be ruled out; however, there is conflicting evidence on the relationship of age.[18,19] Plant-eating is not considered pica, unless it is extreme. Studies in dogs showed that those that did not appear ill before eating plants did not vomit, so plant-eating is not necessarily related to illness, nor related to diet or anthelminthic treatment.[20] While no peer-reviewed studies exist for cats, preliminary results demonstrate that the same holds true for cats.[21]

Diet can have an effect on pica. It was noted that cats that were fed *ad libitum* were less likely to display pica.[19]

A subset of pica is fabric/wool sucking and/or eating, which is proposed to be seen most frequently in cats that have not been weaned properly and in Oriental-type breeds; however, it is unclear about an age predilection. In one study there was a demonstrated significant correlation between sucking and ingesting fabric, so those that are noted to suck on it should be closely monitored for potential ingestion.[19] See Figures 9.6, 9.7 and 9.8 for examples.

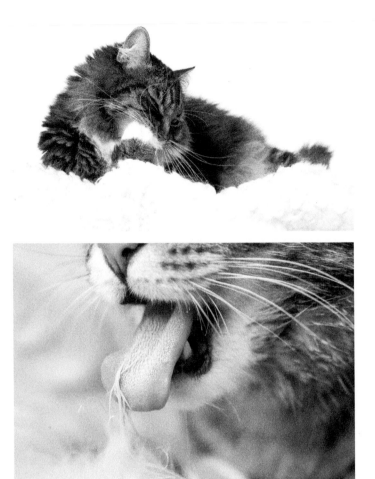

Figures 9.6 and 9.7   Cats who suck on fabrics have a high likelihood of also ingesting fabrics and should be carefully monitored. Lema-lisa / Adobe Stock and Spring / Adobe Stock

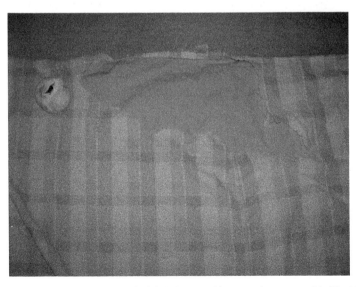

Figure 9.8   Image of hole in fabric ingested by a cat. Image provided by Melissa Bain.

Displacement Behaviors

Displacement behaviors are those behavioral responses to an external stimulus, such as a sound, confinement, or aggression that are performed out of context in response to the trigger. Often these triggers cause anxiety or overarousal, which can precipitate the displacement behaviors.[22,23] Overgrooming, yawning, and pacing are behaviors that are often described as displacement behaviors. Over time, if the behaviors become practiced, and even inadvertently rewarded, they can morph into compulsive behaviors.

Attention-seeking Behaviors

These are behaviors for which an animal receives a reinforcement. Another name is "audience-affected behavior." An owner may let a cat outside in response to chasing its tail, or may feed the cat after it meows repeatedly. Sometimes just an owner making eye contact with the cat is enough of a reinforcement for the animal to continue to perform the behavior. Even something like a verbal reprimand may be considered by the cat as reinforcing.

Stereotypic Behaviors

These are repetitive, unvarying behavior patterns with no apparent goal or function, commonly displayed by animals living in a barren environment, primarily displayed by captive wildlife, production animals, and animals in laboratory settings, and rarely by domesticated cats.

Treatment

When working with owners to develop a treatment plan, one should consider the diagnosis and prognosis, along with the ability of the owners to adhere to a treatment plan.[24] There are few safety risks when treating repetitive behaviors, other than those due to potential side effects due to medications. More risks lie in not treating the cat, as the cat's welfare may suffer.

One way to develop a treatment plan is to work within five general steps: management; tools; training and behavior modification, including desensitization (DS) and counterconditioning (CC) to triggers; and medications and alternative therapies. There are parts of these steps that overlap (i.e. a tool can be utilized in management, medications help DS/CC proceed more smoothly). Aside from behavioral components of the treatment plan, it is important to treat and/or manage any underlying physiological condition contributing to the problem. See Table 9.5 for an overview.

Surgery, Medications, and Other Related Therapies

There are no known surgeries to prevent or treat these problem behaviors. There are reports of cats having their tail amputated in order to treat tail chasing behavior. Unless there is a physiological problem causing the tail chasing, amputation is not recommended as a treatment for this problem. Surgery or endoscopy would be indicated to remove a foreign body if a cat is displaying pica, wool, or fabric sucking that caused ingestion of material. Of course medical treatment would be indicated to treat or manage any underlying medical condition. Neutering is not known to have an effect on these behaviors; however, owners should be counseled against breeding a cat with compulsive behaviors as there could be a genetic predisposition for these behaviors.

Table 9.5   Overview of treatment of repetitive behaviors in cats.

Physical health	Rule out and treat any underlying and concurrent medical conditions
Management	Avoid triggers that can instigate repetitive behaviors
	Avoid triggers that can cause stress or anxiety triggering displacement behaviors
	Provide environmental enrichment to improve overall welfare
Tools	Avoid the use of laser pointers
Training/Behavior modification	Systematic desensitization and counterconditioning to triggers that can instigate repetitive behaviors, or those that cause stress or anxiety
Medications and alternative therapies	Selective serotonin reuptake inhibitors or tricyclic antidepressants:
	● To address an underlying compulsive disorder
	● To help ameliorate signs of stress and anxiety
	Other anxiolytics (gabapentin), nutraceuticals, or pheromones to help ameliorate signs of stress and anxiety
	Treatments for underlying physiological conditions

Management

Owners should be counseled on the importance of managing the environment so that the cat is less likely to continue to perform the behavior. This can be broken down to avoidance of potentially dangerous items that a cat can ingest, should it have pica, wool, or fabric sucking, and avoidance of triggers that cause anxiety or overarousal.

Avoidance can be very difficult, as some cats are very driven to perform these behaviors. Owners should limit access to targeted nonfood items via containment or by removing items from the environment. This may be done by creating a safe room in the house that does not contain the targeted items. If the cat is not used to confinement, then confinement training must be implemented. If the cat is attracted to electrical cords, these must be unplugged or adequately protected from the cat with covers or made inaccessible. Correct any dietary deficiencies and make sure the pet is on the proper amount of a complete and balanced diet for their life stage.

In homes with multiple cats, make sure each has safe access to its food and the opportunity to eat undisturbed. This may mean separating pets during feeding times, which also allows owners to verify food consumption. If outside cats trigger the patient to display displacement repetitive behaviors, owner can discourage cats from entering the yard by removing bird feeders, as well as block the sight of the outside cats with something like window film. If a cat is reactive to sounds, owners can play either classical music or white noise to help block out the sounds.

Owners should not punish their cat for unwanted behaviors, should they be repetitive behaviors or others. Not only does this not address the underlying cause of a behavior, it also can cause an increase in anxiety and aggression and leads to poor welfare for the cat. Yelling, swatting, hitting, and spraying with water are commonly thought of as punishing; however, punishment is in the eye of the beholder. What one cat considers tolerable another finds punishing.

Not only should the owners avoid the items that can be dangerous or cause anxiety, they should provide attractive alternatives and sufficient mental and physical exercise. The perception of control is essential for well-being, and vital in helping to decrease stress in animals. It is important to provide foundations to cats to maintain a quality of life. These include: a stable, consistent environment that enhances learning; a safe environment free from fearful stimuli that allows exploration without harm; and satisfactory nutrition delivered in a way that the cat chooses to ingest it.[25]

Increasing mental and physical stimulation, especially for indoor-only cats, is one way in which owners can positively affect their cats' well-being. There are many ways that this can be done, ranging from visual and olfactory enrichment, to interactive play, to food-dispensing and foraging toys.

If a cat isn't stressed by looking outside, an owner can put a perch by a window, or even design an outside catio that the cat can visit. Some cats are reported to watch television or play games on an iPad or tablet. Olfactory enrichment can be accomplished with such things as catnip and silvervine.

Owner involvement and interaction with their cat is important, as cats are social animals that for the most part enjoy at least some interaction with their owners. This can range from something simple like petting and brushing, to interactive and vigorous play sessions with wand-type toys with feathers attached. Playing with laser pointers should be discouraged for those cats who display compulsive behaviors. As with punishment, it is up to an individual cat to determine whether or not something is rewarding or aversive.

Food-dispensing toys help to motivate the cat to engage with its environment in a meaningful manner, allowing a cat to display more species-typical behaviors of eating multiple times per day. There are many examples of food-dispensing toys, either purchased or homemade. The website www.foodpuzzlesforcats.com presents a multitude of ideas.

Desensitization and Counter-Conditioning (DS/CC)

Behavior modification is primarily focused on systematic desensitization and counterconditioning (DS/CC) toward the trigger that causes the animal to feel distressed and display unwanted behaviors.[26] This is a process in which a conditioned emotional response (CER) such as fear is extinguished by exposing the animal in a graduated manner to the fear-eliciting stimuli, and replaced with an alternative, competing response by pairing it with an eliciting stimulus that will trigger an opposing emotional or physiologic response. When creating a program for systematic DS/CC, a stimulus hierarchy is created which ranges from a level that elicits no discernable response to a level that elicits an extreme response. The animal is exposed to the first step in this hierarchy, where it shows a very mild response, such as noticing that the trigger is present, until the mild response is no longer being displayed. Once this occurs, the animal is exposed to the next step on the stimulus hierarchy. All the while the animal is presented with something that will change the emotional response to one that is favorable toward the trigger, such as a high-value treat.

DS/CC is of limited benefit for a cat with an underlying medical condition causing the behavior, as well as those with a true compulsive disorder, as it is more internally driven. However, some cats with a compulsive disorder may still have external triggers that continue the behavior. Cats diagnosed with a displacement behavior, perpetuated by an external trigger, can be desensitized and counterconditioned to these triggers slowly over time.

Hallmarks of DS/CC are finding the balance between the cat noticing the trigger but not being overwhelmed by it, developing a plan to gradually increase the intensity of the trigger, and find something that the cat finds rewarding that it only gets in the presence of the trigger. If the trigger is a sound, the owner should attenuate the sound by either having it on a recording and playing it at a low volume, having the cat a room (or two) away from the sound, and/or playing classical music or a white noise machine to help block out the sound, and gradually increase the volume over time. If the trigger is another cat in the household, the owner should keep the cats at a distance and gradually bring them closer. While the trigger is present, the owner should be giving the cat something that it finds pleasurable (canned food, treats, play, petting), and when the trigger is either out of sight from the cat or the volume is turned down, the pleasurable reward stops. Each session is only two to three minutes at a time. During these sessions the owner should keep track of the cat's response (desirable or undesirable), so that they can identify trends over time.

Medications and Alternative Therapies

Medications play an important part in treating cats with repetitive behaviors in one of two main ways. They are utilized to decrease anxiety and stress that lead to displacement behaviors, as well as to decrease the underpinnings of compulsive behaviors. Medications work best when combined with management and behavior modification, and do not offer a cure.

Selective serotonin reuptake inhibitors (SSRIs) such as fluoxetine and paroxetine are recommended to decrease anxiety and arousal, as well as decrease the desire to perform compulsive behaviors.[27,28] The dose of fluoxetine, as well as paroxetine, is 0.5 to 1 mg/kg once daily. These medications, along with tricyclic antidepressants/antianxiety medications (TCAs) like clomipramine, take up to six weeks to see the full effect[29]. Quick-to-onset medications, such as gabapentin (100 mg per CAT up to twice daily), can be utilized to decrease anxiety, but have little likelihood to decrease compulsive behaviors.[30]

Other products, such as nutraceuticals and pheromones, have some limited evidence that they can be helpful in decreasing anxiety and stress in cats. It should be noted that medications are not indicated to treat attention-seeking behaviors as the sole cause of repetitive behaviors.

Prevention

Truly compulsive behaviors are difficult to prevent, especially if there is a strong genetic component to the behavior. Veterinarians should counsel owners on breed predispositions toward particular repetitive behaviors, as well as how to interview breeders to avoid purchasing a cat from an affected line.

Owners should provide a cat with appropriate outlets for their species-typical behaviors, places in which to hide, and adequate numbers of resources. These actions can help alleviate stressors that can add to a cat's level of worry. They also should be provided with information on how to identify problems early on. Veterinarians should make a point of asking behavior questions at each appointment in order to discover problems at an earlier stage.

Summary

Repetitive behaviors are due to any of a number of behavioral and physiological problems. Veterinarians should focus on identifying the problem as early as possible, rule out and treat medical problems, and prescribe behavior modification and/or psychotropic medications for the best possible outcome.

References

1 Wassink-van der Schot AA, Day C, Morton JM, Rand J, Phillips CJC. Risk factors for behavior problems in cats presented to an Australian companion animal behavior clinic. *J Vet Behav.* 2016;14:34–40.

2 Bamberger M, Houpt KA. Signalment factors, comorbidity, and trends in behavior diagnoses in cats: 736 cases (1991–2001). *J Am Vet Med Assoc.* 2006;229(10):1602–1606.

3 Horwitz DF. Differences and similarities between behavioral and internal medicine. *J Am Vet Med Assoc.* 2000;217(9):1372–1376.

4 Seibert LM, Landsberg GM. Diagnosis and management of patients presenting with behavior problems. *Vet Clin North Am Small Anim Pract.* 2008;38(5):937–950.

5 Roshier AL, McBride EA. Veterinarians' perceptions of behaviour support in small-animal practice. *Vet Rec.* 2013;172(10):267.

6 Roshier AL, McBride EA. Canine behaviour problems: Discussions between veterinarians and dog owners during annual booster consultations. *Vet Rec.* 2013;172(9):235.

7 Shaw JR. Evaluation of communication skills training programs at North American veterinary medical training institutions. *J Am Vet Med Assoc.* 2019;255(6):722–733.

8 Cornell KK, Coe JB, Shaw DH, Felsted KE, Bonvicini KA. Investigation of the effects of a practice-level communication training program on veterinary health-care team members' communication confidence, client satisfaction, and practice financial metrics. *J Am Vet Med Assoc.* 2019;255(12):1377–1388.

9 Nibblett BM, Ketzis JK, Grigg EK. Comparison of stress exhibited by cats examined in a clinic versus a home setting. *Appl Anim Behav Sci.* 2015;173:68–75.

10 Palestrini C, Minero M, Cannas S, Rossi E, Frank D. Video analysis of dogs with separation-related behaviors. *Appl Anim Behav Sci.* 2010;124(1–2):61–67.

11 Waisglass SE, Landsberg GM, Yager JA, Hall JA. Underlying medical conditions in cats with presumptive psychogenic alopecia. *J Am Vet Med Assoc.* 2006;228(11):1705–1709.

12 Denerolle P, White SD, Taylor TS, Vandenabeele SIJ. Organic diseases mimicking acral lick dermatitis in six dogs. *J Am Anim Hosp Assoc.* 2007;43(4):215–220.

13 Siracusa C, Landsberg G. Psychogenic diseases. In: Noli C, Colombo S, eds. *Feline dermatology: Springer.* New York City, NY, USA: Springer; 2020:567–581.

14 Hewson CJ, Luescher UA, Ball RO. The use of chance-corrected agreement to diagnose canine compulsive disorder: An approach to behavioral diagnosis in the absence of a 'Gold Standard'. *Can J Vet Res.* 1999;63(3):201–206.

15 Overall KL, Dunham AE. Clinical features and outcome in dogs and cats with obsessive-compulsive disorder: 126 cases (1989–2000). *J Am Vet Med Assoc.* 2002;221(10):1445–1452.

16 American Psychiatric Association. Obsessive-compulsive disorder. In: *Diagnostic and statistical manual of mental disorders V*, 5th ed. Washington, DC: American Psychiatric Association; 2013. doi:10.1176/appi.books.9780890425596.dsm06 (accessed April 8, 2022).

17 Seksel K, Lindeman M. Use of clomipramine in the treatment of anxiety-related and obsessive-compulsive disorders in cats. *Aust Vet J.* 1998;76(5):317–321.

18 Bradshaw JWS, Neville PF, Sawyer D. Factors affecting pica in the domestic cat. *Appl Anim Behav Sci.* 1997;52(3–4):373–379.

19 Demontigny-Bédard I, Beauchamp G, Bélanger M-C, Frank D. Characterization of pica and chewing behaviors in privately owned cats: A case-control study. *J Feline Med Surg.* 2016;18(8):652–657.

20 Sueda KLC, Hart BL, Cliff KD. Characterisation of plant eating in dogs. *Appl Anim Behav Sci.* 2008;111(1–2):120–132.

21 Hart BL, Hart LA, Thigpen AP, eds. Characterization of plant eating in cats. *ISAE (International Society of Applied Ethology) 2019: 53rd congress of the ISAE.* Bergen, Norway: Wageningen Academic Publishers; 2019.

22 Beaver B. *The veterinarian's encyclopedia of animal behavior.* Ames, IA: Iowa State University Press; 1994.

23 Bain MJ, Fan CM. Animal behavior case of the month. *J Am Vet Med Assoc.* 2012;240(6):673–675.

24 Casey RA, Bradshaw JW. Owner compliance and clinical outcome measures for domestic cats undergoing clinical behavior therapy. *J Vet Behav.* 2008;3(3):114–124.

25 Buffington CAT, Bain M. Stress and feline health. *Vet Clin Small Anim Pract.* 2020;50(4):653–662.

26 Poggiagliolmi S. Desensitization and counterconditioning: When and how? *Vet Clin Small Anim Pract.* 2018;48(3):433–442.

27 Pryor PA, Hart BL, Cliff KD, Bain MJ. Effects of a selective serotonin reuptake inhibitor on urine spraying behavior in cats. *J Am Vet Med Assoc.* 2001;219(11):1557–1561.

28 Ogata N, Dantas LMdS, Crowell-Davis SL. Selective serotonin reuptake inhibitors. In: Crowell-Davis SL, Murray TF, Dantas LMdS, eds. *Veterinary psychopharmacology,* 2nd ed. Hoboken, NJ: Wiley Blackwell; 2019:103–128.

29 Crowell-Davis SL. Tricyclic antidepressants. In: Crowell-Davis SL, Murray TF, Dantas LMdS, eds. *Veterinary psychopharmacology,* 2nd ed. Hoboken, NJ: Wiley Blackwell; 2019:231–256.

30 Crowell-Davis SL, Irimajiri M, Dantas LMdS. Anticonvulsants and mood stabilizers. In: Crowell-Davis SL, Murray TF, Dantas LMdS, eds. *Veterinary psychopharmacology,* 2nd ed. Hoboken, NJ: Wiley Blackwell; 2019:147–156.

10

Aggression Toward Humans
Elizabeth Stelow

Introduction

Feline human-directed aggression is defined as a cat engaging in posturing, vocalizing, stalking, scratching, biting, or related behaviors toward one or more people.[1] This type of behavior is reported in somewhere between 13.5% and 32% of household cats.[2-5] Roughly 95% of the time, the behavior is directed toward owners, rather than strangers or veterinarians.[2] In one study, nearly half (25/58 cats) of the human-directed aggression displayed by cats was seen as play related; another large percentage (23/58 cats) was labeled petting-induced.[3] Finally, one study showed that 35% of kittens adopted from a humane society had shown aggression toward people by 1 year of age.[6]

Feline aggression can be of great concern to owners, especially those who are most at risk for being physically injured or contracting a zoonotic disease, such as children or the elderly.[1]

The seriousness of feline aggression toward people should not be underestimated.[7] Aggression is one reason given when cats are relinquished to shelters.[8] And one study asserted that 71% of cats relinquished had been reported to have bit a person.[9]

What is Normal?

A behaviorally healthy cat with an appropriately satisfying home life should rarely show signs of aggression (defensive body postures with hissing, growling, scratching, and/or biting). This is not to say that a cat will not occasionally be startled enough to become defensive in its body posture; but it should not feel like the circumstances require it to become offensive as well. In addition, people and dogs passing by the house may elicit mild signs of aggression from cats indoors or in the yard.

What is normal but often unacceptable?

Growling, hissing, scratching, and biting are perfectly normal self-defense behaviors under intensely frightening or stressful situations. Some owners misinterpret the motivation behind the behavior and, instead of finding ways to decrease stress, will assign more negative motivations (vengeance, spitefulness, etc.) rather than fear.

What is abnormal but often acceptable?

Owners may be perpetually tolerant of a cat that growls or hisses at them in certain situations but does not escalate beyond growling or hissing. Some owners may find it humorous

---

(Continued)

(Continued)

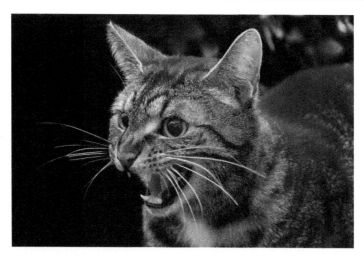

Figure 10.1   Cat owners are often tolerant of a cat that hisses, as long as it doesn't escalate. Photo courtesy of strh / pixabay.

that their cat "talks back" or may not be aware that the cat could escalate at any time, if the situation becomes more stressful. They also may not realize that these behaviors are often indicative of a fearful or stressed cat and that the situations causing them should be addressed. See Figure 10.1.

Kittens that are allowed to play with human body parts (hands, feet, hair) may develop play-related aggression that is capable of hurting someone; but, owners may find these behaviors acceptable in kittens.

What is abnormal and typically unacceptable?

Owners usually are not comfortable with a cat that attacks people. So, cats that bite and scratch people are often rehomed, euthanized, or presented to the veterinarian as a behavior problem.

How to Diagnose

Before the Appointment

Because of the extent of the information required to make an accurate behavioral diagnosis, it is most useful to ask owners to complete a detailed history form and obtain videos of their home and cat(s).

Written Historical Information

To help make things more efficient for the clinician and their staff, they can use a history form (see website) that the owner can fill out and submit before the appointment, giving the team time to review the information beforehand. The clinician will also want any medical records from previous veterinarians, especially if they may have treated this cat for its aggression.

Owner-Provided Video

It is highly unlikely that the clinician will see the aggression toward the owner in their exam room. If such behavior is seen, it is unlikely to be the same behaviors displayed at home. Therefore, video is a good supplement to a thorough written or oral history. When the owners make an appointment, they should be asked to obtain a few types of video:

1) The layout of the home. This can give the clinician an idea of ways to manage the problem, the level of enrichment offered, and other aspects of home life that may be helpful in making the most appropriate diagnosis or treatment plan.

2) The cat in its environment: eating, resting, playing. This can give the clinician a sense of how comfortable the cat is in his environment. The clinician may see some subtle behaviors that will not be present during the appointment. It will also show the clinician how the cat responds to the owner's presence.

3) The circumstances under which aggression is likely to occur. Owners should not be asked specifically to get a video of the aggression happening, both to keep people safe and to avoid triggering the behavior intentionally. Asking for the circumstances, however, allows the clinician to see what may be triggering the aggression. The clinician may also be able to see if any owner is inadvertently behaving in a triggering manner.

During the Appointment

Please refer to the Introduction to this book, which summarizes the questions that should be asked for a thorough behavioral history.

Prompted by a history form and on questioning by the clinician, the owners should be able to provide a list of things that have historically triggered their cat's aggression. They can also gauge the intensity and frequency of the aggression incidents, how the cat behaves between incidents, and what types of things they've tried to resolve the problem. All of this can be useful in determining the motivation and the areas of focus of a treatment plan.

But, to truly diagnose the motivation behind the aggression, it is often essential to know the ABCs – antecedents, behavior, and consequences – of the cat's aggression.

- **Antecedents** are the circumstances before an aggressive event occurs. If the behavior is new, the owners may not have a good sense of "what's usually happening" right before the aggression. But, most owners can be talked through the key episode that brought them in to seek help.
- **Behavior** is what the cat and people are doing during an incident. It's important to ask about body language of the cat, since that can be the key to determining motivation.
- **Consequences** are the things that happen to or around the cat after an incident.

With careful exploration of specific incidents, the clinician may find more than one motivation or more than one type of aggression.

Gathering Incident Information

Ideally, the history form will ask the owners to give details about two or three specific incidents that can be explored more fully during the appointment. When the clinician is exploring, it is useful to break each incident into its ABCs.

For instance, let's say that the patient, Fluffy, attacks visitors to the home. Two incidents are described briefly on the form: one toward a friend of the teenage daughter and one toward a refrigerator repair technician. The clinician can then follow an investigative path like this one:

Table 10.1   Incident information.

- Frequency, intensity, and severity of one or more incidents
- Antecedent to behavior: what was happening around the cat before aggression
- Behavior of the cat during the incident: body language, vocalizations, interaction with people
- Consequences for the cat: responses of persons present, including victim
- A list of all known triggers[10]
- How the cat is between episodes[10]
- Treatments that owner has tried; outcomes

- "Let's look specifically at the incident when the friend was visiting."
    - What were the girls doing just before Fluffy went after the friend? (responses may include sitting quietly, playing with Fluffy, doing something loud or very active, previously sitting but suddenly in motion, ...)
    - What had Fluffy been doing prior to that? (responses may include resting in another room, being vigilant while sitting on the stairs, stalking the friend, attempting to hide, ...)
    - What did the girls say Fluffy looked like when she went after the friend (body language, including ears, eyes, tail) and did she vocalize?
    - What did she do when she made contact? (bite, scratch, etc.)
    - What did the girls do then?

With this last question, the clinician is looking for typical human responses to being attacked, but also any type of punishment (yelling, hitting, etc.) or reinforcement (people running away) that may have occurred.

Repeat a similar set of questions for the other incident given. Compare and contrast Fluffy's triggers and actions. What do they have in common? What's different? See Table 10.1 for information.

The clinician can then use this information to explore further to finalize their diagnosis.

Making a Diagnosis

Once the clinician has gathered the information from the form and interviews with the owners, they are ready to diagnose this aggression. Below are the medical problems they should be prepared to rule out, followed by the most common behavior motivations for feline aggression toward people. The behavioral motivations are paired here with diagnostic criteria; for the diagnostic guidelines for medical problems, please see the appropriate medical textbooks or online resources.

Medical Differentials

While this list is not exhaustive, these differentials should be on the list when diagnosing feline aggression.[11–17]

Degenerative: loss of vision, loss of hearing
Developmental: lissencephaly, hydrocephalus
Anomalous: Feline ischemic encephalopathy
Metabolic: uremic encephalopathy, hepatic encephalopathy, hyperthyroid
Neoplastic: intracranial neoplasia, cerebral infarct

Neurologic: psychomotor or partial seizure, peripheral neuropathy

Nutritional: thiamine deficiency, taurine deficiency, tryptophan deficiency

Infectious: Rabies, pseudorabies, toxoplasma, *Neospora caninum*, feline immunodeficiency virus, feline infectious peritonitis

Inflammatory/Pain: feline interstitial cystitis, granulomatous meningioencephalitis, arthritis

Toxins: lead, zinc, methylphenidate, heavy metal toxicity

Traumatic: brain injury, causes of pain

Vascular: cerebral infarct

Behavioral Differentials

There are many different motivations for aggression, including fear, inappropriate play, petting-induced, redirected, and pain. Development of the best-fit treatment plan requires determining the actual motivation for the aggression. The motivation can often be determined based on the situational factors and body language associated with the reported incidents. (19Curtis) The specific motivations for feline aggression discussed here are fear, play, petting, and redirected. Although others exist, they are less common.

Fear-Related Aggression

Fear is a common motivation for feline aggression toward people. While a cat may show overt signs of fear during aggressive incidents, they need not be present to commit to this diagnosis. Typical findings in the history may include the cat first trying unsuccessfully to retreat from a fear-inducing trigger. When avoidance or escape is not possible, the cat may show defensive postures and vocalization. It may hiss or growl (even spit) and its body posture will likely be reported as low or crouched, with ears flattened back against its head.[18] (See Figure 10.2) If the threat display is not sufficient to stop the trigger, the confrontation may become physical.[13]

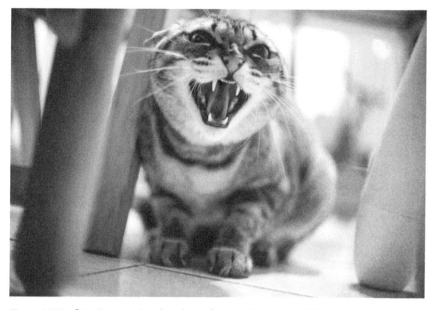

Figure 10.2 Cats that are showing signs of aggression from a defensive location are typically frightened. Photo courtesy of pixabay (YM fang).

Even if the client does not describe these signs of fear, ask whether the cat used to display them earlier in the progression of aggression. With practice, especially when signs of fear did not help minimize the appearance of triggers, the cat may have abandoned fearful body language as unsuccessful. But, the fear is still present.

Triggers and other predisposing factors:

- The owners are often able to identify specific triggers, like punishment (yelling, spraying, swatting), restraint or handling, strangers entering the house, a particular owner doing a particular activity, and veterinary visits.[13] If so, these triggers can be worked on as part of the treatment plan.
- There may be a history of scary events associated with a particular person or item.[19]
- Clients may also describe a cat that is nervous or timid even when not aggressive. Fear may stem from genetic or environmental factors in the cat's history. Studies have shown that "personality," whether fearful or confident, is linked to paternal factors.[20,21]
- A history of the cat having been feral or poorly socialized as a kitten is not uncommon in fear aggression cases.[19,22]

Inappropriate or Misdirected Play Aggression

As noted above, inappropriate play is the second most common type of feline aggression toward people. Despite the harmless sounding name, this type of aggression is anything but harmless.

Risk factors for this type of aggression include

- Young cat (often under two years of age)
- Orphaned and raised without littermates[23]
- Early weaned[24]
- Singly housed, or housed with older cats that don't play
- Kept indoors[25]
- Often limited opportunity to play
- One or more people in the household encouraging rough play. This happens frequently with kittens, as people play with their hands; they wish the cat to stop the behavior as it grows[23,26] Figure 10.3 shows this type of handling.

Characteristics often reported as part of inappropriate play aggression reflect a common play behavior sequence of lying in wait, stalking (as shown in Figure 10.4), chasing, pouncing, and grabbing (Figure 10.5). Ambushes are common[23] and vocalization is at a minimum.[18] While these behaviors should be directed toward a toy or prey animal, they are carried out toward a moving person.[10] The targets are typically the person's hands or feet; and, once contact is made, the cat may bite, scratch, or both.[27] The victim may be a single family member or more indiscriminate.

Key behavioral differentials for this diagnosis include fear-based aggression, redirected aggression, and attention-seeking.[23]

Petting-Induced or Handling-Induced Aggression

Petting-induced or handling-induced aggression is a common problem reported by owners. It is the reason given for up to 40% of the aggression seen by specialists.[3,10]

Characteristics often found in the history for petting-induced aggression include the following: A cat may actively solicit attention by approaching, bunting (head-butting), rubbing, or other invitation to interact. After some amount of petting, the cat will then turn and bite the hand petting it (Figure 10.6).

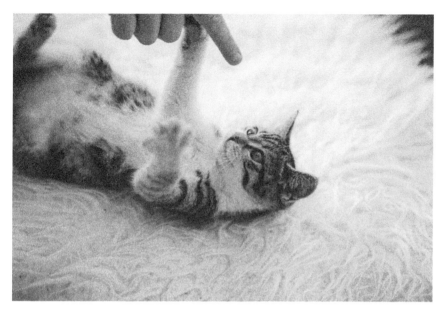

Figure 10.3   Playing with a kitten with hands is a risk factor for play-related aggression. Photo courtesy of pixabay.

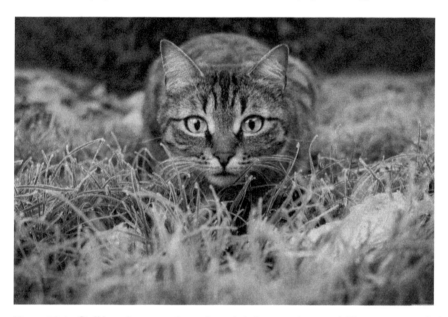

Figure 10.4   Stalking often precedes a play-related aggression attack. Photo courtesy of pixabay.

Risk Factors: It has been theorized that each cat may be responding to one of more of these scenarios:

1) The cat is overstimulated, and early signals given by the cat are not recognized by the person.
2) The cat is trying to control the situation and decides when the petting should end.
3) Human petting, while similar to feline allogrooming, is often performed with long strokes, rather than the short strokes typical of another cat's tongue; it may be that the cat wants something more like allogrooming and is frustrated by what it gets.[28]
4) The session is longer than the cat chooses to tolerate.[10]

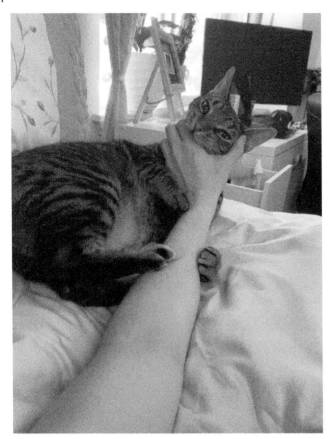

Figure 10.5 One feature of inappropriate play aggression is grabbing the person's arm and biting between the thumb and forefinger. Photo courtesy of Katrina Larkin.

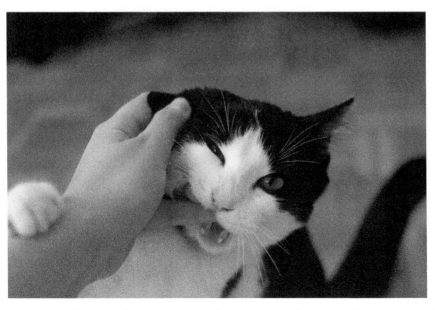

Figure 10.6 Even friendly cats may have a limited tolerance for petting. Photo courtesy of pexels.

The cat, as it becomes increasingly intolerant during a petting episode, will likely start with a tail flick or twitch, fidgeting, muscle tenseness, and leaning away from the petter. If ignored, body language may escalate to tail lashing, rotating ears back, and dilated pupils before biting.[1]

Handling-related aggression is similar, but specific to just being handled, such as restraint during veterinary visits, or during bathing, brushing, or nail trimming.

Redirected Aggression

Redirected aggression is aggression directed at a target that is different from the one eliciting the aggressive response. The actual trigger can be nearly anything that arouses or frightens the cat, including passing dogs or stray cats seen through windows, vacuum cleaners and other "scary" appliances, visitors to the home, or loud sounds.[10,22] Frustration of not being able to get to – or intense fear that prevents the cats from approaching – the actual trigger causes redirection onto an owner or others.

Triggers: In one study of feline aggression, a reaction to a loud noise or an interaction with another cat was determined to be the trigger in 95% of redirected aggression incidents. This same study showed that approximately 65% of these cats redirected toward people, most often their owner. Redirected aggression can also be directed toward the owner after a fight with a household cat, especially if the owner tries to break up a fight.

It is crucial to identify the actual trigger, as it will need to be considered in the treatment plan.

Other Types of Feline Aggression

The types of feline aggression described above are the most common types presented for treatment. Other types have been reported. These include maternal, status, confidence, pain-induced, and others. If an aggressive feline patient does not meet the diagnostic criteria for any of the types of aggression presented here, the clinician is encouraged to consult available literature for other differentials.

Treatment

A treatment plan should be tailored to the specific motivations and triggers that lead to the episodes of aggression. For the owner's convenience, the clinician should organize the plan into large categories: management, relationships, behavior modification, and medications and other related therapies. Within each category, the details for each element can be outlined for presentation to the owner. The clinician may find that, for a given case, she may have overlap or not use all elements.

Below are general guidelines for treatment of behavior issues. This overview is summarized in Table 10.2. These are followed by specific recommendations for the diagnoses presented above.

General Treatment Plan Components

Management: This represents the "What can be changed now to help the cat avoid its triggers?" Perhaps, the fearful cat can be put away (in a room with food toys and white noise) when strangers visit. Or, maybe the owner can stash appropriate toys around the house to distract the play-aggressive cat. How and where should the cat be fed to maximize hunting and keep the cat from attacking the owner for food?

Within the context of aggression cases, management encompasses two major sub-categories: Safety and Avoidance and Environmental Enrichment, each with a different goal.

Table 10.2   Overview of treatment of feline human-directed aggression.

Physical health	Rule out or treat underlying medical conditions Castrate or spay, as deemed appropriate	
Management	*Safety and avoidance*	Avoid relevant triggers (varies by diagnosis): <ul><li>Block visual access to passing dogs or outdoor cats</li><li>Put cat away while vacuuming or strangers visiting</li><li>Do not force cat to move from furniture</li><li>Block access to places from which cat ambushes people</li><li>Distract cat while moving through room</li><li>Avoid punishment</li><li>Do not assume cat wants to be held/petted</li></ul>
	Environmental enrichment	<ul><li>Optimize:Feeding routines</li><li>Litter box numbers, locations, and maintenance</li><li>Number and placement of perches and resting spaces</li><li>Number and placement of scratching posts and facial rubbing stations</li><li>Access to outdoors</li><li>Access to self-play toys</li></ul>
Relationships	Consent tests for petting Training of new skills Interactive play with appropriate toys	
Behavior modification	Desensitization and counterconditioning	
Medications and related	Medications are discussed in Appendix 1.	

Safety and Avoidance

It is important that owners avoid the situations in which their cat has shown aggression. This gives the cat a break from the stress of facing its triggers, prevents the cat from practicing behavior the owners would like to change, and protects people from being injured. Owners may struggle to avoid some common triggers and may balk at avoiding others; so, they should be helped to understand that the avoidance is temporary and can be relaxed when behavior modification and/or medications reduce the cat's response to these triggers.

For all motivations for aggression, explain to owners that they should avoid all types of punishment.[24,28] They may already have noticed that it escalates the aggression. But, many owners continue to do it because they feel they should.

Environmental Enrichment

Cat owners should be helped to appreciate the role of environmental enrichment in reducing the threat of aggression toward people.[27] Indoor cats face a number of stressors originating from lack of control over their diet and how it's presented, household population density, specific housemates (people and other pets), home size and layout, resources offered and their locations, litter box options, sleeping or hiding spaces, and many other aspects of comfort in their lives.

When a cat is not provided with everything that helps them live a comfortable life, the stress may worsen aggression. They may not be able to retreat when they want, avoid encounters with others, or fully engage in species-specific activities within the lifestyle provided. A review of the history form and any videos provided should highlight opportunities for improvement in the household enrichment. Some options include:

- Food toys for hunting play; there are commercial products as well as opportunities for owners to make these from toilet paper cardboard rolls or empty plastic bottles.
- Timed feeder options to remove the owner from the feeding process overnight.
- Perches and hiding spaces, including towers, wall shelves, den spaces, etc.
- Scratching posts and facial rubbing stations. These will encourage cats to mark with their claws or by facial rubbing (bunting) to increase "happy" pheromones it may be helpful to provide attractive scratching posts of sisal rope, corrugated cardboard or fabric, and rubbing devices.
- Sufficient number and placement of litter boxes of adequate size, with appropriate substrate, and suitable hygiene.
- Plenty of well-placed water stations that provide clean water.
- Opportunities for outdoor exploration. Many people have found ways for their cats to spend time outdoors safely. There are safety fences (search the Internet for "cat fence" for ideas), outdoor rooms, and other items available; or owners can design their own. Access to the outdoors can reduce inter-cat tension, boredom, and other contributors to inappropriate urination and aggression.
- Self-play toys that are alternated frequently.

For more ideas and details to share with owners, please see Chapters 3 and 4 on prevention and play, as they both focus on different aspects of keeping cats happy indoors.

Relationships: This includes positive interactions with people and other pets.

How will people in the home (or visitors) be asked to interact with the cat? Would it help everyone for the cat to be trained to get off furniture by itself or allow the owner to instill ear medications without a struggle? Should the owners be playing with the cat differently/more? How much does this cat like to be petted? Answers to these types of questions will help to formulate the "Relationships" category of the treatment plan. Specific elements may include:

Increased interactive play. Wand toys and tossed toys can encourage cats of any age to exercise, keep their brains active, and expend their need for hunting behaviors. This exercise is especially helpful before bedtime or any time the can gets "amped up" on a regular basis. See Chapter 4 for more details.

Training. One way to interact positively with a cat is to reward it for learning new behaviors. In Box 10.1, this chapter presents two specific cues of "Touch" and "Sit." But owners can teach their cats to do many skills and tricks. Throughout the "How To" sections, we recommend when to use the "marker" word of "Yes." The marker word tells the cat the specific moment it did what the owner was looking for and that a reward is coming. This is a crucial step, since it's not usually possible to get a treat to the cat at that precise moment. Alternatively, the owner can use a clicker, if they already know – or want to explore – how to use it properly.

Box 10.1   Useful cues and how to teach them

The Touch Cue: This cue will teach a cat to follow the owner's outstretched fingers like a lure to show it where to go. This cue functions as a redirection process: if the owner wants to call the cat away from something, they can show the cat where they would prefer it to go. Additionally, it can function as a "come" cue.

How to Train Touch: The owner can start with the cat on an elevated surface – such as a table or cat tree. The owner will then put two fingers out toward the cat and stop about an inch from its nose. When the cat investigates the fingers, it will accidentally touch its nose to the owner's fingers. The owner should say "yes" and give a treat. When the owner feels a nose, they say "yes," then feed. They will repeat this process several times for two minutes 1–2 times a day. Once the cat is regularly touching its nose to the owner's fingers from a close distance, they can try offering their fingers a little farther away. Once the cat is comfortable moving toward the owner's fingers, they can add a cue of "Touch" or "Come." The owner will say the verbal cue then offer their fingers near the cat. If the cat moves toward the fingers, the owners say "Yes," then give a reward when the cat touches the owner's fingers.

Sit: This is a great behavior for a cat to be taught, since a cat that is sitting isn't engaged in some other, less desirable, activity.

How to Train Sit: This cue is best taught by "capturing" the target behavior: rewarding the cat every time the owner sees it go from a standing position to a sitting position. When the owner observes the cat moving from stand to sit, they should say "yes" and give a treat. With timely reinforcement, the cat will get the idea that sitting is a positive behavior and will do it more often. The owner can then put a verbal cue to it.

Other tricks: Once the owner gets the knack of teaching the cat to do certain things on cue, they can capture any behavior they'd like to see the cat perform again and again simply by rewarding it.

Behavior modification: Desensitization and counterconditioning can be very useful in acclimating a cat to things that frighten (therefore, trigger) it. Please see the website for the general guidelines for desensitization and counterconditioning.

Desensitization and Counter-Conditioning (DS/CC)

Desensitization and counter-conditioning is the most common type of behavior modification. Desensitization (DS) is the gradual exposure of a trigger stimulus below the threshold of an animal's reactivity. Counterconditioning (CC) is the pairing of the trigger with something that is rewarding for that animal, usually delicious food; the goal is for the animal to make a positive association between the formerly fear-inducing stimulus and the reward.

Medications and Other Related Therapies

For cats with aggression that stems from fear, stress, and anxiety, medications and nutriceuticals can be a key part of the treatment plan.

Medications: For fear-related, redirected, and play-related aggression, medications may help facilitate implementation of the treatment plan, particularly behavior modification.

Below are specific treatment suggestions for the four most common motivations for feline aggression toward people. For the best efficacy, these suggestions should be selected carefully to match the particulars of the history presented by the owner. This helps to avoid a "one size fits all" treatment plan.

When preparing and delivering a comprehensive treatment plan, the clinician should consider the owner's ability and willingness to follow instructions. It pays to check in frequently with owners to make sure that they share the clinician's understanding of each element of the plan. Ask them to repeat what they have heard. It's a valuable exercise to ask owners to volunteer ways they envision implementing elements of the recommended plan, so that the clinician can assess how thoroughly the owners comprehend what they will be doing once they get home.

Fear-Related Aggression: Treatment

In addition to general treatment plan elements for feline aggression, the following should be considered in cases of fear-related aggression:

For **Management**, make a list of things that frighten the cat. Brainstorm with the owner how these things can be avoided. If the cat is frightened by household or outside noises, the clients may wish to try white noise machines. If the cat is fearful of strangers, the clients should put the cat away before visitors arrive. If bottlenecks in traffic flow in the house cause the cat to feel cornered easily, the clients can look at ways to rearrange the furniture layout or where key resources are kept. It should be made absolutely clear that the cat should never be forced to interact with any person, particularly those who may have caused fear in the past.[27]

Depending on the patient's level of overall arousal or reactivity, **Medications** may be considered. These medications may be viewed as a tool to allow DS/CC to proceed more quickly, especially if the cat is not likely to remain under threshold in the presence of its fear triggers.[1,17]

Inappropriate Play: Treatment

In addition to general treatment plan elements for feline aggression, the following should be considered in cases of inappropriate play aggression:

For **Management**, clients should ensure that the environment does not offer places for the cat to lie in wait to ambush its victims. Should a client be ambushed, they should stand completely still until the cat disengages; this strategy leads to the lowest level of injury to the victim and reduces the amount of reinforcement the cat gains from the encounter.[27] Clients should also be counseled to avoid punishment for their cat's behavior, as it will most likely increase arousal without decreasing the likelihood that the behavior will recur.[18,27]

Victims might benefit from the cat wearing a collar with one or more bells on it, reducing the chances of the person being surprised by an ambush.[1]

As part of cat-client **Relationships**, clients should provide ample opportunity for appropriate play.[1,27] These clients can explore the cat's interest in wand toys, food toys, and self-propelled/battery-operated toys that the cat can chase and attack. Some cats also enjoy attacking stuffed toys like the Kong Kickaroo and others (Figure 10.7). Please see Chapter 3 for more information.

Because being a single cat is one of the risk factors for this type of aggression, clients may consider adding a second cat.[19,27] They may choose to foster a cat from a rescue group, in case the resident cat is not accepting of the newcomer.

It is possible that **Medications** will be advisable or necessary to decrease the cat's arousal to the point that other elements of the treatment plan will work. The most commonly used drug classes

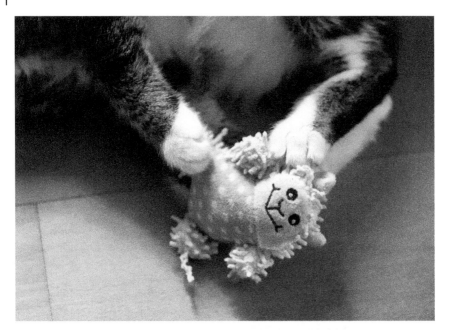

Figure 10.7   Cats should be encouraged to tackle stuffies instead of hands. Photo courtesy of pixabay.

for this diagnosis are selective serotonin reuptake inhibitors and tricyclic antidepressants, although there is good support for any appropriate medication that decreases arousal. Please see Appendix 1 for more information.

Petting-Induced Aggression: Treatment

In addition to general treatment plan elements for feline aggression, the following should be considered in cases of petting-induced aggression:

Management is key to resolving petting-induced aggression. First, the owner should not assume that the cat that sits on or near to a person wishes to be petted. Simply using the human's impulse control to avoid petting reduces the need for the cat to become aggressive to stop the petting.[27] Two very useful management elements to discuss with owners are:

Understanding Body Language. Owners should learn their cat's body language, especially as it relates to the early signs of frustration or aggression. Please see Chapter 1 for more information.

Consent Testing for Petting. Owners of a cat being treated for petting-induced aggression will avoid many mishaps if they get into the habit of "consent testing" the cat each time they start to pet it. To do this, they allow the cat to approach their relaxed but slightly extended hand. They can then pet the cat two or three times in an area of the body the cat has tolerated some petting in the past. After those two to three pets, the person returns his hand to the relaxed but slightly extended position. If the cat bunts or rubs the hand again, the person can pet two or three more times. This is repeated until the cat walks away or the person is tired of petting the cat. This way, owners can learn the limits of a particular cat's petting tolerance and pet accordingly.[19]

In the realm of **Behavior Modification**, it may be possible to make petting more positive for the cat using DS/CC.[18,27]

Medications. For cats that are afraid to be touched or whose tolerance for petting is unnaturally low, medications, pheromones, or other non-pharmaceutical supplements may be warranted. Please see Appendix 1 for more information.

Redirected Aggression: Treatment

In addition to general treatment plan elements for feline aggression, the following should be considered in cases of redirected aggression:

For the **Management** of redirected aggression, it is very important to identify the triggers to be avoided.

- If the cat attacks people when it sees passing dogs or outdoor cats, window privacy film will block visual access to those triggers. If the sound of passing dogs is a problem, consider white noise. If the smell of outdoor cats is a trigger, it becomes crucial that owners prevent the approach of these cats to the house. This can be accomplished with fencing that prevents cats from entering the yard; at least two general designs are available: a netting structure or a series of spinning rods (similar to a coyote roller) that attaches to the top of existing fencing to keep resident cats in and other cats out.
- If the trigger is noises, it important to know which noises. If they are sounds "leaking" into the house from outdoors, white noise might help. If the noises are due to activities inside the house (vacuums or other appliances, certain television programs, children playing, etc.), the cat can be sequestered to quiet spaces in the home while those activities are happening.
- If the trigger is visiting humans or dogs, putting the cat away for the duration of the visit will help.

Part of management for redirected aggression is for the owner not to interact with the cat when it starts to be aroused. It takes at least several minutes (possibly hours to days) for the cat's reactivity to return to normal; during that time, the odds of an attack are increased.[18,19]

For **Behavior Modification**, it may be possible to DS/CC the cat to the triggers that cause it to redirect onto the nearby humans.[27]

Medications. Just as with fear-related aggression, some cats may benefit from a medication that decreases overall anxiety or their fear of the trigger so that DS/CC can be more effective. The most commonly used drug classes for this diagnosis are selective serotonin reuptake inhibitors and tricyclic antidepressants, although there is good support for any appropriate medication that decreases arousal. Please see Appendix 1 for more information.[18]

A Note about Neutering

There is no evidence of a positive effect in decreasing human-directed aggression from castrating or spaying a cat. Castration at any age has been shown to be effective in decreasing cat-directed aggression, spraying, and roaming. Owners and breeders should be advised to refrain from breeding very fearful cats.

Prevention

Whenever, possible, it is preferable to prevent a problem behavior from starting rather than treating it once it starts. Chapter 2 gives many ideas on preventing behavior problems in our house cats before they begin.

For aggression, prevention comes from clients understanding their cats' body language (to notice problems as they are emerging), appropriate enrichment (including ample ways to be away when

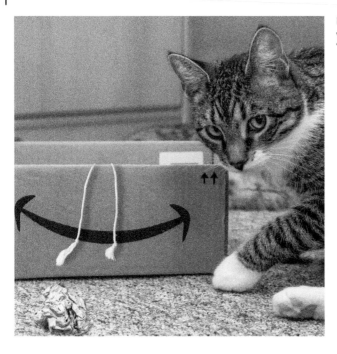

Figure 10.8 Clients should know when their cat's body language says "stay away." Photo courtesy of pixabay.

concerned), appropriate play outlets, and appropriate handling by the people in the household. Figure 10.8 shows a cat owners might not wish to approach. New cat owners are well served by having conversations about preventative measures at their first veterinary visit with the cat or kitten.

Summary

Feline aggression toward people has a negative – sometimes disastrous – impact on the human–animal bond. Veterinarians and their staff can play an important role in preventing, diagnosing, and treating these problems. The clinician can identify whether the motivation is fear, play, intolerance of petting, or redirected, then create a targeted treatment plan to address the motivation behind the problem.

References

1 Landsberg G, Hunthausen W, Ackerman L. Feline aggression. In: *Behavior problems of the dog and cat*, ed 3. St Louis: Elsevier; 2013:327–343.
2 Bamberger M, Houpt KA. Signalment factors, comorbidity, and trends in behavior diagnoses in cats: 736 cases (1991–2001). *J Am Vet Med Assoc.* 2006;229(10):1602–1606.
3 Amat M, Ruiz de la Torre JL, Fatjó J. Potential risk factors associated with feline behaviour problems. *Appl Anim Behav Sci.* 2009;121:134–139.
4 Ramos D, Reche-Junior A, Hirai Y, et al. Feline behaviour problems in Brazil: A review of 155 referral cases. *Vet Rec.* 2019;186(16):1–3.
5 Tamimi N, Malmasi A, Talebi A, et al. A survey of feline behavioral problems in Tehran. *Vet Res Forum.* 2015;6(2):143–147.

6 Wright JC, Amoss RT. Prevalence of house soiling and aggression in kittens during the first year after adoption from a humane society. *J Am Vet Med Assoc.* 2004;224(11):1790–1795.

7 Houpt KA, Honig SU, Reisner IR. Breaking the human-companion animal bond. *J Am Vet Med Assoc.* 1996;208(10):1653–1659.

8 Salman MD, Hutchison J, Ruch-Gallie R, et al. Behavioral reasons for relinquishment of dogs and cats to 12 shelters. *J Appl Anim Welf Sci.* 2000;3(2):93–106.

9 Scarlett JM, Salman D, New JG, et al. The role of veterinary practitioners in reducing dog and cat relinquishments and euthanasias. *J Am Vet Med Assoc.* 2002;220(3):306–311.

10 Chapman BL. Feline aggression: Classification, diagnosis, and treatment. *Vet Clin North Am Small Anim Pract.* 1991;21(2):315–327.

11 Landsberg GM, Hunthausen W, Ackerman L. Is it behavioral or is it medical? In: *Behavior problems of the dog and cat*, 3rd ed. Edinburgh (Scotland): Elsevier Saunders; 2013:75–80.

12 Overall KL. Medical differentials with potential behavioral manifestations. *Vet Clin North Am Small Anim Pract.* 2003;33(2):213–229.

13 Horwitz DF, Neilson JC eds. Aggression/Feline: Fear/defensive. In: *Canine and feline behavior, Blackwell's Five Minute Veterinary Consult.* Ames (IA): Blackwell Publishing; 2007:117–124.

14 Reisner IR. The pathophysiologic basis of behavior problems. *Vet Clin North Am Small Anim Pract.* 1991;21:207–224.

15 Mills D, Karagiannis C, Zulch H. Stress- its effects on health and behavior: A guide for practitioners. *Vet Clin North Am Small Anim Pract.* 2014;44:525–541.

16 Clarke SP, Bennett D. Feline osteoarthritis: A prospective study of 28 cases. *J Small Anim Pract.* 2006;47:439–445.

17 Klinck MP, Frank D, Guillot M, et al. Owner-perceived signs and veterinary diagnosis in 50 cases of feline osteoarthritis. *Can Vet J.* 2012;53:1181–1186.

18 Seksel K. Behavior problems. In: Little S, ed. *The cat: Clinical medicine and management.* St Louis (MO): Elsevier Saunders; 2012:211–225.

19 Curtis TM. Human-directed aggression in the cat. *Vet Clin North Am Small Anim Pract.* 2008;38:1138–1143.

20 McCune S. The impact of paternity and early socialisation on the development of cats' behaviour to people and novel objects. *Appl Anim Behav Sci.* 1995;45(1–2):109–124.

21 Reisner IR, Houpt KA, Erb HN, et al. Friendliness to humans and defensive aggression in cats: The influence of handling and paternity. *Physiol Behav.* 1994;55(6):1119–1124.

22 Amat M, Manteca X, Brech SL, et al. Evaluation of inciting causes, alternative targets, and risk factors associated with redirected aggression in cats. *J Am Vet Med Assoc.* 2008;233(4):586–589.

23 Horwitz DF, Neilson JC eds. Aggression/Feline: Play related. In: *Canine and feline behavior, Blackwell's Five Minute Veterinary Consult.* Ames (IA): Blackwell Publishing; 2007:141–147.

24 Hart BL, Hart LA. Feline behavioural problems and solutions. In: Turner DC, Bateson P, eds. *The domestic cat. The biology of its behaviors*, 3rd ed. Cambridge: Cambridge University Press; 2014:201–212.

25 Berger J. Feline aggression toward people. In: Little S, ed. *August's consultations in feline internal medicine.* St Louis, MO: Elsevier; 2016:911–918.

26 Overall KL. Undesirable, problematic, and abnormal feline behavior and behavioral pathologies. In: Overall KL, ed. *Manual of clinical behavioral medicine for dogs and cats.* St Louis: Elsevier; 2013:360–456.

27 Amat M, Manteca X. Common feline problem behaviours: Owner-directed aggression. *J Feline Med Surg.* 2019;21(3):245–255.

28 Beaver BV. Feline social behavior. In: Beaver BV, ed. *Feline behavior. A guide for veterinarians*, 2nd ed. St Louis, MO: Elsevier; 2003:127–163.

11

Aggression Toward Other Cats

Sharon Crowell-Davis and Elizabeth Stelow

Introduction

Inter-cat aggression is defined as a cat engaging in posturing, vocalizing, stalking, scratching, biting, or related behaviors toward one or more other cats.[1] Such aggression often presents as feline social conflicts that are consistent, proactive, and frequently out of context of an actual threat.[2]

Such behavior can be directed toward cats outside the home (unfamiliar cats) or inside the home (other household cats). Because aggression toward unfamiliar cats outside the home is primarily a management problem (i.e., reduce the cat's access to unfamiliar cats), this chapter focuses on aggression among cats living in the same household.

The Scope of the Problem

To put inter-cat aggression in perspective, we consider how many households have cats, how many of those have multiple cats, and what percentage of these households experience aggression among the cats. In 2018, there were reported to be over 58 million cats in 31.8 million US households; and on average, each of these households had 1.8 cats.[3]

Inter-cat aggression is reported in somewhere between 30% and 36.4% of these multi-cat households.[4–7] In one study, of the 2,492 multi-cat owners that were surveyed, 31.7% reported their cats to stare at each other daily and 13.6% reported daily hissing.[8] While staring is not necessarily a threatening or aggressive behavior, it certainly can be; and owners can learn to differentiate between cats checking in with each other and agonistic stares.

In a 2000 study, Salman et al. found that "problems with new pet and other pets" was the second most common behavioral reason given for relinquishing a cat to a shelter, just behind house soiling.[9]

A number of studies have looked at the impact of adding a new cat on aggression. One study showed inter-cat aggression when a new cat is added to a household with other cats to be almost 50%.[10] In those houses with new cats added, households that reported fighting early in the introduction period were 38.5 times more likely to have continued fighting than households that did not have early fighting.[10]

Inter-cat aggression can be of great concern to owners, who are concerned about the safety of the cats involved and the loss of peace in the household.

What is Normal?

Cats that are truly "friends" engage in affiliative behaviors, including sleeping nearby or touching, allogrooming, or allorubbing, touching noses in passing. See Images 11.1 and 11.2. Cats showing these signs often have a healthy relationship and are less inclined to show signs of aggression, including defensive body postures with hissing, growling, scratching, and/or biting each other.

What is normal but often unacceptable?

Cats living in close proximity, even those with a comfortable social relationship, will occasionally squabble, often over a resource. This may involve agonistic staring or blocking access to resources (often unnoticed by owners); but hissing or growling may occur. As long as the moment is fleeting and not repeated, the cats likely have moved past the issue. Yet, owners may be concerned that this is the beginning of a social problem between the cats. Some cats play rough with each other; owners may mistake rough play for aggression. Chapter 2 discusses the distinctions between the two.

What is abnormal but often acceptable?

Many owners do not know to look for the affiliative behavior described above between their household cats. Thus, pairs of cats that do not engage in affiliative behaviors will be considered by most owners to be "normal" or "fine together." While a lack of these behaviors may simply mean that the cats are not particularly social, they may indicate social tension or discomfort between the cats, predisposing them to outbursts of passive or active aggression.

What is abnormal and typically unacceptable?

Cats, even when aggressive, should not cause injury to one another. Cats have developed a wide repertoire of postures and auditory communications to resolve disputes without physical contact. When inter-cat aggression reaches the level of injury, owners typically seek intervention.

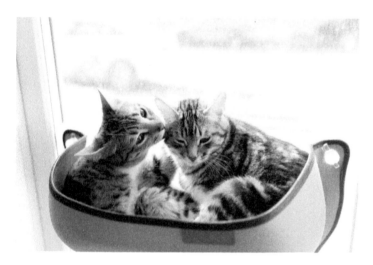

Images 11.1 and 11.2   Cats that have comfortable social relationships are frequently seen to sleep in proximity to each other and groom each other.

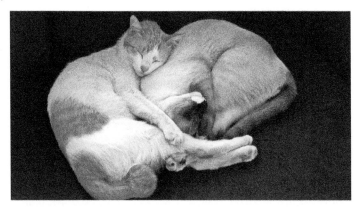

Images 11.1 and 11.2   (Continued).

Characteristics and Risk Factors

Aside from the staring and hissing described above, what does inter-cat aggression look like, and what cats are most at risk?

Characteristics of Inter-cat Aggression

Following are characteristics commonly found in inter-cat aggression:

- Varied Intensity. Inter-cat aggression can range from mild (agonistic staring or hissing) to severe (injury to one or more cats).[1]
- Passive or Active Conflict. Passive signs include staring, blocking access to resources, and posturing. Hissing, swatting, biting, and other types of fighting are active signs.[2,11]
- Fear as Motivator. In one study, 70% (72/107 cats) of the inter-cat aggression displayed by cats was seen as defensive.[5] Image 11.3 shows the defensive body posture (the cat on the right) that owners might notice.
- Sudden or Gradual Onset. Interact aggression may appear suddenly (based on one traumatic event) or evolve gradually (based on many small stressors).[1]

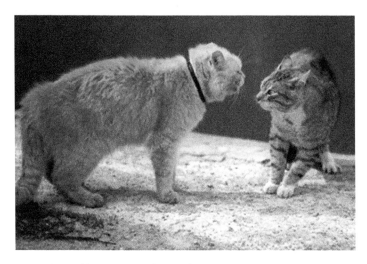

Image 11.3   The cat on the right is displaying defensive body posture that indicates fear.

- "Out of the Blue" Appearance. Aggression may arise *de novo* in cats that have previously not engaged in overt aggression.[1]

Clearly, not all cases presented for inter-cat aggression will have all these characteristics; but they are common.

Risk Factors and Triggers

The knowledge of what predisposes household cats to fight or begin to show conflict, both in the form of risk factors and as triggers, aids in both prevention and treatment of aggression.

- Genetics and Previous Social Experience: These likely both play a role.[1]
- Big Household Changes: People or pets moving in or out of the household may predispose cats to new or worsened tension. Aggression may arise after a move to a new home or other large environmental change.[1]
- Today's Veterinary Visit: Tensions may climb if one cat returns from a veterinary visit or hospitalization, especially if sedated or smelling from a treatment or procedure. "Group scent" cannot be underestimated in its role in promoting positive relationships between cats.[1,12]
- Pain: Acute or chronic pain may trigger new aggression.[1]
- Maturation: Social tension may start or worsen due to the maturation (into social maturity at 2–4 years of age) or aging (into senior years) of one of the cats; such changes in social status can change the social structure in the home.[1,2]
- Lack of Social Adhesion: Cats use affiliative behavior to strengthen the social group bond. It stands to reason, then, that cats who have not displayed consistent affiliative behaviors may be more likely to experience aggression as a means to establish different core areas of the home and live as separate social groups.[12,13]
- Early Weaning: Cats weaned in adulthood were less likely to be aggressive than those weaned earlier.[14]
- Social Incompatibility: Tension may arise due to one cat not accepting the other cat's unwillingness to engage with it.[2]
- Redirected Aggression: An incident of redirected aggression is a common catalyst for inter-cat aggression and can alter a previously stable relationship.[11] In one study of feline aggression, a reaction to a loud noise or an interaction with an outside cat (Image 11.4) was determined to be the trigger in 95% of redirected aggression incidents and approximately 29% of these cats redirected onto the other household cat.[5,15]

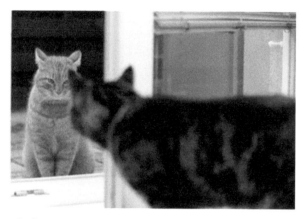

Image 11.4   Redirected aggression can be caused by a cat being faced with a passing outdoor conspecific.

Noticeably absent as a risk factor is "the number of cats in the household." In studies of feline stress as measured by glucocorticoid metabolites, the number of household cats does not appear to increase stress. In fact, the highest levels were measured in young, singly housed cats.[6]

Causes

While variations in the genetics and experiences of the cats involved may change how it presents, inter-cat aggression in the home is caused by a disruption in feline social structure. It's important to note the reasons for those disruptions. Specifics will vary by case; but a few general principles are important, too.

Chapter 2 presents Normal Feline Social Behavior and it is crucial to understand the social needs of a cat in order to appreciate the pressures of living in multi-cat households. Most importantly, indoor cats face a number of stressors originating from lack of control over:[12,13]

- their diet and how it's presented
- household population density
- specific housemates (people, cats, and other pets)
- home size and layout
- resources offered and their locations
- litter box options
- sleeping or hiding spaces

and many other aspects of comfort in their lives. When a cat is not provided with everything that helps it live a comfortable life, the stress may worsen aggression. They may not be able to retreat when they want, avoid encounters with other cats or people, or fully engage in species-specific activities within the lifestyle provided. Image 11.5 shows a cat that is uncomfortable, likely about the population density around what appears to be a single feeding station.

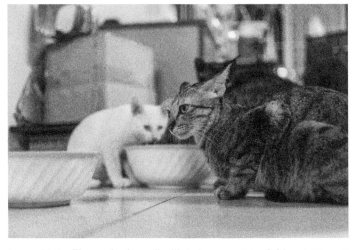

Image 11.5   The ear-back, pupils dilated appearance of this cat suggests discomfort, perhaps about sharing resources.

How to Diagnose

The clinician will need to gather extensive information about the problem to know how to diagnose and treat it. The process of diagnosing is broken into stages of information gathering and assessment.

Before the Appointment

Because of the extent of the information required to make an accurate behavioral diagnosis, it is most useful to ask owners to complete a detailed history form and obtain videos of their home and cats.

Written Historical Information
To help make things more efficient for the clinician and their staff, they can use a history form (see website) that the owner can fill out and submit before the appointment, giving the team time to review the information beforehand. The clinician will also want any medical records from previous veterinarians, especially if they may have treated this cat for its aggression.

Owner-Provided Video
It is important to keep cats from fighting in the examining room so that the clinician may observe body language, etc. Therefore, video is a good supplement to a thorough written or oral history. When the owners make an appointment, they should be asked to obtain a few types of video:

1) The layout of the home. This can give the clinician an idea of ways to manage the problem, the level of enrichment offered, and other aspects of home life that may be helpful in making the most appropriate diagnosis or treatment plan.
2) The cats in their environment: eating, resting, playing, sleeping. This can give the clinician a sense of how comfortable each cat is in his environment. The clinician may see some subtle behaviors that will not be present during the appointment. It will also show the clinician how each cat responds to the owner's presence and the presence of the other cats.
3) The circumstances under which aggression is likely to occur. Owners should not be asked specifically to get a video of the aggression happening, so as not to trigger the behavior intentionally. Asking for the circumstances, however, allows the clinician to see what may be triggering the aggression.

During the Appointment

Please refer to the Introduction to this book, which summarizes the questions that should be asked for a thorough behavioral history.

Prompted by a history form and on questioning by the clinician, the owners should be able to provide a list of things that have historically trigger their cats' aggression. They can also gauge the intensity and frequency of the aggression incidents, how the cats behave between incidents, and what types of things they've tried to resolve the problem. All of this can be useful in determining the extent of the problem and the areas of focus of a treatment plan.

But, to truly diagnose the extent and causes of the aggression, it is often essential to know the ABCs – antecedents, behavior, and consequences – of incidents of aggression.

- *Antecedents* are the circumstances before an aggressive event occurs. Most owners can be talked through the key episode that started the aggression between the cats or brought them in to seek help.
- *Behavior* is what the cats are doing during an incident. It's important to ask about body language of both cats, since that can be the key to determining the triggers and severity of the problem.
- *Consequences* are the things at happen to or around the cats after an incident.

With careful exploration of specific incidents, the clinician may find more than one motivation or more than one type of aggression.

Gathering Incident Information

Ideally, the history form will ask the owners to give details about two or three specific incidents that can be explored more fully during the appointment. Table 11.1 shows some of the topics to be explored. When the clinician is exploring, it is useful to break each incident into its ABCs.

For instance, let's say that the patient, Dion, sometimes attacks his littermate, Poke. Two incidents are described briefly on the form: one in which Poke just returned from the veterinarian and another when a stranger visited the home. The clinician can then follow an investigative path like this one:

- "Let's look specifically at the incident when Poke returned from the vet visit."
  - What medical procedures had been done (anything that involved sedation, rubbing alcohol might change how Poke responds or smells to Dion)?
  - How was Poke acting on the car ride home?
  - Where was Dion when you brought Poke in?
  - Where did you release Poke from his carrier?
  - What specifically did Dion do to Poke and how did Poke respond?

Repeat a similar set of questions for the other incident given. Compare and contrast Dion's triggers and actions. What do they have in common? What's different?

The aggressor may stare, block access to resources, raise hackles/hiss/growl/swat, pursue, monitor the location and actions of the victim. The victim may choose to avoid/hide from his aggressor or fight back (leading to paired threats).[2]

The clinician can then use this information to explore further to finalize their diagnosis.

Behavioral Differentials

A few possible motivations exist for cats to begin fighting with one another.

- Sudden social tension or overt fear may be the motivation if the aggression involves a newcomer or returning cat. The "returning cat" may have just been to the vet or groomer but, due

Table 11.1   Incident information.

- Frequency, intensity, and severity of one or more incidents
- Antecedent to behavior: what was happening around the cats before aggression
- Behavior of each cat during the incident: body language, vocalizations, interaction with people
- Reaction of the victim cat
- Consequences for the aggressor cat: responses of persons present
- A list of all known triggers[16]
- How the cats are with each other between episodes[16]
- Treatments that owner has tried; outcomes

---

to changes in its appearance or smell, present as a new cat to the one who stayed home. See Image 11.6.

- Redirected aggression can be triggered by indoor or outdoor stimuli to which one or both cats react. Indoor triggers include vacuum cleaners, among others (Image 11.7).
- Social-status aggression may result if one cat reaches either social maturity or old age, changing the social dynamics, and tipping what might have been tolerance between the cats to more overt aggression.
- Finally, pain can trigger aggression.

While it is good to know which of these is most likely, the treatment plan varies little among these diagnoses.[1]

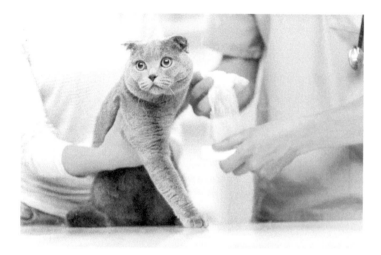

Image 11.6 This cat may smell like the vet and have other household cats respond badly to it when it gets home.

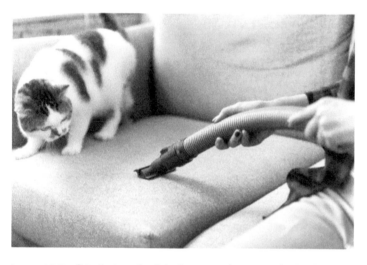

Image 11.7 Cats that are fearful of vacuum cleaners and other household items may direct their fear aggression on housemate cats.

Medical Differentials

Once the clinician has gathered the information from the form and interviews with the owners, they should rule out medical causes for their findings. While this list is not exhaustive, these differentials should be on the list when diagnosing feline aggression toward other household cats.[17–23]

Degenerative: loss of vision, loss of hearing
Developmental: lissencephaly, hydrocephalus
Anomalous: Feline ischemic encephalopathy
Metabolic: uremic encephalopathy, hepatic encephalopathy, hyperthyroid
Neoplastic: intracranial neoplasia, cerebral infarct
Neurologic: psychomotor or partial seizure, peripheral neuropathy
Nutritional: thiamine deficiency, taurine deficiency, tryptophan deficiency
Infectious: Rabies, pseudorabies, toxoplasma, *Neospora caninum*, feline immunodeficiency
  virus, feline infectious peritonitis
Inflammatory/Pain: feline interstitial cystitis, granulomatous meningioencephalitis, arthritis
Toxins: lead, zinc, methylphenidate, heavy metal toxicity
Traumatic: brain injury, causes of pain
Vascular: cerebral infarct

Most of these should be easy to eliminate based on signalment or the presentation of the behavior; others may require a minimum database or specialty diagnostics. Pain is often the most challenging one to rule out, given a cat's tendency to appear stoic.

Prognosis

Prognosis depends on the severity of the attacks, the likelihood that the cats will fight when they see each other, and the amount of patience the clients have for the aggression and implementation of the treatment plan. Some cats lack the social experience or adaptability to remain in a shared home. Others have some medical or emotional pathology that precludes learning to form social bonds. Poor prognosis is typically addressed with either rehoming or humane euthanasia of one cat.

Treatment

A treatment plan should be tailored to the circumstances that lead to the episodes of aggression and the severity of the worst bouts of aggression. For the owner's convenience, the clinician should organize the plan into large categories: Management, Behavior Modification, and Medications and Other Related Therapies. Within each category, the details for each element can be outlined for presentation to the owner. The clinician may find that, for a given case, she may have overlapped or not used all elements.

Below are general guidelines for treatment of intercat aggession. This overview is summarized in Table 11.2.

Table 11.2   Overview of treatment of inter-cat aggression.

Physical Health	Rule out or treat underlying medical conditions	
	Castrate or spay, as deemed appropriate	
Management	*Safety and Avoidance*	Avoid relevant triggers (varies by case):
		● Block visual access to passing dogs or outdoor cats
		● Put cats away while vacuuming or strangers visiting
		● Minimize loud noises
		Separate cats, if needed
	Environmental Enrichment	Optimize: Feeding routines
		● Litter box numbers, locations, and maintenance
		● Number and placement of perches and resting spaces
		● Number and placement of scratching posts and facial rubbing stations
		● Access to outdoors
		● Access to self-play and predatory play toys
Behavior Modification	● Desensitization and counterconditioning to each other and to triggers	
	● Gradual reintroduction, if separated	
Medications and Related	Medications, nutraceuticals, and pheromones. Please see Appendix 1.	

Treatment Plan Components

Management: This represents the "What can be changed now to help the cat avoid its triggers?" Perhaps, the aggressor cat can be put away (in a room with food, toys, and white noise) when strangers visit or it's time to vacuum. Or maybe the cats would feel more comfortable in the home with an added cat tower or additional litter box.

Within the context of aggression cases, management encompasses two major sub-categories: Safety and Avoidance, and Environmental Enrichment, each with a different goal.

Safety and Avoidance

It is important that owners avoid the situations in which their cat has shown aggression. This gives the cat a break from the stress of facing its triggers, prevents the cat from practicing behavior the owners would like to change, and protects the other cats and the owners from being injured. Owners may struggle to avoid some common triggers and may balk at avoiding others; so, they should be helped to understand that the avoidance is temporary and can be relaxed when behavior modification and/or medications reduce a cat's response to these triggers.

If the triggers cannot be avoided and the aggression is severe and frequent, the cats should be separated.[1] This may mean separating completely until they can be gradually brought together, or separating them when they can't be supervised. The completeness of the separation will be based on the needs of the cats and the clients. Strategies for re-integrating the cats are presented below under "Gradual Reintroduction of Separated Cats."

Explain to owners that they should avoid all types of punishment toward the aggressor cat.[24,25] They may already have noticed that it escalates the aggression. But, many owners continue to do it because they feel they should.

Other safety strategies include:

- If one cat attacks the other cat when it sees passing dogs or outdoor cats, window privacy film will block visual access to those triggers. If the sound of passing dogs is a problem, consider white noise.
- If the smell of outdoor cats is a trigger, it becomes crucial that owners prevent the approach of these cats to the house. This can be accomplished with fencing that prevents cats from entering the yard; at least two general designs are available: a netting structure or a series of spinning rods (similar to a coyote roller) that attaches to the top of existing fencing to keep resident cats in and other cats out.
- If the trigger is the victim cat returning from a vet visit, keep the cats separated until the effects (smells, sedation, etc.) of the visit have worn off (maybe overnight) and bring the cats back together with treats or a play session.
- Put one or more bells on the cats so that they cannot sneak up on each other.[2]
- Intervene with the cats when they are still at the "passive aggression" stage to avoid escalation.[26]
- To avoid injury to owners, separate fighting cats using a noise, blankets, or heavy gloves rather than bare body parts.[26]
- If breaking up a fight, owners should avoid interacting with either cat for a while. Cats can have an increased reactivity to stimuli for from several minutes to a few days.[11]

Help the owners manage other triggers that may be uncovered during history taking.

Environmental Enrichment

Cat owners should be helped to appreciate the role of environmental enrichment in reducing the threat of aggression.[27] In fact, mild cases of inter-cat aggression may resolve simply by creating a home environment with ample resources for each cat.[1] A review of the history form and any videos provided should highlight opportunities for improvement in the household enrichment.

At a minimum, each distinct feline social group in the home should have an area of the house containing all their resources so that social groups have less need to mix.[26]

The treatment plan should consider:

- Food toys for hunting play; there are commercial products as well as opportunities for owners to make these from toilet paper cardboard rolls or empty plastic bottles.[28]
- Perches and hiding spaces, including towers and wall shelves for vertical space, as well as boxes and tunnels as den spaces.[26] Images 11.8–11.10 show different types of hiding spaces for cats.
- Scratching posts and facial rubbing stations. These will encourage cats to mark with their claws or by facial rubbing (bunting) to increase "happy" pheromones, it may be helpful to provide attractive scratching posts of sisal rope, corrugated cardboard or fabric, and rubbing devices.
- Sufficient number and placement of litter boxes of adequate size, with appropriate substrate, and suitable hygiene.[28]
- Plenty of well-placed water stations that provide clean water.[28]
- Opportunities for outdoor exploration. Many people have found ways for their cats to spend time outdoors safely. There are safety fences (search the Internet for "cat fence" for ideas), outdoor rooms, and other items available, or owners can design their own. Access to the outdoors can reduce inter-cat tension, boredom, and other contributors to inappropriate urination and aggression.[28]

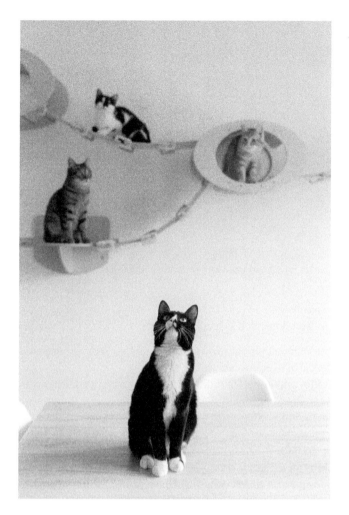

Image 11.8 Perches allow for use of vertical space.

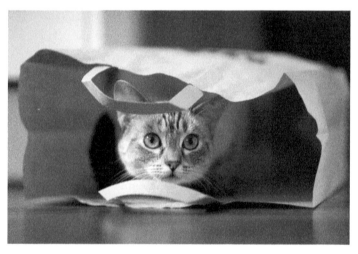

Image 11.9 Even a simple paper bag allows a cat a bit of time out of the flow of social traffic.

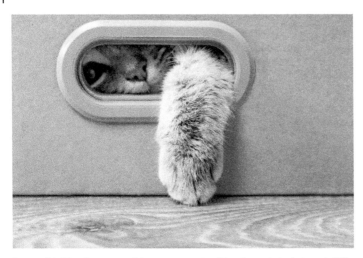

Image 11.10   Boxes provide easy opportunities for cats to interact differently with their environments.

- Self-play toys that are alternated frequently.
- Respect for the feline sense of smell when choosing household products.[28]

For more ideas and details to share with owners, please see Chapters 3 and 4 on prevention and play, as they both focus on different aspects of keeping cats happy indoors.

Behavior modification: Desensitization and counterconditioning can be very useful in acclimating a cat to things that frighten (therefore, trigger) it. Please see the website for the general guidelines for desensitization and counterconditioning.

Desensitization and Counterconditioning (DS/CC)

Desensitization and counter-conditioning is the most common type of behavior modification. Desensitization (DS) is the gradual exposure of a trigger stimulus below the threshold of an animal's reactivity. Counterconditioning (CC) is the pairing of the trigger with something that is rewarding for that animal, usually delicious food; the goal is for the animal to make a positive association between the formerly fear-inducing stimulus and the reward. Ideally, it would be possible to DS/CC the cat to the triggers that cause it to redirect onto the other household cats, as well as to the cats themselves.[27]

Gradual Reintroduction of Separated Cats

If cats have been completely separated, they will likely need to be reintroduced gradually to encourage a harmonious relationship. In many ways, they are in a more challenging social situation than two cats meeting for the very first time. They have a history of negative interactions that may flavor even their initial responses to each other.

For a planned gradual reintroduction, please follow the tenets of DS/CC (cats remaining under threshold, positive interactions only). The following steps are often presented as a suitable plan:[1]

1) Allow each cat to explore the common living areas when the other cat is not present to sustain the familiarity of each cat with all living spaces.
2) To mingle the scent of the two cats, groom cats alternately with the same towel; include facial scent glands. Take care in the event that the cat being rubbed reacts with aggression to the scents of the other cat.

3) Allow the cats to approach the door that separates them. Feeding both cats (assuming they are relaxed enough to eat) makes this exposure more rewarding. See Image 11.11.
4) Periodically replace the solid barrier with a screen/baby gate barrier so that the cats can see each other. Continue to use food or play time to make these exposures more positive.
5) Hang an interactive a toy from the baby gate in such a way that it will move from one side of the barrier to the other as one of the cats plays with it. This may create mutual play.
6) Begin to allow supervised time in the same space with no barrier; increase time with ongoing success.

Cats that show no improvement during gradual reintroduction may require medications. Another option includes rehoming.

Medications and Other Related Therapies

Some cats may benefit from a medication that decreases overall anxiety or their fear of the trigger so that DS/CC can be more effective. The most commonly used drug classes for this diagnosis are selective serotonin reuptake inhibitors and tricyclic antidepressants, although there is good support for any appropriate medication that decreases arousal. Please see Appendix 1 for more information.[11]

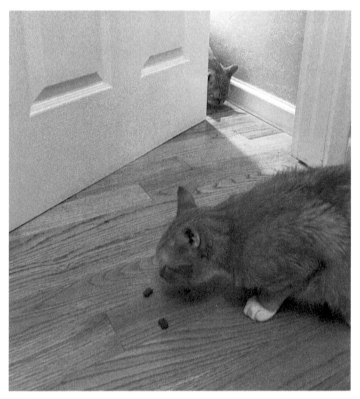

Image 11.11   Cats can be reintroduced gradually and rewarded with tasty food for being calm in each other's presence. Photo courtesy of Liz Stelow.

Prevention

Whenever, possible, it is preferable to prevent a problem behavior from starting rather than treating it once it starts. Chapter 2 gives many ideas on preventing behavior problems in our house cats before they begin.

For aggression, prevention comes from clients understanding their cats' body language (to notice problems as they are emerging), appropriate enrichment (including ample ways for cats to be away when concerned), appropriate play outlets, and appropriate handling by the people in the household. New cat owners are well served by having conversations about preventative measures at their first veterinary visit with the cat or kitten.

Summary

Most cats living in multi-cat households manage to exist without significant tension and inter-cat aggression. Tension, however, can exist "under the radar" of the average cat owner if the signs are passive and relatively subtle. Those tensions can flare in times of stress, leading to overt aggression. Prevention (introducing cats gradually, providing ample resources, and monitoring body language) is preferable to treatment of aggression. But treatment can be successful with desensitization and anxiolytic medications.

References

1 Landsberg G, Hunthausen W, Ackerman L. Feline aggression. In: *Behavior problems of the dog and cat*, 3rd ed. St Louis: Elsevier, 2013:327–343.

2 Overall KL. Undesirable, problematic, and abnormal feline behavior and behavioral pathologies. In: Overall KL, ed. *Manual of clinical behavioral medicine for dogs and cats*. St Louis: Elsevier; 2013:360–456.

3 American Veterinary Medical Association. *2017-2018 US pet ownership & demographics sourcebook*. 2020. www.avma.org/resources-tools/reports-statistics/us-pet-ownership-statistics. Accessed August 2, 2022.

4 Bamberger M, Houpt KA. Signalment factors, comorbidity, and trends in behavior diagnoses in cats: 736 cases (1991–2001). *J Am Vet Med Assoc.* 2006; 229(10):1602–1606.

5 Amat M, Ruiz de la Torre JL, Fatjó J. Potential risk factors associated with feline behaviour problems. *Appl Anim Behav Sci.* 2009; 121:134–139.

6 Ramos D, Reche-Junior A, Hirai Y, et al. Feline behaviour problems in Brazil: A review of 155 referral cases. *Vet Rec.* 2019; 186(16):1–3.

7 Tamimi N, Malmasi A, Talebi A, et al. A survey of feline behavioral problems in Tehran. *Vet Res Forum* 2015; 6(2):143–147.

8 Elzerman AL, DePorter TL, Beck A, Collin JF. Conflict and affiliative behavior frequency between cats in multi-cat households: A survey-based study. *J. Feline Med Sur.* 2020; 22(8):705–717.

9 Salman MD, Hutchison J, Ruch-Gallie R, et al. Behavioral reasons for relinquishment of dogs and cats to 12 shelters. *J Appl Anim Welf Sci.* 2000;3(2):93–106.

10 Levine E, Perry P, Scarlett J, Houpt KA. Intercat aggression in households following the introduction of a new cat. *Appl Anim Behav Sci.* 2005;90(3–4):325–336.

11 Seksel K. Behavior problems. In: Little S, ed. *The cat: Clinical medicine and management.* St Louis (MO): Elsevier Saunders; 2012:211–225.

12 Bradshaw JWS, Casey RA, Brown SL. Undesired behaviour in the domestic cat. In: *The behaviour of the domestic cat*, 2nd ed. CABI: Oxfordshire, UK; 2012:190–205.

13 Bradshaw JW. Sociality in cats: A comparative review. *J Vet Behav.* 2016;11:113–124.

14 Ahola MK, Vapalahti K, Lohi H. Early weaning increases aggression and stereotypic behaviour in cats. *Sci Rep.* 2017;7(1):1–9.

15 Amat M, Manteca X, Brech SL, et al. Evaluation of inciting causes, alternative targets, and risk factors associated with redirected aggression in cats. *J Am Vet Med Assoc.* 2008;233(4):586–589.

16 Chapman BL. Feline aggression: Classification, diagnosis, and treatment. *Vet Clin North Am Small Anim Pract.* 1991;21(2):315–327.

17 Landsberg GM, Hunthausen W, Ackerman L. Is it behavioral or is it medical? In: *Behavior problems of the dog and cat*, 3rd ed. Edinburgh (Scotland): Elsevier Saunders; 2013:75–80.

18 Overall KL. Medical differentials with potential behavioral manifestations. *Vet Clin North Am Small Anim Pract.* 2003;33(2):213–229.

19 Horwitz DF, Neilson JC, eds. Aggression/feline: Fear/defensive. In: *Canine and feline behavior, Blackwell's five minute veterinary consult.* Ames (IA): Blackwell Publishing; 2007:117–124.

20 Reisner IR. The pathophysiologic basis of behavior problems. *Vet Clin North Am Small Anim Pract.* 1991; 21:207–224.

21 Mills D, Karagiannis C, Zulch H. Stress- its effects on health and behavior: A guide for practitioners. *Vet Clin North Am Small Anim Pract.* 2014;44:525–541.

22 Clarke SP, Bennett D. Feline osteoarthritis: A prospective study of 28 cases. *J Small Anim Pract* 2006; 47:439–445.

23 Klinck MP, Frank D, Guillot M et al. Owner-perceived signs and veterinary diagnosis in 50 cases of feline osteoarthritis. *Can Vet J.* 2012; 53:1181–1186.

24 Hart BL, Hart LA. Feline behavioural problems and solutions. In: Turner DC, Bateson P, eds. *The domestic cat. The biology of its behaviors*, 3rd ed. Cambridge: Cambridge University Press; 2014:201–212.

25 Beaver BV. Feline social behavior. In: Beaver BV, ed. *Feline behavior. A guide for veterinarians*, 2nd ed. St Louis, MO: Elsevier; 2003:127–163.

26 Heath S. Intercat conflict. In: Rodan I, Heath S., eds. *Feline behavioral health and welfare.* St. Louis, MO: Elsevier Health Sciences; 2016:357–373.

27 Amat M, Manteca X. Common feline problem behaviours: Owner-directed aggression. *J Feline Med Surg.* 2019 Mar;21(3):245–255.

28 Heath SE. Keynote presentation: A multimodal approach to resolving tension between cats in the same household: A practical approach. In: *Proceedings of the 11th International Veterinary Behaviour Meeting* 2017 August; 45:39. CABI.

12

Nuisance/Destructive/Unruly Behaviors

Rachel Malamed and Karen Lynn C. Sueda

Nuisance/destructive/unruly behaviors

a) Attention seeking/"pestering" the owner
b) Food seeking
c) Scratching of objects
d) Climbing on objects

Relevance:

- Most are normal behaviors but inappropriate for owners
- May result in relinquishment or euthanasia
- Can be prevented or treated

Introduction

Nuisance behaviors such as attention seeking, begging/food-seeking, scratching, and climbing on objects are often normal behaviors that owners find problematic. The owner's perception of what is "appropriate" may negatively impact the human–animal bond and result in relinquishment or euthanasia for behavioral reasons.[1,2] Since these are normal behaviors, they cannot and should not be eliminated. By gaining insight into species-typical behaviors, owners can adjust their expectations. Primary-care veterinarians play an important role in educating clients regarding early detection and prevention.

The Introduction to this volume presents questions to be used to gain a general behavior history. The following sections each include questions targeted to gather information specifically regarding those possible nuisance behaviors.

Attention Seeking/"Pestering" the Owner

Attention-seeking behavior is a normal behavior that may either be acceptable and invited by an owner, or may be perceived as a nuisance behavior. Whether or not a behavior is perceived as "appropriate" may depend on how the cat seeks attention, the intensity of the behavior, and owner factors such as tolerance level and the strength of the human–animal bond.

Clinical Handbook of Feline Behavior Medicine, First Edition. Edited by Elizabeth Stelow.
© 2023 John Wiley & Sons, Inc. Published 2023 by John Wiley & Sons, Inc.
Companion Website: www.wiley.com/go/stelow/behavior

Common manifestations of attention-seeking behavior include:

- Excessive vocalization
- Allorubbing or weaving in and out of the owner's legs repeatedly
- Pacing (e.g. in front of the TV or computer screen)
- Pawing and scratching
- Play based behaviors (pouncing, chasing). See Figure 12.2
- Biting or aggressive play
- Licking and chewing (self and/or human-directed)
- Nocturnal activity and waking owners
- Climbing
- Destructive behavior (chewing/biting furniture or household objects)

Cats are social animals and solicitation of attention is a means to acquire specific physical or behavioral needs. If the animal learns that the behavior effectively elicits a desirable response, the behavior is reinforced and is therefore likely to occur again in the future (see Figure 12.1).

Although some cats may hide or become avoidant, increased attachment, "clinginess" or vocalization may be an attempt to seek comfort in response to general illness, pain, and discomfort. Such behaviors may be overlooked as a cause for concern and simply perceived as "more affectionate." However, sudden behavioral change or deviations from "normal" may be a non-specific sign of illness or an anxious response to environmental stressors. An examination by a veterinarian is recommended whenever a behavioral change occurs.

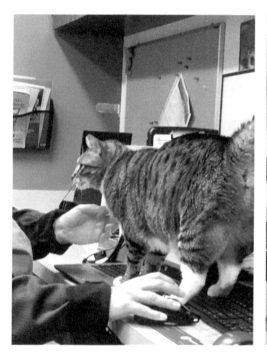 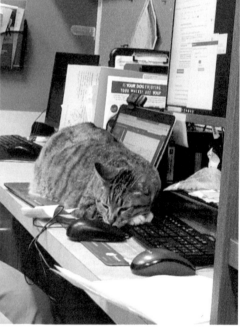

Figure 12.1   Cats commonly walk in front of computer or TV screens inserting themselves in the person's line-of-sight. They may settle on the keyboard for warmth or as a means to get attention. Photos courtesy of Karen Sueda.

Occasionally, a lack of attention may result in frustration, agitation, or aggressive arousal, which could lead to other problem behaviors such as biting. Solicitations in the form of nipping, biting, and aggressive play that are persistent may be either normal or abnormal but can become a serious health and safety concern particularly for children, elderly, or immune-compromised people.

A poorly enriched indoor environment that lacks complexity and novelty may result in boredom or frustration, causing the cat to exhibit unwanted behaviors including attention-seeking behaviors. The importance of feline enrichment and its many benefits have been demonstrated, including its impact on health and welfare. Environmental enrichment satisfies the cat's innate physical, social, and mental needs. While attention-seeking behavior is most often "normal," it could also be reflective of fewer opportunities to engage in a variety of other behaviors such as hunting, playing, climbing, and scratching.

Genetic variation and heritability of both social and non-social behaviors exist amongst cat breeds.[3] For example, excessive vocalization is more common in oriental breeds and is highly innate.[4] In terms of social behavior, Persians have been ranked low in attention seeking and sociability,[5] and in one study had the highest probability for low contact to people.[3] Breed differences in the expression of vocalization, activity, and social behavior toward humans may alter expectations and owner perception of what is "normal" or "abnormal" for the individual cat.

Diagnosis

Attention-seeking behavior may be obvious based on description as well as context in which the behavior occurs. The presence of a behavior that occurs exclusively in the owner's presence, not when alone, can be confirmed by video. Direct observation of body language by the clinician may also help to discern motivations. The vocalizations and body postures of a cat that is anxious or in a state of aggressive arousal differ from a cat that is relaxed and soliciting attention or play.

Diagnostic recommendations will depend on the specific behavior. A physical examination and lab work including a complete blood count, serum biochemistry panel, total thyroid level and urinalysis are recommended as a minimum database to rule out obvious underlying medical issues. Neurologic examination, CSF tap, and advanced imaging may be considered where there is a higher index of suspicion for intracranial disease such as when there are acute behavioral changes, particularly in geriatric animals, and those exhibiting cognitive or neurologic signs.

Differential Diagnosis

While some forms of attention-seeking behavior are clearly more playful and affectionate, e.g. allorubbing and solicitations to be petted, others behaviors such as pouncing (Figure 12.2), chasing, scratching, and biting must be differentiated from aggression stemming from fear, territoriality, redirection, high arousal, or predatory behavior. Excessive vocalization that resolves, at least momentarily, with the provision of food or attention is likely a normal form of communication or attention-seeking behavior.

Learned behaviors are powerfully reinforced by intermittent reinforcement schedules. A person that tries to ignore vocalizations but inadvertently reinforces them may yield more intense or frequent vocalizations as the cat learns that persistence pays off. Intermittent reinforcement occurs when a reward is not administered every time the desired response is performed. This differs from continuous reinforcement in which a reward is delivered each time the behavior or response is performed.

Table 12.1   General history questions for feline nuisance behaviors.

1) Description of the problem. The goal is to obtain an objective description of the problematic behavior, rather than an anthropomorphic explanation
   a) Client description of the problem
      i) Video recording of the behavior is extremely helpful in providing a more accurate representation of the behavior
   b) Cat's body language or behavior when it engages in the problematic behavior
      i) Are there any signs of fear or anxiety, pain or discomfort, etc.?
   c) Location(s) where the problem behavior occurs
   d) Time of day or days of the week when the problem behavior occurs
   e) Frequency of the problem behavior (e.g. five times a day; once a week)
   f) Change or development of the problem over time
      i) How long has this behavior been going on for?
         1) When did the behavior first start?
         2) Event(s) that may have occurred around that time
      ii) Description of the behavior when it first started if different from current behavior
2) Antecedent events. This question may help determine the cat's motivation and/or factors that predict when the problem behavior may occur
   a) Location and time of day as above
   b) Presence or absence of other pets or human household members
   c) Situational events (e.g. if food is left out; when the client is on the computer; after seeing an outdoor cat)
3) Client's response (past and current). The client's past and current reaction to the cat may reveal whether the client has consciously or inadvertently reinforced the behavior
4) Treatment attempts (past and current) and client perception of efficacy. The clinician can focus on treatments that seem to work and provide strategies that the client has not already tried
5) Client concerns, expectations and/or goals. Generally speaking, nuisance behaviors may either be normal but unacceptable to the client (i.e. client-related problem) or abnormal expressions of normal behaviors (i.e. cat-related problem). It is therefore essential for the client to understand WHY the cat engages in these behaviors and to ACCEPT that engaging in these behaviors, at least occasionally, is necessary for the cat to express normal, species-specific behavior. To obtain client "buy in," it is important to address client concerns as well as discuss and manage their expectations.
6) Comorbid behavior problems. Nuisance behaviors may be clinical signs of other behavioral problems
7) General information
   a) Household demographic information
      i) Human household members or people who have frequent contact with the cat
      ii) Other animals (e.g. cats, dogs) within or outside the household with whom the cat has frequent contact
   b) Living environment
      i) Indoor, outdoor, indoor/outdoor, access to "catio" (enclosed outdoor space), etc.
      ii) Description of the home or floorplan showing locations where the problem behavior occurs, food/water, litterboxes, resting areas, etc.
   c) Medical history including recent diagnostic test

Petting, providing food or treats, talking to the cat or simply making eye contact may reward and reinforce undesirable attention-seeking behaviors. For some cats, any form of recognition, even verbal or physical confrontation such as scolding or spraying the cat with water can inadvertently reinforce undesirable behavior. These aversive responses may diminish the human–animal bond and result in conditioned fear of the person administering punishment.

Table 12.2 Medical and behavioral differential diagnoses will depend on the specific behavior.

Behavior	Behavioral differential	Medical differential
		Neuropathies, cognitive dysfunction, and conditions causing pain/discomfort (orthopedic, dermatologic, etc.) are differentials for excessive vocalization, nocturnal activity, and destructive behaviors

Excessive vocalization	Type of vocalization (meow vs. hiss) may assist diagnosis
	Meow
	  • Solicitation for food, attention, etc.
	  • Play
	  • Inadequate enrichment/boredom frustration
	  • Learned/reinforced
	  • Compulsive disorder
	  • Anxiety-related
	Growl/Hiss
	  • Aggressive arousal
		• Conditions causing polyphagia
		• Hyperthyroidism
		• Cognitive dysfunction
		• Visual or auditory impairment

Licking/chewing/sucking on owner clothing/hair/skin	• Attention seeking behavior • Play • Pica • Compulsive disorder or displacement behavior • Other anxiety • Normal/non-nutritive suckling	• Gastrointestinal disease • Conditions causing polyphagia or negative energy balance
Nocturnal activity/waking owners	• Food or attention-seeking behavior • Hunger (e.g. cats placed on weight-loss diet) • Anxiety based or response to environmental stimuli (noises) • Territorial arousal • Play • Boredom/frustration due to lack of enrichment • Excessive sleep or inactivity during the day	• Hyperthyroidism
Destructive behavior	• Self-reinforcing behavior – normal exploration/play or scratching • Re-directed aggression/displacement behavior • Boredom/lack of enrichment • Attention-seeking behavior	

An environment with insufficient outlets for normal behavioral expression may support boredom or a lack of enrichment as a motivation for certain behaviors. Destructive behavior such as knocking over or chewing on objects may be self-reinforcing or normal exploratory behavior that manifest when other outlets are unavailable.

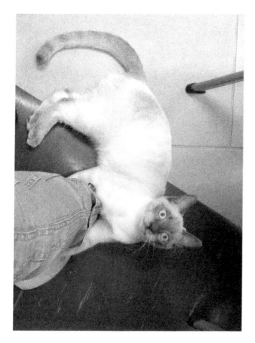

Figure 12.2 This six month old kitten refused to be ignored and would pounce on feet and climb up pant legs to solicit play and attention. Photo courtesy of Karen Sueda.

New or sudden behaviors at any age may indicate underlying pathology (see Table 12.2). Conditions causing pain/discomfort (e.g. orthopedic and dermatologic disease), cognitive dysfunction, sensory decline (visual or auditory), endocrine (hyperthyroidism), metabolic, neoplasia, or neurologic disease should be considered. Age-related conditions such as cognitive dysfunction might contribute to behaviors such as excessive vocalization often misinterpreted as a normal solicitation for attention.

Excessive licking of surfaces has been associated with underlying gastrointestinal disease in canines.[6] Although data for felines is lacking, the possibility of underlying gastrointestinal disease can be considered, particularly if other clinical signs are suggestive of gastrointestinal disease. Licking or non-nutritive sucking of human skin or hair may be a normal and self-reinforcing behavior, compulsive, or comfort-seeking behavior. Frequent consumption of non-food items or pica may be compulsive in nature, but medical issues should first be ruled out.

Sample History Questions

In addition to the questions in Table 12.1, other areas of inquiry include the following:

- Activity level: Is the cat very active or more sedentary? A kitten or young adult cat may be more likely to display playful solicitations for attention compared to a geriatric cat.
- Enrichment: Is the cat an indoor or outdoor cat? What types of enrichment are available, and what is the cat most motivated by (food, attention, play, toys)?
- What are the cat's typical daily routines and activities, including type and frequency of interactions with people or other pets? What times of the day is the cat most active?
- Owner schedule how much time does the cat spend alone? Has there been a change in anyone's schedule?
- Human–cat bond: How bonded is each family member with the cat? How often do they interact with or play with the cat?
- Have there been changes to the environment such as the introduction of new people/animals?
- Are any household members at increased risk for injury or infection (children, elderly, immunocompromised) as a result of cat bites or scratches?
- How do various household members respond to the behavior? Was the cat rewarded with petting/touching, play/toys, or food? Was it positive punishment (verbal/physical reprimand)?
- What attempts were made to extinguish the behavior and with what consistency and duration? If ignored, was it with passive avoidance (e.g. not responding to behavior) or active avoidance (e.g. leaving room)?
- What was the pet's behavioral response to these interventions (change in frequency and/or intensity, increased aggression or arousal, etc.)?

Treatment Options

- *Address medical concerns and underlying anxiety*
  Treatment depends on the actual diagnosis. Please see Chapter 8: Anxiety/Stress/Fear Behaviors for more information.
- *Avoidance and management strategies*:
  Avoid and reduce environmental stressors that may be causing anxious or "clingy" behaviors. Inappropriate items should be safely stowed away to avoid reinforcement of destructive behaviors. Useful tools may include cord protectors to prevent chewing or museum putty to prevent cats from knocking items off shelves. Areas or objects that are frequently knocked over can be blocked off to minimize opportunities for unwanted behaviors.
- *Environmental enrichment*:
  Prevent boredom and frustration by ensuring outlets for normal feline behaviors. The pet owner can be referred to online educational resources such as The Ohio State University's Indoor Pet Initiative website for enrichment ideas.
- Special games, motorized toys, food, or other highly motivating opportunities for independent play can be provided during times when the cats may be expected to seek attention or when household members cannot give attention. For example, additional outlets for play in the evening and before bedtime, and food toys available during the night, may be helpful for cats that exhibit nocturnal vocalization or activity.
- Food-dispensing toys and puzzle games offered throughout the day may reduce the frequency of food-seeking behavior while keeping the pet occupied in natural hunting behaviors (see Figure 12.3). The frequency of play, structured interactions with owners (e.g. training) and petting can be built into the daily routine and offered at various points throughout the day, particularly at times when the pet tends to be more active. The addition of another pet may help in some cases but not others. Owners should be counseled accordingly.
- *Positive reinforcement for desirable behavior*
  Remove reinforcers for attention-seeking behavior (e.g. attention, petting, or feeding on demand) and reward calm behaviors that are incompatible with the undesirable behavior. For example, the cat is fed when sitting quietly or in response to a command, rather than when vocalizing. A conditioned reinforcer such as a clicker can be used to remotely reward calm behavior and teach commands such as a "go to place" cue.
- *Negative punishment*:
  Ignore or remove attention at the onset of behavior. This can be passive (non-response) or active (physically leaving the room). It may be necessary to move away or leave the room if the behavior is persistent or could result in some level of injury toward owner such as a scratch or bite.

Prepare owners for an initial "extinction burst." During an extinction burst, the frequency or intensity of the behavior (e.g. vocalization) will increase as the cat may try harder to get the desired response. Intermittent reinforcement during the extinction burst can serve to intensify the response and must be

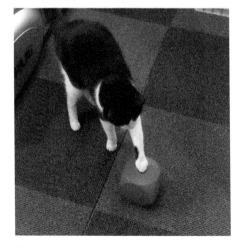

Figure 12.3   Cat plays with a Buster Food Cube, a food-dispensing marketed for dogs but readily used by cats. Photo courtesy of Karen Sueda.

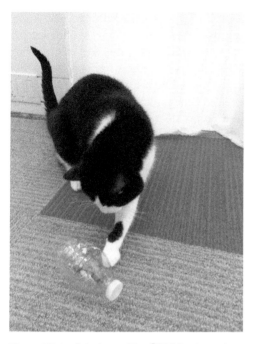

Figure 12.4 Cat plays with a "DIY" food puzzle toy made from an empty water bottle with small holes cut out of the sides. Photo courtesy of Karen Sueda.

avoided. Owners may not recognize subtle responses such as eye contact as being rewarding to the cat. Therefore, an explanation of specific reinforcers should be detailed. An "extinction burst" will usually diminish if the pet is consistently ignored. If disruptive to human sleep, consider placing the cat in a separate area with ample resources, including food toys or a timed feeder.

- An interruptive stimulus or remote punishment can be used as long as the stimulus does not cause fear or distress. For example, a cat who is vocalizing or demonstrating destructive behavior can be interrupted with a loud audible noise such as hand clapping or ultrasonic alarm. When calm, the cat can then be rewarded.
- *Medications*
  Psychotropic medications are not indicated for attention-seeking behaviors. The use of medications in conjunction with behavior modification may be considered as treatment for an anxiety-based condition that has been identified as a behavioral component. See Appendix 1 for further information.

Food-Seeking Behavior

Food-seeking behavior is a normal adaptive behavior that communicates when the pet is hungry (see Figure 12.5). When excessive, this may be perceived as a nuisance or deemed unacceptable if exhibited frequently or at inconvenient times. At times, this may reflect underlying pathology. Emotional or stress induced overeating and the influence of other factors besides hunger, has been documented in humans and other animals.[7] Research by Moesta et al. suggests a relationship between impulse control and overeating in cats, similar to findings in humans.[8,9]

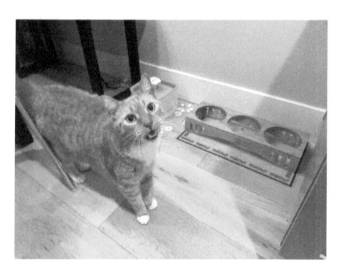

Figure 12.5 Cat vocalizing to be fed dinner. A scheduled meal or interaction may inadvertently reinforce attention-seeking behaviors that precede it. (Photo Courtesy of Dr. Poorna Chowdry and Paul Beldan).

Nocturnal activity or persistent vocalization even after feeding or during early morning hours may be learned through feeding schedules and owner response (see Chapter 5 re: species-specific feeding schedules). Activity and solicitations in the form of pacing, meowing, and purring may increase in anticipation of feeding. A pet that is successful in solicitations for food learns that specific people serve as a consistent source of food dispensation. The pet will continue to beg for food. Often, reinforcement occurs during mealtime when soliciting human food from the table or the cat inadvertently acquires a morsel of food dropped on the floor. Similar to other attention-seeking behaviors, intermittent reinforcement (particularly during an extinction burst) powerfully maintains the behavior and owners may find it difficult to consistently ignore food-seeking behavior.

Food-seeking behavior can manifest as begging or vocalizing for food at the table, jumping on counters where food is accessible, aggression or destructive behavior such as chewing into bags or knocking over trash bins and food containers (see Figure 12.6).

Food seeking may occur if the cat receives insufficient calories to support metabolic needs and this may be accompanied by weight loss or poor body condition. Metabolic energy requirements may vary depending on breed, age, sex, life stage, and activity level as well as individual variance in metabolism and interest in food. However, highly palatable food may encourage food-seeking even if caloric requirements have been met[10] and may be accompanied by weight gain.

Cats are predatory animals that naturally hunt for their food. Kane et al. demonstrated that cats will choose to consume small, frequent meals (between 8 to 16 feedings of a commercial diet) in a 24-hour period. In the field, cats spend ample time hunting prey and will continue to kill prey before consuming previously killed prey.[11,12] Play and predatory behavior are closely related.[13]

Despite the tendency for cats to hunt and work for their food (contrafreeload), research by Delgado and colleagues showed that, unlike other tested species, cats do not show a strong preference to contrafreeload when offered food puzzles in the home environment, compared to freely accessible food.[14] However, this study also suggests a relationship between hunger and effort as those cats that consumed more food in general were also more likely to consume food from a puzzle and the authors determined that this was due to hunger. Similarly, other research demonstrates that hunger does increase play and predatory behaviors, although it is not necessary for either behavior to occur.

Meal feeding from bowls does not engage a natural predatory sequence of food acquisition or the "appetitive" component of feeding behavior. The addition of food-dispensing toys or puzzle toys helps to satisfy this behavior with the added benefit of allowing the cat to graze and acquire food frequently throughout the day (see Figure 12.4).

Dantas et al. noted behavioral and health-related benefits after implementation of food puzzles along with other forms of behavior modification.[15] These benefits included weight loss, decreased aggression toward humans and other cats, reduced anxiety and fear, cessation of attention-seeking behaviors, and resolution of litter-box avoidance behavior.

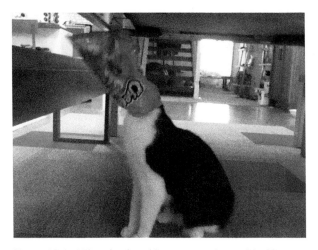

Figure 12.6 When food-seeking gets you in trouble. Photo courtesy of Karen Sueda.

Diagnosis

Clients may complain that their cat is "begging" for food or recognize that food-seeking is the underlying motivation for another undesirable behavior. However, the primary complaint may be "jumping on counters," "keeping us up at night," etc. and it is up to the clinician to determine that food-seeking is the underlying cause.

As with other behavioral issues, feeding behaviors are evaluated with video capture and observation, behavioral and medical history, physical examination, and laboratory diagnostics. However, it is particularly important to gather information regarding the cat's diet and feeding habits as well as the presence or absence of other physical clinical signs to rule out diseases that may be causing polyphagia.

A thorough history includes information about diet and dietary changes, caloric intake, and metabolic energy requirement (MER) calculations. The activity level, concurrent medical conditions and age of cat are needed to determine energy requirements. Food seeking may occur when the cat's diet is changed, especially for medical reasons (e.g. regular to weight-loss diet; dry to canned food to increase water consumption; highly palatable to less palatable specialized diet; elimination of treats or snacks, etc.).

The presence of clinical signs such as weight loss, weight gain, obesity, alternations in appetite, polyuria, polydipsia, gastrointestinal signs, and dental or oral pain causing dysphagia, should also be noted.

Food seeking may manifest as, or be accompanied by excessive vocalization, destructive behavior, or climbing on counters (refer to other sections). Food or attention-seeking motivations can be confused with anxiety related conditions as well as cognitive decline or sensory decline that manifest as vocalizations and aimless wandering at night. A pet that vocalizes persistently may be in discomfort and conditions causing pain should be ruled out.

Questions regarding appetite may reveal a sudden increase in appetite or ravenous appetite despite sufficient caloric intake. A range of medical conditions that cause polyphagia should be ruled out (see Table 12.3). A complete and current list of the pet's medications is needed to rule out iatrogenic causes (e.g. corticosteroids or benzodiazepines).

Table 12.3 Behavioral and medical differentials for food-seeking behavior.

	Behavioral	Medical

Food-seeking behavior	• Learned/owner reinforced
	• Boredom/frustration/insufficient outlets for hunting
	• Conflict/competition with other animals over food
	• Compulsive disorder/pica
	• Attention-seeking behavior
	• Anxiety-based
	• Cognitive decline
		Polyphagia
		• Endocrinopathy
		  – Diabetes Mellitus
		  – Hyperadrenocortism
		  – Hyperinsulinism
		  – Hyperthyroidism
		• Gastrointestinal disease/malabsorption (infectious, inflammatory, neoplastic)
		• Intracranial disease (neoplasia)
		• Pregnancy/lactation
		• Growth
		• Inadequate caloric intake or poor quality food (or difficulty prehending food secondary to oral disease/pain)
		• Increased exercise
		• Low temperatures
		• Iatrogenic

A complete blood count (CBC), serum biochemistry panel, T4 and urinalysis are recommended as a minimum database in most cases. Abdominal and thoracic radiographs, ultrasound, gastrointestinal panels, endoscopy, and biopsy may be indicated.

Sample History Questions

In addition to the questions in Table 12.1, other areas of inquiry include the following:

- Dietary history including type (wet or dry), brand, and quantity as well as energy composition of food. Treats and human food items should be included.
- List of current medications.
- What is the cat's daily feeding schedule and strategy including location (private or high traffic area), frequency (meal feeding vs. ad libitum), and receptacle (food toys, bowls, hand-feeding, or automatic feeders)?
- Does the cat receive table food? Is food left on countertops or other areas accessible to pet? How is food stored and secured?
- Are other animals present and do they compete for food?
- Have there been any changes in household composition (new people, pets, etc.), schedules, or interaction with individuals in the household?
- Has the pet's diet been changed? For example, was a regular adult-maintenance diet switched to weight-loss diet or prescription diet? Has there been a switch from canned to dry food or vice versa? Were additions made to increase palatability of food since the onset of behavior?

Treatment Options

- *Address underlying physiologic or pathological causes for food-seeking behavior (see Table 12.3).* Ensure that nutritional and caloric needs are being provided and address underlying medical issues. If caloric intake is increased, the cat should be re-weighed at appropriate intervals to achieve ideal body condition and to monitor for excessive weight gain or weight loss if intended.
- *Remove reinforcers for food-seeking behavior:* Once physiologic needs have been met, reinforcers for the behavior should be removed. This includes not feeding the cat on demand and ignoring early morning solicitations. Food should be kept in a secure container that is not accessible to the cat. Knowledge that physiologic needs are being met is often reassuring to cat owners who can then more confidently ignore food-seeking behaviors (see earlier discussion on negative punishment and extinction bursts).
- Owners may need to be conscientious of not leaving food out on counters or where cats may eat it. Food can be kept in cat-proof containers or in another room. In some cases, cats may need to be confined away from owners and provided with enrichment if they tend to steal food from the table. See other sections if the cat is climbing to get food or being vocal.
- *Modify feeding routine and receptacles:* Food and feeding routines should be dissociated from the owner to avoid reinforcement throughout the day or at specific times. If food is not provided on demand, the cat will learn to look elsewhere. Food can be provided on a set schedule or during calm, quiet behavior. Automatic or timed feeders can be set to dispense food before the cat normally wakes owners and the time of dispensation can be gradually moved to establish a more acceptable feeding schedule not connected to the human. Automatic feeders allow for timed feeding of more frequent, small meals, which is most congruent with observed preferences.[16-18] Alternately, food-dispensing toys can be left out for the cat to graze and hunt "as needed" through the night and day and meal

feeding from bowls minimized or eliminated. This, in addition to other forms of enrichment can be offered regardless of what is motivating the behavior.

- *Reduce competition amongst household cats*:
  If competition from other animals is preventing the cat from acquiring enough food, eating too quickly, or seeking excessive amounts of food, the food should be moved to a quiet area away from animals such as a closed room or gated area that is only accessible to that particular cat (magnetic gate). A "house of plenty" provides ample resources for all cats including multiple feeding station to reduce competition. If inter-cat aggression or anxiety-based conditions exist, these should also be addressed.

Undesirable Scratching Behavior

Scratching objects with their front claws is a fundamental aspect of normal feline maintenance behavior which fulfills both physical and behavioral needs. Kittens begin scratching at as young as 5 weeks of age[19] and the behavior continues throughout a cat's lifetime. As the cats' claws grow, the outer keratinized sheath loses its blood supply and sheds, revealing a newer and slightly sharper nail underneath. Scratching loosens and removes these outer, dead sheaths, effectively exfoliating, sharpening, and conditioning the claws at the same time. Older cats that are unable to scratch may develop thick, overgrown claws that are brittle, prone to breaking, and more difficult to retract. The physical act of scratching – reaching, grasping, and pulling – stretches tendons and tones muscles and may provide an upper-body workout for the cat.

Scratch marking is also a form of communication. When cats scratch, they leave both a visual mark and deposit pheromones from interdigital scent glands. Scratching helps cats define their territory and manage social spacing by leaving "calling cards" to inform conspecifics as to who has been there in the recent past. Some authors have also suggested that scratching may also help cats orient to its environment or help discriminate safe from unsafe locations.[19] In free-ranging cats, scratch marking occurs more along frequently used pathways than at the periphery of territories.[19]

Cats may choose to scratch one object and not another based on personal preference for both the type or texture of scratched material and its positioning. When appropriate scratching substrates are offered, cats <10 years old preferred rope over other materials such as cardboard, carpet, and wood. However geriatric cats between 10–14 years old preferred carpets.[20] Fabric (typically furniture) and carpets were the most common inappropriate substrates scratched by cats.[21]

Cats may also prefer scratching vertical versus horizontal objects. Generally speaking, cats tend to prefer scratching vertically on both appropriate (e.g. cat trees, simple vertical posts)[20] and inappropriate (e.g. side of the sofa)[21] objects. Both appropriate[20] and inappropriate[21] horizontal surfaces were used less often. Angled objects and hung or wall-mounted posts were least frequently used. [20,21]

When appropriate scratching posts are offered, cats tended to use shorter (<3 feet tall) posts more often than taller (>3 feet) posts. However, inappropriate scratching behavior was less frequent in homes that provided taller posts versus shorter posts.[20] Given that cats prefer to scratch large, fabric covered furniture (e.g. sofa, chairs) versus loose fabric (e.g. curtains), stability of the scratching item may also play a role.[21]

Diagnosis

Scratching of objects considered to be inappropriate by cat owners is extremely common. In one survey, 83.9% of cat owners reported that their cat scratched inappropriate items.[2] Additionally, inappropriate scratching behavior has been associated with increased risk of relinquishment.[2]

Diagnosis is based on the client conveying that they have witnessed their cat scratching unacceptable objects or finding damage after the fact (see Figure 12.7). The clinician must determine if scratching is comorbid with another behavioral problem (e.g. inter-cat aggression, generalized anxiety) or if the cat is simply expressing normal maintenance behavior but in a way deemed unacceptable to the client.

In multi-cat household, it may be difficult to determine what cat or cats are the culprits. More than one cat may be involved with multiple cats scratching the same object or different cats scratching different objects. Video recording rooms where objects have been scratched over a period of several days may help determine which cats require intervention.

Although objectionable scratching behavior is not associated with any particular physical illness, a decrease in scratching may be a general sign of illness or discomfort, especially arthritis or a claw disorder (e.g. nail avulsion, paronychia). Any change in behavior warrants examination by a veterinarian.

Sample History Questions

The goal of history taking is to determine the cat's underlying motivation for scratching objects that are unacceptable to the client. Thoughtful investigation may reveal whether scratching is secondary to a behavioral disorder or if the client's objection to scratching is due to lack knowledge of typical feline behavior and husbandry requirements. Understanding the client's tolerance for scratching behavior is also important since this will affect prognosis and treatment outcome.

In addition to the questions in Table 12.1, other areas of inquiry include the following:

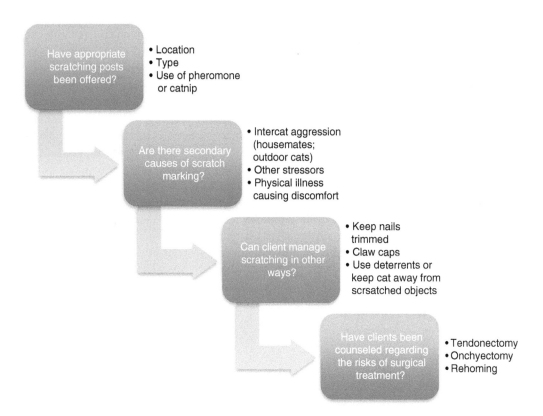

Figure 12.7   Decision-tree once unacceptable scratching behavior has been identified.

- Description of what the cat is scratching. Photographs of the object may be useful to determine the extent of damage as well as identify the type of material (e.g. fabric, wood, carpet, etc.) and object position (e.g. vertical, horizontal) being scratched.
- Location of the scratched object(s), especially in relation to other socially significant areas such as favorite resting areas, food and water, litter box, etc. These may be indicated on a floor plan of the house.
- Circumstances associated with the cat scratching (antecedent events). Does the cat scratch on the object during a play session or after an altercation with another cat, for example.
- Provision of objects that are acceptable for the cat to scratch (e.g. scratching posts), their description (e.g. height, material), where they are located and how often the cat uses them.
- Treatments that have been tried in the past and perceived efficacy.
- Comorbid behavior problems. Unacceptable scratching may be a clinical sign of another behavioral problems, especially problems related to anxiety.
  - Inter-cat aggression
  - Generalized anxiety
  - Attention-seeking behavior
- Client concerns and expectations. Answers to the above questions above may reveal gaps in the client's feline husbandry knowledge. They may not realize that scratching is a normal behavior, that cats vary in the type of substrate they like to scratch or that indoor/outdoor cats may still want to scratch objects indoors. Additionally, the degrees to which clients tolerate scratching behavior varies from person-to-person and depend on what objects were scratched. For some clients, any damage to a cherished object, even if minimal, is not acceptable. For example, a client may complain that their cat has snagged the upholstery of their new sofa yet refrained from reporting that the same cat scratched their previous sofa for years prior to replacement. Other clients may have an excellent grasp of feline husbandry but are unable to clip their cat's nails or express concern that their cat may scratch and injure a person.

Treatment

Scratching is essential to maintaining normal feline physical and behavioral health and therefore clients must provide cats with an acceptable outlet to scratch. The goal of treatment is to redirect scratching onto an object the client finds acceptable.

- *Provide an acceptable scratching post.* Cat owners may not realize that they need to provide an appropriate scratching post for their cat. In one survey, almost a quarter of owners (23.9%) did not provide a scratching item for their cat.[21] Some owners may think that a cat with access to the outdoors do not need a scratching post; however, outdoor cats will still scratch indoors and when a scratching post is provided, will often use it.[19]

  Most cats prefer a vertical scratching post <3 feet high made of rope. However, a fair number of cats (49.5%) also used a horizontal post on the floor or a post at an angle (24%).[20] Similarly, a quarter of cats ≤9 yo and cats >10 yo preferred carpet rather than rope.[20] It is therefore worthwhile to provide different types of scratching posts to determine an individual cat's preference. The characteristics of the inappropriately scratched object may provide a clue to the type of substrate and positioning the cat desires.
- *Place the scratching post near the scratched area.* In free-ranging cats, scratch marking occurs more along frequently used pathways than at the periphery of territories.[19] Appropriate scratching posts placed in frequented areas of the house may be used more often than out-of-the-way locations at

the periphery. Although having a scratching post near the inappropriately scratched object does not necessarily deter the behavior,[20,21] it at least provides an acceptable, accessible alternative.

- *Enhance the desirability of the scratching post.* Increasing the attractiveness of the scratching post over that of the inappropriate substrate is beneficial. Rubbing catnip or silvervine on the scratching post may draw the cat to it and encourage use.

  Feliscratch by Feliway™ is a synthetic form of the feline interdigital semiochemical (FIS) cats deposit when scratching. In addition to the FIS, Feliscratch also contains a dye to mimic the visual signal component. Application of Feliscratch as directed on a new scratching post placed near a previously scratched area or near the cat's sleeping area resulted in resolution of undesirable vertical scratching in 74% of cats and a significant reduction in undesirable horizontal scratching over the four-week study.[22]

- *Reward the cat for using the scratching post.* Behaviors that are reinforced are more likely to occur in the future. Cats may be encouraged to use the scratching post by rewarding them with treats, play, or praise/attention when they do so. Owner that rewarded their cat for using their scratching post were more likely to report that their cat used the post at least once daily versus owners that never rewarded scratching.[20]

- *Remove access to or deter the cat from using unacceptable areas.* Preventing the cat from scratching inappropriate objects prevents practicing the undesirable behavior. Besides limiting access to rooms, deterrents such as double-sided sticky tape, vinyl carpet protector, static shock mats, motion-activated compressed air canisters, etc. may punish cats when they scratch. Whenever positive punishment-based training methods are used, care must be taken to prevent anxiety or generalization of the aversive.

- *Trim the cat's claws.* While trimming a cat's claws won't prevent scratching behavior, keeping claws short may lessen the extent of damage scratching may cause. Clients should be taught the proper way to trim a cat's nails utilizing rewards and patience. Every new kitten examination should include a brief talk and demonstration of nail trimming training.

- *Address any underlying reasons for scratching.* Because scratching is a form of communication, scratching (especially if it is treatment-resistant) may be a sign of a larger behavioral problem such as inter-cat aggression, generalized anxiety, etc. A more thorough behavioral history should be obtained or referral to a veterinary behaviorist considered.

  A synthetic feline pheromone complex with high affinity for vomeronasal organ binding sites (FELIWAY® Optimum, Ceva Sante Animale) was developed to address multiple behavior disorders in cats. In an open-label, uncontrolled trial, treatment with FELIWAY® Optimum resulted in significant reductions in problem scratching, as well as problem urination, fear and inter-cat conflict, after four weeks of use.

- *Claw caps.* Plastic claw caps (e.g. Soft Claws®) may be applied to both front paws. Similar to trimming a cat's claws, caps do not prevent scratching behavior but may prevent damage to furniture. Caps may be difficult to apply if the cat is uncooperative and may not last long.

- *Onychectomy.* "Declawing" is avoidable in the vast majority of cases and should only be considered as a last resort after all other treatment options have been explored.

  There is considerable controversy surrounding the ethics, practice, and short- and long-term outcomes of declawing. Mills et al. provides a review of the topic including post-operative pain management and short- and long-term complications.[23] In regards to behavioral sequelae following onychectomy, various studies provide contradictory results. While some studies indicate an increased frequency of behavioral problems in declawed cats (biting, barbering,[24] and house-soiling[24,25]), others show no association between declawing and an increased incidence of behavioral problems.[26,27] Interestingly, one study found the number of declawed cats in a Seattle, Washington, shelter was significantly lower than the general population but that declawed cats stayed in the shelter significantly longer than non-declawed cats, even though there was no correlation between being declawed and euthanasia.[26]

Climbing and Jumping up on Objects

Climbing and jumping up on objects are normal behaviors which clients find unacceptable depending on where the cat wants to go (e.g. cat tree okay; countertop not okay) and whether it inconveniences the client (e.g. jumping on the mantle is okay, but not when the cat blocks the view of the TV above the mantle). Common irritants include climbing on people or objects (e.g. curtains, screen door, furniture) and jumping up on elevated surfaces (e.g. counters, tables, shelves). Unacceptable climbing and jumping may result in destructive behavior such as torn curtains, scratched or ripped furniture, or items knocked over and broken. Additionally, clients may express health concerns regarding the practice of cats jumping on counters and tables where food is prepared or eaten.

Climbing and jumping are defining characteristics of feline behavior and anatomy (see Figure 12.8). Cats evolved in a world where they were both hunters and prey to other animals. *Felis silvestris lybica*, the African wildcat from whom the domestic cat evolved, have been observed to leap to capture birds mid-flight and are excellent climbers who use trees for both escape and rest (see Figure 12.9).[28] Domestic cats' powerful hind limbs also allow them to leap vertically, up to a height of 1.6 meters (5.2 feet) in one experiment.[29]

Selective breeding has altered both the physical ability and relative motivation for climbing and jumping. Cat breeds with short legs, such as the Munchkin, can jump but may not be able to jump as high as other cats depending on the relative length of their hind legs.[30] Some cat breeds are more active than others and therefore may be more prone to climbing and jumping; these include

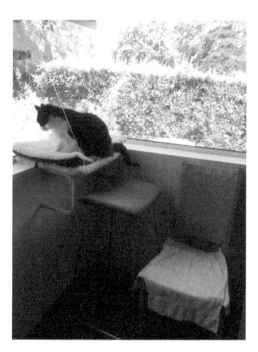

Figure 12.8 Despite suffering from arthritis, a senior cat's favorite resting spot was still his window perch. Chairs of various heights were added as he got older to facilitate access. Courtesy of Karen Sueda.

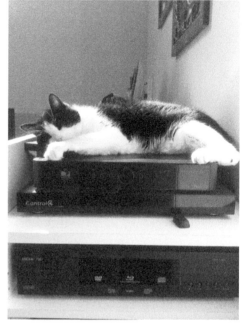

Figure 12.9 Elevated locations, particularly when they are located near a window or are warmed by electricity, are favorite resting areas for cats.

Bengals, Abyssinians, Siamese, and Oriental breeds. Persians, Ragdolls, Maine Coons, and Sphinx cats rank low on activity.[31]

Cats may possess an instinctive drive to climb and jump, making these behaviors inherently rewarding to perform. Climbing and jumping are also motivated by either gaining access to something rewarding located up high (positive reinforcement) or escaping from something undesirable located below (negative reinforcement). The most interesting items in the house (e.g. food, knickknacks) are typically found on elevated surfaces (e.g. tables, counters, shelves). Since object play by adult cats is stimulated both by smaller size[32] and novelty,[33] cats may be attracted to small items kept out of reach. Similarly, cats may have learned that social interactions with people are more likely if they jump up on the desk or counter to get to human eye level.

It may be a natural instinct for cats to seek elevation as a defensive strategy. Cats may climb or jump up to escape from undesirable situations at floor level. This may include agonistic interactions with other pets in the case of inter-cat or interspecific aggression, inanimate objects (e.g. vacuum) or people (e.g. crawling baby, visitors, client trying to catch the cat to go to the vet).

Diagnosis

Diagnosing undesirable climbing or jumping behavior is typically straightforward and based on client observation and communication to the clinician that they find the behavior to be problematic (see Figure 12.10). In some cases, the client may not have witnessed the cat, but instead found

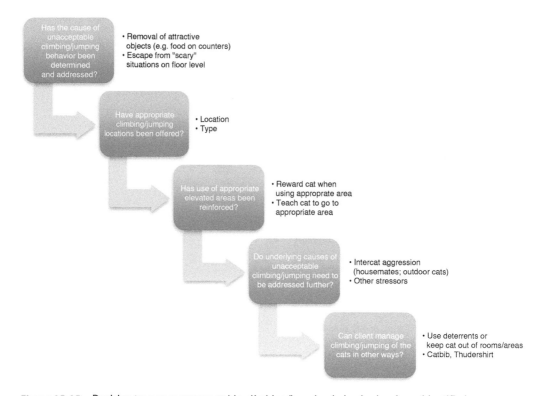

Figure 12.10 Decision tree once unacceptable climbing/jumping behavior has been identified.

items knocked over or destroyed. In multi-pet households, video recording using a security camera may be helpful in determining which pet(s) is/are at fault.

Although there are no specific medical differentials for unacceptable climbing and jumping, hyperthyroidism or toxicities that result in hyperactivity or agitation may cause a cat to engage in these behaviors uncharacteristically. Diseases that cause polyphagia may motivate a cat to seek out food on counters or cabinets. Cats that are ill may become reclusive and try to hide in closets or on top of cabinets.

A decrease in frequency or ability to jump (or climb) may be of greater and more commonplace concern. Difficulty in jumping or decreased use of elevated areas may be a sign of illness including, but not limited to, osteoarthritis or neuropathy, especially in older cats.

Sample History Questions

Since climbing and jumping are normal behaviors, but unacceptable to the client, the clinician must decide what motivates the cat to engage in the behavior and use this knowledge to devise a treatment plan that allows the cat to engage in normal, species-specific behavior but in a way that is acceptable to the cat's owner.

In addition to the questions in Table 12.1, other areas of inquiry include the following:

- Specific location and description of where or on what the cat is climbing or jumping.
- Cat's behavior once it climbs or jumps up to these areas. This may help determine the cat's motivation. For example, does the cat eat food on the counter, stare at the other cats below, hide for the rest of the day, meow to get attention, etc.
- What is near these location(s). Areas may be inherently rewarding (e.g. windows, sunny spot in the late morning, food on counters) or have social significance (e.g. in front of the TV, where another cat resource guards the litter box).
- Items that are acceptable for the cat to climb or jump up on (e.g. cat tree, shelves), their description (e.g. height, material) and where they are located.
- Circumstances that cause the cat to jump up on these locations (antecedent events). For example, the cat might climb the screen door when it sees an outdoor cat or jump up on the counter when the client is preparing food.
- Treatments that have been tried in the past and perceived efficacy.
- Comorbid behavior problems. Unacceptable climbing or jumping may be a clinical sign of another behavioral problems.
  - Inter-cat aggression: climbing or jumping to get away or get to another cat
  - Generalized anxiety: attempt to get to a hidden, safe spot
  - Attention-seeking behavior: getting in front of the owner to get their attention
- Client concerns and expectations. The client's specific concerns should be acknowledged and addressed. For example, a client who cares for an immune-compromised family member may be particularly worried about disease transmission if the cat jumps on a food-preparation area. The owner of an elderly cat may worry that the cat will fall if he jumps up on a ledge.
- Circumstance in which the cat is allowed to climb or jump up on these areas. A client may encourage his cat to sleep on his desk when he is surfing the internet but not when he is trying to work. Inconsistent "rules" may perpetuate undesirable behavior.

Treatment Options

Because jumping and climbing is instinctive, it's impossible to completely eliminate this behavior. The goal of treatment is to redirect the cat's jumping behavior to acceptable locations while decreasing the cat's motivation to jump on unacceptable surfaces.

- *Client education.* The foundation of all treatment plans begins with an explanation of the cat's behavior and how the treatment plan addresses the underlying motivation for the behavior. This is also an opportunity to address misconceptions and client factors that may impede success.
  - *Discuss WHY this particular cat climbs or jumps.*
  - *Discuss the cat's prognosis keeping in mind the client's expectations.* Generally speaking, the prognosis for decreasing unacceptable climbing or jumping behavior is fair to good, as long as the client understands that this is a normal behavior that cannot be eliminated completely, and that the success of treatment depends on the client's ability to adhere to the treatment plan.
  - *Discuss the importance of consistency.* Cats learn best when rules are consistently applied by everyone in the household. Clients may be inconsistent in regard to when it is acceptable or unacceptable for cats to be in certain locations. A client may feed his cat on the counter to prevent the dog from eating the cat food, but not want the cat to be on counter while they are cooking dinner for the family. In this case, a new feeding location should be found if the client doesn't want the cat on the counter, period.
- *Provide acceptable elevated areas.* Set the cat up for success by providing elevated surfaces he wants to jump up on. These acceptable surfaces and location should satisfy the same underlying motivation for jumping on the unacceptable location. For example, if the cat was jumping on the mantle in front of the TV to get attention, a cat tree may be placed close to the couch where the owner can pet the cat while watching TV. If the cat was knocking items off a shelf when he jumped up there to get away from the dog, the shelves could be cleared of items and a cat bed placed there instead. Acceptable elevated options might include cat trees, window perches, cat shelving, or designated pieces of furniture. Offer several locations throughout the house; cats may want to perch in different areas at different times of day.
- *Encourage and reward use of acceptable elevated areas.* Placing elevated areas near windows or leaving treats or toys on perches motivates cats to explore them. For cats that jump on counters to look for food, clear a shelf or top of a credenza off near the kitchen or place a cat tree nearby and consistently leave cat treats on it. This may encourage the cat to forage in that location instead of the countertop. If you see the cat using the perch reward her with attention or a treat. Cats may also be taught to go to a location (e.g. a cat bed or rung on a cat tree) on cue. When the client observes the cat about to climb or jump on a unacceptable area, the cat may be redirected to an acceptation location (e.g. "Go to your perch") and rewarded.
- *Make unacceptable places difficult to access or undesirable.* Don't tempt your cat to jump on counters or tables by leaving food or "fun" items on them. You may also block access by making the landing surface small or irregular or removing access to "intermediate levels" that are used to jump to higher locations (e.g. push in chairs so it's harder for the cat to get on the table). Deterrents such as upside-down (nubby side up) vinyl carpet protector, motion-activated compressed air canisters, static shock mats, or alarms (audible or ultrasonic) may be used to punish incursion into unacceptable areas. These should be used judiciously and with the aim of increasing the likelihood that cats will use acceptable elevated areas, which can then be reinforced. Spray bottles or other types of punishment directly inflicted by the client (e.g. hitting,

swatting, scruffing) may stop the cat from jumping up for the moment, but often result in the cat simply learning to climb or jump only when the owner is *not* present.

Additional Information

General Information

- Clicker Training for Cats by Karen Pryor
- Decoding Your Cat by DACVB
- Basic Indoor Cat Needs: The Indoor Pet Initiative – The Ohio State University: https://indoorpet.osu.edu/cats/basic-indoor-cat-needs

Additional Information

- Scratching Educational Resources by the American Association of Feline Practitioners: https://catvets.com/content/scratching-resources
- AAFP Position Statement: Declawing: https://catvets.com/public/PDFs/PositionStatements/2017-DeclawingStatement.pdf
- Basic Indoor Cat Needs: Scratching; The Indoor Cat Initiative – The Ohio State University: https://indoorpet.osu.edu/cats/basicneeds/scratching
- 8 Steps to Fear Free Nail Trims for You and Your Cat: https://fearfreehappyhomes.com/8-steps-fear-free-nail-trims-cat
- FeliScratch by Feliway: https://www.feliway.com/us/Products/feliscratch-by-feliway

Climbing and Jumping

- Basic Indoor Cat Needs: Perches. The Indoor Pet Initiative – The Ohio State University: https://indoorpet.osu.edu/cats/basicneeds/perches
- "How can I train my cat to go to a mat" (YouTube Video): https://www.youtube.com/watch?v=8LcK-UXIMeo

References

1 Salman MD, Hutchison J, Ruch-Gallie R, et al. Behavioral reasons for relinquishment of dogs and cats to 12 shelters. *J Appl Anim Welf Sci.* 2000;3(2):93–106.
2 Patronek GJ, Glickman L, Beck A, et al. Risk factors for relinquishment of cats to an animal shelter. *J Am Vet Med Assoc.* 1996;209:582–588.
3 Salonen M, Vapalahti K, Tiira K, et al. Breed differences of heritable behaviour traits in cats. *Sci Rep.* 2019;9:7949.
4 Landsberg G, Hunthausen W, Ackerman L. Unruly behaviors, training, training and management – cats. In: *Handbook of behavior problems of the dog and cat*, 2nd ed. Oxford: Elsevier Saunders Ltd; 2003:323.
5 Duffy DL, de Moura RTD, Serpell JA. Development and evaluation of the Fe-BARQ: A new survey instrument for measuring behavior in domestic cats (Felis s. catus). *Behav. Processes.* 2017;141:329–341.
6 Bécuwe-Bonnet V, Bélanger MC, Frank D, Parent J, Hélie P. Gastrointestinal disorders in dogs with excessive licking of surfaces. *J Vet Behav.* 2012;7(4):194–204. Mugford RA. External influences on the feeding of carnivores. In: Kare M, Maller O, eds. *The chemical senses and nutrition.* 1977;25–50.

7   McMillan FD. Stress-induced and emotional eating in animals: A review of the experimental evidence and implications for companion animal obesity. *J Vet Behav.* 2013;8:376–385.

8   Moesta A, Bosch G, Beerda B. Choice impulsivity and not action impulsivity may be associated with overeating in cats Paper presented at: Proceedings of the 12th International Veterinary Behavior Meeting. 2019.

9   Giel KE, Teufel M, Junne F, et al. Food-related impulsivity in obesity and binge eating disorder—a systematic update of the evidence. *Nutrients.* 2017;9:1170.

10 Denenberg S. Begging: canine and feline. In: Horwitz DF ed. *Blackwell's five-minute veterinary consult clinical companion: canine and feline behavior*, 2nd ed. Wiley-Blackwell; 2017:736.

11 Leyhausen P. *Cat behaviour.* New York, NY: Garland; 1979.

12 Adamec RE. The interaction of hunger and preying in the domestic cat (Felis catus): An adaptive hierarchy? *Behav Biol.* 1976;18:263–272.

13 Witzel AL, Bartges J, Kirk C, et al. Nutrition for the normal cat. In: Little S ed. *The cat: Clinical medicine and management.* St Louis (MO): Elsevier Saunders; 2012:243–254.

14 Delgado M, Bain MJ, Buffington T. A survey of feeding practices and use of food puzzles in owners of domestic cats. *J Feline Med Surg.* 2019;22(2):193–198.

15 Dantas LM, Delgato M, Johnson I, Buffington T. Food puzzles for cats: Feeding for physical and emotional wellbeing. *J Feline Med Surg.* 2016;18(9).

16 Beaver BV. *Feline behavior: A guide for veterinarians.* St. Louis, MO: Saunders; 2003:212–246.

17 Bradshaw J, Casey R, Brown S. Feeding behaviour. In: *The behaviour of the domestic cat.* Wallingford, UK: CABI Publishing; 2012:113–127.

18 Mugford RA. Feeding of Carnivores. In: Kare MR, ed. *The chemical senses and nutrition.* Elsevier Inc; 1977:25. https://www.sciencedirect.com/book/9780123978509/the-chemical-senses-and-nutrition#book-info

19 Mengoli M, Mariti C, Cozzi A, Cestarollo E, Lafont-Lecuelle C, Pageat P, Gazzano A. Scratching behaviour and its features: A questionnaire-based study in an Italian sample of domestic cats. *J Feline Med Surg.* 2013;15(10):886–892.

20 Wilson C, Bain M, DePorter T, Beck A, Grassi V, Landsberg G. Owner observations regarding cat scratching behavior: An internet-based survey. *J Feline Med Surg.* 2016;18(10):791–797.

21 Moesta A, Keys D, Crowell-Davis S. Survey of cat owners on features of, and preventative measures for, feline scratching of inappropriate objects: A pilot study. *J Feline Med Surg.* 2018;20(10):891–899. 1098612X17733185.

22 Beck A, De Jaeger X, Collin JF, Tynes V. Effect of a synthetic feline pheromone for managing unwanted scratching. *Int J Appl Res Vet Med.* 2018;16(1):13–27.

23 Mills KE, von Keyserlingk MA, Niel L. A review of medically unnecessary surgeries in dogs and cats. *J Am Vet Med Assoc.* 2016;248(2):162–171.

24 Martell-Moran NK, Solano M, Townsend HG. Pain and adverse behavior in declawed cats. *J Feline Med Surg.* 2018;20(4):280–288.

25 Gerard AF, Larson M, Baldwin CJ, Petersen C. Telephone survey to investigate relationships between onychectomy or onychectomy technique and house soiling in cats. *J Am Vet Med Assoc.* 2016;249(6):638–643.

26 Fritscher SJ, Ha J. Declawing has no effect on biting behavior but does affect adoption outcomes for domestic cats in an animal shelter. *Appl Anim Behav Sci.* 2016;180:107–113.

27 Patronek GJ. Assessment of claims of short- and long-term complications associated with onychectomy in cats. *J Am Vet Med Assoc.* 2001;219(7):932–937.

28 Herbst M. *Behavioural ecology and population genetics of the African wild cat, Felis silvestris Forster 1870, in the southern Kalahari* (Doctoral dissertation, University of Pretoria) 2010. https://repository.up.ac.za/bitstream/handle/2263/28963/Complete.pdf?sequence=6 (accessed February 27, 2022).

29 Zajac FE. Thigh muscle activity during maximum-height jumps by cats. *J Neurophysiol.* 1985;53(4):979–994.

30 MunchkinCat. Can munchkin cats jump? *Munchkin Cat Guide* 2019. https://www. munchkincatguide.com/can-munchkin-cats-jump (accessed July 26, 2020).

31 Hart BL, Hart LA. *Your ideal cat: Insights into breed and gender differences in cat behavior.* Purdue University Press; 2013.

32 Hall SL, Bradshaw JW. The influence of hunger on object play by adult domestic cats. *Appl Anim Behav Sci.* 1998;58(1–2):143–150.

33 Hall SL, Bradshaw JW, Robinson IH. Object play in adult domestic cats: The roles of habituation and disinhibition. *Appl Anim Behav Sci.* 2002;79(3):263–271.

13

The Senior Cat

Gina Davis and Ilana Halperin

Introduction

What is a "senior" cat and why do we need a chapter devoted entirely to their behavior problems?

The American Animal Hospital Association/American Association of Feline Practitioners (AAHA/AAFP) guidelines suggest that cats be classified as "mature" at 7–10 years and "senior" at over 10 years of age.[1] As our understanding of the medical and social needs of cats has progressed, we are better able to care for our feline companions, keeping them healthier for a longer period of time; thus, the aging companion feline population is growing. In 2016, it was estimated that there were 58.4 million pet cats in the US.[2] Over 18% of these cats were over 11 years of age. This finding represents an increase in geriatric (>11 years old) cat ownership compared to prior years (10.6% in 1987, 11% in 1991, 13.3% in 1996, 16.8% in 2001) and a slight decrease compared to 2011 (20.4%).[2] This same study found that 76% of respondents view their pet cats as "family members," 20% viewed them as "companions," and only 4% see them as "property." [2] An understanding of the specific needs of geriatric cats is increasingly necessary to better serve this cherished population.

How can we know which of these aging cats is struggling in some way? We know that, as seen in Figure 13.1, a cat may appear "normal" to the owner and still be experiencing challenges. As with any other animal, we explore their situations through careful history taking! We have been trained to use the behavior of companion animals to provide us clues about their general health. While some history questions are more objective and factual, such as, "How many times did she vomit?" other questions rely on observations of the animal – "What is your cat doing when it wanders around the house? And how often does that happen?" When we gather the information from our history and physical exam, then compile a problem list and differential diagnoses, we can expect to see multifaceted and overlapping information.

Is It Medical or Behavioral?

When considering a senior pet, it is especially important to avoid the pitfall of asking the question: Is this problem medical *or* behavioral? The answer will usually be "both."

That said, there are conditions that may be medical with behavioral manifestations. Identifying and addressing these medical conditions is critical in the management of the geriatric feline patient. Most of the commonly seen medical conditions present a complex array of behavioral clinical signs, some of which overlap with primarily behavior-based conditions. Failure to identify

Clinical Handbook of Feline Behavior Medicine, First Edition. Edited by Elizabeth Stelow.
© 2023 John Wiley & Sons, Inc. Published 2023 by John Wiley & Sons, Inc.
Companion Website: www.wiley.com/go/stelow/behavior

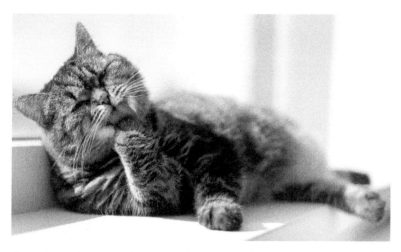

Figure 13.1   Older cats deserve special consideration as we examine them for medical and behavioral issues. Iakov Kalinin / Adobe Stock

these medical conditions which underlie behavior changes, and thereby failure to take advantage of opportunities to initiate appropriate medical therapy leaves the clinician at a disadvantage.

A change in behavior is often the client's first indication that a change in health has occurred. The presence of specific behaviors can guide the clinician toward consideration of differential diagnoses and can aid in selection of appropriate diagnostics. Common medical diseases of senior cats that have predominantly behavioral manifestations include osteoarthritis, chronic kidney disease, cognitive dysfunction, dental/periodontal disease, hyperthyroid disease, neoplasia, and loss of vision and hearing.[3] The most common behavioral problems reported in cats are inappropriate house soiling, anxiety, aggression, excessive vocalization, and changes in mentation/personality.[3-6] As always, appropriate treatment requires investigation into the presenting clinical signs to identify the underlying cause.

This chart compiles many of the common medical or physical problems that afflict senior cats and the behavior presentations that owners report.

Medical diagnosis	Behavioral signs
Osteoarthritis	Hiding, decreased grooming (may be localized), reduced activity, reduced climbing and jumping, changes in frequency and character of vocalizations
CKD	Loss of house training (along with increased drinking, increase volume and frequency of urination), increased vocalizations
Feline cognitive dysfunction	Disorientation, reduce social interactions, sleep–wake cycle disturbances, loss of housetraining, increased anxiety
Dental/Periodontal disease	Reduced grooming, reduced socialization, reduced appetite/food prehension
Hyperthyroid disease	Increased vocalization, increased activity/agitation, increased appetite, possible loss of house training, (along with increased drinking, increased volume and frequency of urination).
Diabetes mellitus	Reduced jumping, loss of house training (along with increased drinking, increased volume and frequency of urination).

(Continued)

(Continued)

Medical diagnosis	Behavioral signs
Systemic hypertension	Nighttime vocalization, disorientation, lethargy, seizures
Neoplasia	Pain = restlessness, vocalization, aggression, self-trauma, and altered sleep cycles
	Intestinal Lymphoma = house soiling and restlessness (from nausea and diarrhea)
	Meningioma = altered consciousness, seizures, vestibular dysfunction, compulsive behaviors, unprovoked aggression, disorientation, fear, anxiety, loss of learned behaviors, house soiling, altered activity, vocalization, and altered sleep cycles
	Renal Tumors = pain signs (above), loss of house training
Loss of vision	Disorientation, reluctance to jump, unwillingness to go outside, loss of house training, anxiety, changes in cognition, aggression, and nighttime vocalization

This chart lists the most common behavior problems reported in senior cats, along with the medical differentials that should be considered.

Behavioral diagnosis	Common medical differentials
Anxiety	Pain (arthritis, dental, neoplasia, etc.), loss of special senses, feline cognitive dysfunction, hyperthyroid disease, loss of vision or hearing
Excessive vocalization	Hyperthyroid disease, pain
Aggression	Pain, neoplasia
House soiling	Any medical cause of polyuria/polydipsia, osteoarthritis, history of lower urinary tract disease

This chapter presents:

- An approach to the geriatric feline veterinary visit, with a focus on history taking, the actual physical examination, and diagnostics to consider
- The most common medical problems with behavioral manifestations in senior cats
- The most common primary behavior issues in senior cats, along with their medical differentials.

Approach to the Geriatric Feline Visit

The overall approach to examining the senior cat is not markedly different from that of other age groups or other species. What bears emphasizing, however, is those medial and behavioral problems that are considerably more common in this age group than in others.

Client Interview/Patient History

As with all patients, a thorough history is an essential first step when a senior cat presents for behavior changes. American Animal Hospital Association (AAHA) and American Association of Feline Practitioners (AAFP) have published senior care guidelines recommending that practitioners include behavioral history as part of the visit.[6,7] Therefore, additional investigation into the following areas is recommended when evaluating the senior feline patient:

- For all senior patients, ask about changes in:
  - Sleep/wake patterns
  - Sleeping locations
  - Play behavior
  - Changes in vocalization – tone and frequency or pattern
  - Appetite – probe for not only how much the patient eats, but when and how they eat, and if modifications need to be made to the diet to ensure that a full meal is ingested. The need for addition of dressings or treats to encourage a patient to ingest a complete meal may be overlooked if clients simply respond "yes" or "no" to whether the pet is eating as much as usual.
  - Mobility (ability to jump onto surfaces, climb into boxes, navigate stairs, etc.)
  - Socializing with people and other pets
- Senior patients with a specific presenting complaint
  - Age of onset of the condition
  - Progression of the condition
  - Interventions attempted and their results

One way to assess these factors is to provide the clients with a questionnaire to complete at each visit. It would contain the types of changes that are most likely to occur in a senior cat and could be compared from visit to visit to look for changes. A second questionnaire can screen specifically for cognitive dysfunction.

Physical Exam

While a complete physical exam is recommended for all patients, the exam for senior cat patients should emphasize the following:

- Orthopedic exam to uncover possible osteoarthritis, skeletal pain
- Careful evaluation of hydration status. This can be difficult in underconditioned animals; include mucous membrane moisture, tear film evaluation where necessary
- Palpation of cervical region for thyroid nodules
- Evaluation of muscle mass to determine Muscle Condition Score in addition to Body Condition Score, since sarcopenia is common in older cats.

Diagnostics

In addition to a complete blood count, serum biochemistry panel, and urinalysis, the minimum database for senior cats should include blood pressure measurement. A total T4 should be considered, depending on the history and physical exam findings. Further, a B12 assay should be considered, as hypocobaliminemia may be an indication of emerging or current infiltrative bowel disease.[8,9]

Urinalysis obtained via cystocentesis and urine culture are essential in ruling out urinary tract infection and should be considered depending on patient presenting complaint (periuria, dysuria, hematuria) and presence of concurrent diseases; patients with neoplasia or diabetes mellitus are predisposed to urinary tract infection.[10,11] Urine sediment analysis should ideally be used in conjunction with urine aerobic culture and sensitivity to help confirm suspicion of infection, identify antimicrobial resistant bacteria, and document the type of bacteria found, which is helpful in differentiating between reinfection and relapse when treating subsequent infection.[10] Patient history is used to differentiate between UTI and bacteriuria or pyuria without clinically significant infection.[10]

Imaging (abdominal ultrasound or thoracic radiographs) may be indicated based on presenting complaints, history, physical exam findings, and minimum database results.

Specific Medical Diagnoses with Behavioral Signs

As previously noted, the most common causes of behavior changes in the senior cats are osteoarthritis, cognitive dysfunction, hypertension/chronic kidney disease, hyperthyroidism, diabetes mellitus, loss of special senses, and meningiomas.[4] These, along with dental disease, are discussed below, with a focus on the behavioral presentations.

Osteoarthritis

Osteoarthritis is one of the most common age-related feline diseases. One study of 100 client-owned cats found that 61% of cats over the age of 6 years had osteoarthritis in the appendicular skeleton.[12] This same study found that 48% of the surveyed cats had osteoarthritis in more than one joint.[12] Another study found that 90% of cats greater than 12 yo had radiographic evidence of degenerative joint disease.[12,13]

Osteoarthritis may go underrecognized in cats in comparison to dogs due to the challenges presented in performing a complete mobility assessment of a cat in the hospital. We often do not have the opportunity to observe feline patients ambulating, as the cat in Figure 13.2 is doing, in the exam room. Diagnosis is further complicated by both the typically gradual onset of clinical signs related to osteoarthritis and frequent lack of overt lameness in the cat.[13–15]

Another obstacle to identification of osteoarthritis is client perception that these signs may be due to "normal aging."[16,17] Additionally, cats can be inactive for up to 80% of the day,[18] leaving little opportunity for the owners to observe changes in their cat's mobility.

Behavior-Related Signs

Typical behavior-related clinical signs reported by owners of cats with osteoarthritis include:

- Hiding
- Urination and defecation outside the litter box or on furniture
- Decreases in overall grooming or increased grooming of particular areas
- Changes in the manner of claw-sharpening (e.g., on horizontal instead of vertical surfaces)
- Poorer mood
- Change in frequency (both increased and decreased) of interactions with family members
- Decreased play and tolerance of interactions with other household animals and reduced independent play and hunting behaviors

Figure 13.2 Cats with osteoarthritis are prone to many behavioral changes. Roman / Adobe Stock

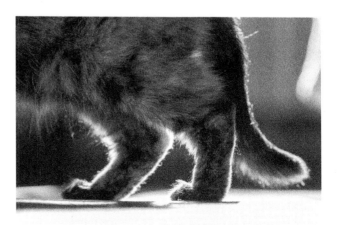

- Changes in character and frequency of vocalizations
- Reduction in head- or body-rubbing behavior.[17,19]

Another study demonstrated associations between presence of osteoarthritis and increased time spent sleeping, reduced willingness to go outside, reduced appetite, reduced time spent grooming, increased sociability with people, decreased sociability with other animals, increased agitation/irritation, and increased vocalization both at night and during the day.[20]

Diagnostic Criteria

These findings suggest that clinicians may improve the rate of identification of feline osteoarthritis by means of completing a thorough behavioral history, including targeted questions investigating the cat's grooming, scratching behavior, as well as interactions with humans and other pets in the household, and toileting behaviors.

While cats are notoriously skilled at compensating for and hiding signs of chronic pain,[13,19] and a complete mobility exam may be hampered by feline patients' tendency to be reluctant to ambulate in the exam room, a careful orthopedic examination, followed by radiographs when indicated by examination findings, are key in aiding in identification of feline osteoarthritis.[11,19,21]

Treatment

Once osteoarthritis has been identified, appropriate pain management may improve unwanted behaviors. Environmental modifications such as lowering litter-box edges may assist cats with osteoarthritis who have difficulty entering a litter box and therefore may reduce unwanted toileting behaviors.[1] In addition, a high-sided box with a low entrance will contain the urine of a cat whose osteoarthritis prevents it from crouching while eliminating.

Chronic Kidney Disease

Incidence of chronic kidney disease (CKD) has been reported to be from 28% in cats over 12 years of age to 80.9% in cats over 15 years of age.[22,23]

Behavior-Related Signs

Most clinicians are familiar with typical signs of CKD including weight loss and polyuria/polydipsia. One study found a statistically significant association between CKD and the following:[20]

- increased vocalization both during the day and the night
- increased house-soiling
- increased agitation/irritation
- decreased sociability with other animals
- being more sociable with people
- a decrease in willingness to go outside.

There are several reasons that polyuria and polydipsia can lead to toileting issues.[1,20,24] Cats with renal disease produce more urine; if cat owners do not keep up with litter box cleaning duties, this will create an unfavorable litter-box environment. With more rapid bladder filling, urgency and urge incontinence may contribute to house soiling. This may be exacerbated by the presence of osteoarthritis, which may cause decreased mobility and reluctance to enter challenging litter boxes (see previous section) in individuals affected by both osteoarthritis and renal disease (see Figure 13.3).

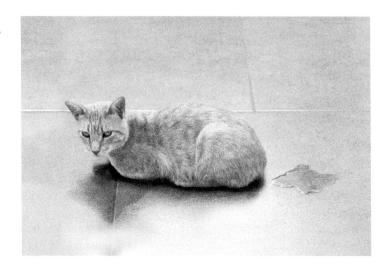

Feline Cognitive Dysfunction Syndrome

Cognitive Dysfunction Syndrome (CDS) is a progressive neurodegenerative disease. Brain changes include loss of neurons, amyloid deposits, cerebral atrophy, and ventricular enlargement. While CDS is considered a diagnosis of exclusion, it may be comorbid with other medical and behavioral diagnoses.[25–28]

Behavior-Related Signs

Signs of cognitive decline may start in the early senior years; but owners may not recognize these mild signs. It is important for clinicians to obtain a thorough history for every senior cat, regardless of the presenting complaint. The most noted clinical signs are changes in the sleep–wake patterns, changes in the social relationship of the cat and other members of the household, increased vocalization, changes in elimination habits, signs of disorientation or confusion, and changes in activity levels.[4,29]

Demonstration of clinical signs is more apparent in the older cat. As many as 50% of cats older than 15 years of age will show signs of cognitive decline, compared to 28% of cats between 11–14 years of age.[4,30] The list given above is a comprehensive list of common clinical signs for cats with CDS, but these signs can vary by age. The most common signs in the older group of cats are alterations in activity and excessive vocalization; the most common sign in the younger group of cats is an alteration in social interactions.[30]

Diagnostic Criteria

Purina Institute created an informational brochure and questionnaire for clinicians and owners to be able to recognize and document signs of cognitive impairment. It can be used to track the progression of signs over time when assessed at each semi-annual exam. The categories for DISHAA are as follows:

- (D)isorientation
- Social (I)nteractions
- (S)leep/Wake Cycles
- (H)ouse soiling, Learning, and Memory
- (A)ctivity
- (A)nxiety

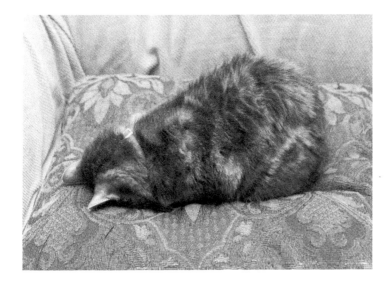

Figure 13.4 Signs of feline cognitive dysfunction may be subtle (see Figure 13.4) and are often noted as behavior changes rather than any specific troubling behavior.

With specific questions in each section, these are given a number score from none (0) to severe (3). The tabulated results will allow the clinician to assess the cat's level of cognitive decline from mild to moderate to severe. With early identification, the clinician and owner can work together to slow the progression of the decline and improve the cat's quality of life.[30]

Treatment

Treatment is designed to address the specific clinical signs that the cat is manifesting and is adjusted as necessary over time. Management strategies should be created to help with any changes or restrictions in mobility or activity levels; these include use of stairs or ramps to help with climbing, or baby gates to prevent access to areas where confusion or lack of stability could result in an injury. Litter boxes may need to be moved or altered to manage house soiling issues. Environmental enrichment and attention to schedules will be important to help with learning and memory, social interactions, and anxiety. Purposeful engagement with the cat throughout the day will provide mental stimulation and help to maintain appropriate daytime/nighttime sleeping schedules.[2,4,25,29]

There are no approved medications for the treatment of cognitive dysfunction in cats. But, there are two drugs approved for dogs that can be used for cats in an off-label fashion:

- *Selegiline* is a selective irreversible inhibitor of monoamine oxidase B (MAOB) approved for use in North America. The mode of action in dogs is not clear. It cannot be used with drugs or supplements that may increase serotonin such as SSRIs, TCAs, Tramadol, Buspirone, and most narcotics. Off label use in cats has shown beneficial results in the areas of disorientation, vocalization, and decreased interest in affection at a dose of 0.5 to 1 mg/kg per day.[25]
- *Propentofylline* is a xanthine derivative which may improve microcirculation. It is licensed for use in some countries (not in North America) for signs of senility which may include lethargy, tiredness, and mental dullness. Anecdotally it has been used in cats at a dose of 12.5 mg orally every 12 hours.[4,25,26]

Natural supplements labeled for cats may be preferable, given the lack of approval or extensive use of the above medications.

- Diets for cats >7 years of age aim to address oxidative stress and damage. Clinicians may consider recommending diets which are supplemented with fish oil, ascorbic acid, B vitamins, antioxidants, and arginine to slow the progression of cognitive decline.[4,25]
- Senilife is an ingredient blend labeled for use in cats that contains phosphatidylserine which is an important building block of cell membranes that may facilitate neuronal signal transduction and enhance cholinergic transmission.[25,29] This supplement has been shown to improve cognition in dogs in both clinical and laboratory studies. Ginkgo biloba, vitamin E, and resveratrol, and vitamin B6 are additional ingredients in Senilife.
- Activait, another feline labeled supplement, contains phosphatidylserine, omega-3 fatty acids, vitamins E and C, L-carnitine, coenzyme Q, and selenium. Although there are no adequate studies in cats, studies on dogs have shown improvement in the areas of social interactions, disorientation, and house soiling.
- Cholodin-Fel contains choline, phosphatidylcholine, methionine, inositol, vitamin E, zinc, selenium, taurine, and B vitamins.[30]

Dental/Periodontal Disease

Although periodontal and endodontal disease is found in cats of all ages, in patients with a lack of preventive or regular periodontal care, the accumulation of plaque, calculus (see Figure 13.5), and bone loss over time contribute to an increased incidence of dental disease in older cats.[31] One study found that while 50% of cats over age 4 years had periodontal disease affecting at least one tooth, that number increased to 93% of cats over age 8 years.[32]

Behavior-Related Signs

The most common behavior-related clinical signs associated with periodontal disease in cats were:[20]

- reduced time spent grooming
- decreased sociability with other animals
- reduced appetite

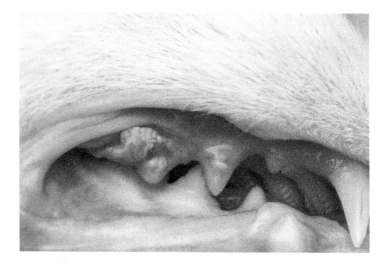

Figure 13.5 Painful dental or periodontal disease can strike at any age; but the senior cat that has lacked routine dental care is most predisposed.

Oral pain can also cause nighttime vocalization.[33] It is important to note that the clinical signs associated with periodontal disease can be subtle and are not exclusive to periodontal disease.[34]

In one author's experience, cats may eat well despite significant periodontal disease; so any patient presenting for evaluation decreased appetite should be thoroughly evaluated, without jumping to the conclusion that periodontal disease, even if present, is the sole cause of the hyporexia. The clinician may be more inclined to move periodontal disease up the rank of the differential diagnoses list for cats presenting with apparently normal appetites, but who have been observed to be hesitant in eating; unable to prehend, masticate, or swallow food; not grooming well; ptyalism; preferentially chewing on one side of the mouth; dropping food from the mouth; or avoiding hard foods.[35]

Diagnostic Criteria

Because multiple age-related diseases may present with the nonspecific signs of reduced grooming and appetite and decreased sociability with other animals, these patients require a thorough workup. Kidney disease, neoplasia, and pain related to osteoarthritis may result in decreased appetite. Osteoarthritis and cognitive dysfunction may cause cats to spend less time grooming, and decreased sociability with other animals can be seen as a result of osteoarthritic pain, kidney disease, neoplasia, cognitive dysfunction, or loss of special senses. Accordingly, evaluation of these patients should include a careful oral exam, orthopedic exam, CBC, chemistry panel, and urinalysis at a minimum.

Hyperthyroid Disease

Hyperthyroid disease is one of the most commonly diagnosed age-related diseases of cats.[36] In the United States, hyperthyroid disease is actually the most common endocrine disorder of older cats, found in 10% of cats over the age of 10 years.[37] In comparison, worldwide, hyperthyroidism is found in 1.5–11.4% of senior cats.[36,37]

Typical clinical signs associated with hyperthyroid disease include weight loss, polyphagia, polyuria, polydipsia, increased vocalization, agitation, increased activity, tachypnea, tachycardia, vomiting, diarrhea, aggression, and an unkempt hair coat.[36,38]

Behavior-Related Signs

As hyperthyroidism manifests in behavioral changes, clients may note:

- Increased nighttime vocalization[33]
- Agitation
- Increased activity
- Elimination outside of the litterbox due to polyuria and polydipsia or diarrhea.

As was discussed in the section devoted to renal disease, a polydipsic/polyuric cat requires more frequent cleaning of the litter box; if cat owners are not keeping up with the cat's increased urination, the result will be an unfavorable litter-box environment. Increased bladder filling may lead to urgency and urge incontinence may contribute to house soiling. The same may be true of diarrhea.

A survey summarizing client responses to a questionnaire about pet feline health, with data gathered from 2010 to 2015, also showed that hyperthyroid disease in cats was associated with increased vocalization during the day and night, polydipsia, reduced appetite, reduced time spent grooming, and less willingness to go outside.[20]

Diagnostic Criteria

If left untreated, hyperthyroid disease can result in thyrotoxic heart disease,[36,39] gastrointestinal disease (typically diarrhea and vomiting),[36,40] and exacerbation or progression of kidney disease via activation of the renin–angiotensin–aldosterone system; increased glomerular capillary pressure and proteinuria in cats with hyperthyroidism may contribute to progression of renal disease.[36,41,42]

Considering how common and how treatable hyperthyroid disease is in older cats – and considering the adverse effects of leaving the disease untreated – ruling out hyperthyroid disease as a potential cause of increased vocalization, toileting issues, reduced time spent grooming, weight loss, or increased activity is an important first step.

Diagnosis of hyperthyroid disease involves demonstration of persistently elevated thyroid hormone concentrations (T4, or T4 plus free T4 by equilibrium dialysis [fT4ed]) along with presence of one or more of the typical clinical signs associated with hyperthyroid disease. Those clinical signs are:[36]

- Weight Loss
- Polyphagia
- Polyuria
- Polydipsia
- Increased vocalization
- Agitation or increased activity
- Tachypnea, tachycardia
- Vomiting, diarrhea
- Unkempt hair coat
- Apathy, inappetence, lethargy

Careful inquiry into activity level and patterns of vocalization, as well as changes in thirst, urination, and presence of vomiting or diarrhea should be included in history collection.

The physical exam in senior cats must include palpation of the thyroid glands. The clinician must take into consideration that lack of a palpable thyroid nodule does not rule out hyperthyroid disease, because ectopic thyroid tissue may be present in approximately 4–9% of hyperthyroid cats.[36,43] One study of 2096 cats with hyperthyroidism found that 3.9% of them had ectopic thyroid tissue.[43] Conversely, palpation of enlarged thyroid glands should raise suspicion of hyperthyroid disease, but is not always indicative of hyperthyroid disease, as cats may have non-functional adenomas.[44–46] Finally, asymmetry of thyroid glands and increasing size of the thyroid nodule are more likely to indicate hyperthyroid disease.[45,46]

Body weight should be recorded at each visit and any notation of weight loss, even if the patient's body condition score is still within normal limits (see Figure 13.6) should always be accompanied by an inquiry into changes in feeding and appetite.[36,47]

Figure 13.6 Hyperthyroid disease is a common cause of behavior changes in geriatric cats. Photo courtesy of Pixabay.

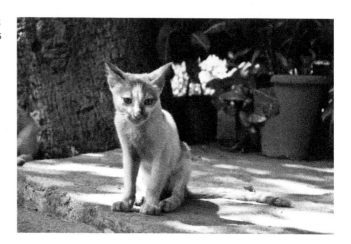

As mentioned previously, suspicion of hyperthyroid disease should be confirmed via careful history and physical exam (body and muscle condition score, cardiac auscultation, palpation of thyroid nodules), evaluation of CBC, Chemistry panel, and Urinalysis, which will provide further information regarding systemic health, and as is important prior to beginning treatment for hyperthyroid disease, a better understanding of renal function.

In terms of specific hormonal testing to rule hyperthyroid disease in or out, total T4 alone is sufficient to confirm hyperthyroid disease in more than 90% of hyperthyroid cats.[42,48,49] If clinical signs and history are consistent with hyperthyroid disease, and a single total T4 measurement is within the normal reference range, it is worth investigating for other underlying diseases and retesting total T4 in several weeks, as normal fluctuations of thyroid hormones or concurrent disease in cats with early or mild hyperthyroidism may cause random total T4 measurements to fall within the reference interval.[36,42] Measurement of free T4 and TSH evaluated in conjunction with total T4 may be necessary in some cases.[36,42]

Because hyperthyroid disease is often accompanied by hypertension, measurement of blood pressure is indicated. Because veterinary-visit related stress may contribute to artificial increases in blood pressure, performing a fundic exam to investigate for hypertensive retinopathy is also helpful.[36]

Diabetes Mellitus

While there are multiple risk factors associated with development of diabetes mellitus, cats over the age of 7 years have been found to be at higher risk.[50]

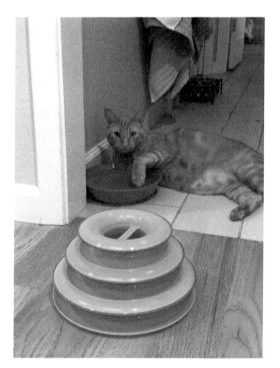

Figure 13.7 Increased water consumption and the volume/frequency of urination are only two of the behavioral signs of diabetes in the older cat. Photo courtesy of Liz Stelow.

Behavior-Related Signs

Behavioral changes may include:

- Signs of polyuria/polydipsia
- Reduced jumping
- Reduced litter-box use

Cat owners may report changes in resting places (see Figure 13.7), if the diabetic cat's ability to jump has been impaired by diabetic distal neuropathy.[51] As discussed in the section on chronic kidney disease, polyuria and polydipsia can lead to urination outside of the litter box.[8] Diabetes can also contribute to house soiling issues if the diabetic cat develops diabetic distal neuropathy, which can make it difficult for cats to climb into high sided litter boxes.[51]

Diagnosis

For cats presenting to the veterinarian with the above behavioral signs, the possibility of diabetes mellitus can be investigated by including the following:

- Thorough history and physical examination including questioning about toileting habits and changes in activity level and inquiries

into whether the cat is able to jump and if the cat is spending time in different areas of the house, as well as gait analysis to assess for plantigrade stance
- Serum biochemistry and evaluation of blood glucose
- Complete urinalysis, ideally with culture (especially if there is an active sediment)
- Serum fructosamine if blood glucose levels are not clearly indicative of hyperglycemia
- Serum T4 to rule out hyperthyroidism.[50]

Systemic Hypertension

Systemic hypertension can occur as a primary disease or in association with chronic kidney disease or hyperthyroid disease.[50] Studies have found rates of hypertension in otherwise apparently healthy cats to be 13%,[52] in cats with CKD to be from <25%[53] to 65%,[54] and in cats with hyperthyroid disease to be 10–90%.[55] This wide variety of results may be due to artifact; cats are typically anxious in the hospital setting and this anxiety has been shown to result in elevated blood pressure readings.[53–56]

Behavior-Related Signs

Behavioral signs that may be indicative of hypertension include:

- Nighttime vocalization[33]
- Disorientation
- Lethargy
- Seizures secondary to hypertensive encephalopathy.[57]

For this reason, older cats presenting with these signs should undergo blood pressure measurement as well as screening for common underlying diseases that can cause hypertension: kidney disease and hyperthyroid disease.[55]

Neoplasia

The category of neoplasia encompasses a multitude of conditions. For the purposes of this discussion, it is therefore useful to list clinical signs associated with common types of neoplasia in geriatric cats. Neoplasia may be associated with pain, diarrhea, nausea/vomiting, inappetence, and depression.[33,58–60] Behavioral changes linked to pain from neoplasia include decreased activity, restlessness, vocalization, aggression, self-trauma, and altered sleep cycles.[5]

One of the most common forms of neoplasia in cats is lymphoma, with alimentary lymphoma being the most common form.[61,62] Behavioral changes associated with gastrointestinal disease involving nausea and diarrhea include house soiling and restlessness.[5]

The most common primary brain tumor found in cats is meningioma[63] followed by intracranial lymphoma.[64,65] Clinical signs associated with meningioma include altered consciousness, seizures, and vestibular dysfunction.[64] Unlike dogs, cats are more likely to have partial or complex seizures, which may present as compulsive behavior, unprovoked aggression, disorientation, fear, or anxiety.[65,66] Behavioral clinical signs caused by CNS disease include loss of learned behaviors, house soiling, altered activity levels or consciousness, vocalization, increases in fear or anxiety, and altered sleep cycles.[28,64]

Tumors affecting the urinary tract of cats include renal lymphoma (the most commonly seen urinary tract neoplasm in cats), followed by transitional cell carcinoma,[67] which is rarely seen but warrants mention as it may contribute to lower urinary tract signs and abdominal pain,[67] which may be associated with behavioral changes, as bladder neoplasia may contribute to house soiling.[20]

Diagnosis

Elements in the patient history and physical exam that may lead to a suspicion of neoplasia include weight loss, house soiling, vomiting, diarrhea, masses, decreased energy, or peripheral lymphade-nopathy. Serum biochemistry may reveal hypercalcemia or hyperglobulinemia. CBC may reveal anemia (typically nonregenerative but in the case of a mass that may be bleeding, a regenerative anemia may be identified). Diagnosis of neoplasia can seldom be made based history or physical exam alone. Imaging may begin with thoracic radiographs and abdominal ultrasound to identify lymphadenopathy, effusions, or masses (either primary or metastatic). Endoscopy or laparotomy and biopsy may be needed to diagnose alimentary lymphoma. If bone pain is identified on physical exam, targeted radiographs of those areas may be pursued. Fine needle aspirate or biopsy are necessary for characterization of masses or lymphadenopathy. If bone marrow involvement is sus-pected, bone marrow aspirate or biopsy may be indicated.

Loss of Vision

Reduction or loss in vision can occur at any time; but it is most common in geriatric cats. And the clinical signs are entirely behavioral.

Behavior-Related Signs

Behavioral changes associated with blindness may be reactions to the blindness itself or may be secondary to a primary disease causing blindness such as a forebrain lesion[66] or hypertension that has caused retinal detachment.[67] Changes directly attributable to blindness may include disorien-tation, reluctance to jump,[66,67] or unwillingness to go outside.[66] Cats with behavioral changes attributed to blindness itself may also present with house soiling,[9,66] anxiety, changes in cognition, aggression,[8] and nighttime vocalization.[33] When blindness is secondary to a brain lesion, cat owners may report personality changes, aggression, loss of learned habits, house soiling, restless-ness, and compulsive behaviors.[66] Many of these signs might easily be mistaken for signs of osteo-arthritis, cognitive dysfunction, or seen by cat owners as "just slowing down with age."

Diagnosis

A thorough evaluation of a cat with any of the above presenting complaints involves ruling in or out blindness. This includes measurement of systemic blood pressure, and if hypertension is found, investigating for diseases commonly associated with hypertension (hyperthyroid disease and chronic kidney disease) as described previously. In cats who present with reluctance to jump or go outdoors, a thorough orthopedic exam and, if indicated, radiographs, can help differentiate bet-ween decreased vision and orthopedic disease. Inability to jump may be due to diabetic neurop-athy, as discussed in the section on diabetes mellitus, and thus ruling out that disease for these cats is important. Finally, in order to rule out intracranial disease, a neurologic exam including evalu-ation of mentation, gait, postural reactions, and cranial nerve examination is important.[66]

Specific Behavioral Diagnoses and Their Medical Differentials

As stated before, medical conditions often first become apparent to owners based on changes in behaviors. What, then, of behavior changes that do not appear to have a medical cause? Sometimes behavior changes are caused by motivations that are emotional rather than physiologic in nature. The "behavior" diagnoses considered here include anxiety, excessive vocalization, aggression (toward people or other cats), and house soiling (both toileting and urine marking). Other possible behavior changes, like changes in sleeping or eating habits were considered above, since they are most likely to have medical causes.

Anxiety

Anxiety is a commonly diagnosed behavioral problems affecting dogs and cats.[3,68] Anxiety is defined as the emotional anticipation of an adverse event, i.e. it is the anticipation of something unpleasant that may or may not be real.[69] We often use the term broadly, but it is important to be specific when we are using it for a diagnosis. The pet may have a situational anxiety related to a particular occurrence, such as confinement (crate) anxiety or veterinary visit anxiety, or it may have a broader diagnosis such as separation anxiety or generalized anxiety.

Signs of anxiety in a senior cat include:

- Restlessness or pacing
- Vocalization (whining, crying, hissing)
- Avoidance behaviors (hiding, withdrawn)
- Clingy behaviors (attention seeking, following)
- Irritability (with other individuals, with handling)

Senior cats may develop signs of anxiety later in life, without having had the same concerns previously, or mild and subclinical anxiety may worsen. Physical challenges, decreased comfort, sensory decline, and household changes may lead to decreased adaptability. In the senior cat, pain (regardless of source) is the primary medical cause to be considered. See Chapter 7 for more information.

Owners of senior cats who have never previously addressed anxiety issues, will need to understand the role of environment and household changes in their cat's anxiety. Keeping the environment and routines as consistent as possible will be very important. Acknowledge and reward the desired behaviors and ignore and try to prevent the undesirable behaviors. Medications such as gabapentin, fluoxetine, or benzodiazepines may be considered as well. Please see Chapter 8 for more information.

Excessive Vocalization

Excessive vocalization may be reported by owners when is it especially loud or when it occurs at unacceptable times. The clinician is tasked with determining the cause of this problem. In general, behavioral reasons may include the solicitation of resources such as food or attention, reactions or threats to outside stimuli, or sexual behavior.[70] Top medical rule outs include pain related conditions, sensory changes such as vision or hearing loss, or metabolic diseases such as hyperthyroidism, all of which are addressed above.[4,25]

When medical conditions have been ruled out or otherwise addressed, the clinician will need to consider behavioral causes or comorbidities. Anxiety, cognitive decline, or attention seeking are the most likely diagnoses.[4,25,71] Additionally, even when a medical condition has been successfully treated, the excessive vocalization may persist and will need to be addressed and managed.

History will provide important information to help determine the potential causes. Questions about the time of day, frequency, environment, presence of other household members, and the owner's response provide important details.

If anxiety or CDS appear to be the most likely cause, please see the sections above that address those topics. In addition, the owner should be aware that anxiety about changes in the routine, presence or absence of household members, outside environmental factors, and concomitant medical or sensory changes may be influencing factors for either of those diagnoses.

For the attention-seeking cat, management will be an important part of the treatment plan. Ensure all of the cat's physical needs are being met, including necessary adjustments for physical ability changes. The senior cat may have different social needs compared to when she was younger. Structure and routine are very important for anxious individuals. Consider adjustments for different styles of play and include food toy enrichment options. Take care to avoid unwittingly reinforcing the behavior by giving the cat attention, rather try to anticipate when she may be prone to showing the behavior and try to engage the cat in a desirable activity.[25]

Anxiolytics or medications to help promote sleep may be indicated.

Aggression

When cats display aggression, it may not be readily apparent to the owners. Particularly with inter-cat aggression, silent and intimidating body language directed toward the other household cat(s) may be displayed. Owners commonly misidentify which cat is the bully and which cat is the victim. When the target is a human, the behaviors may be more obvious, but the reasons may be unclear. Please see Chapters 10 and 11 for more information.

Aggression is even more challenging when the first signs develop when the cat becomes a senior. There may be many intersecting factors to consider, including medical conditions causing discomfort or pain, and those that may cause the cat to feel lethargic, nauseated, etc. These medical conditions may lead to increased irritability and decreased tolerance.[68] Less commonly, aggression may result from endocrine imbalances like hepatic encephalopathy or toxic/infection causes like toxoplasmosis or heavy metal ingestion.[38]

Changes commonly experienced with age including physical discomfort, sensory changes or decline, and household changes may cause increased anxiety and fear, leading to aggression in some circumstances.

Even if a physical medical condition has been diagnosed and treated or managed, the clinician will still need to provide guidance for behavioral management and behavior modification ± behavioral medications.

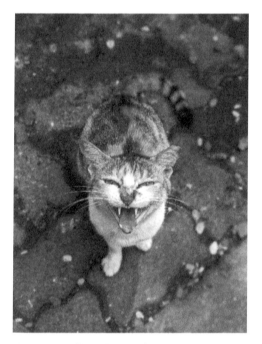

Figure 13.8 Excessive vocalization (see Figure 13.8) in the senior cat has many possible causes – some medical and some behavioral. Photo courtesy of Unsplash.

House Soiling

Elimination outside of the litter box may be a significant behavioral clinical sign of a medical problem for any cat, but particularly important for senior cats. The issue may start because of a medical illness but can persist for behavioral reasons. For example, a cat may have diarrhea that causes frequent and painful defecation and if he experiences pain while inside of the litter box, an aversion to using that box may develop and persist. For this reason, it is important for the clinician to develop a behavior treatment plan in addition to any medical treatments.

Pain is often underdiagnosed in cats. Previous pain while eliminating in a litter box and/or pain related to accessing and using the litter box may lead a cat to choose to eliminate in a different place. The clinician will need to take a thorough history to help the client recognize the impacts pain may have on the toileting problem. Pain management must be incorporated in the behavior treatment plan.

Sensory changes may also impact the proper use of the litter box. As vision declines, it may cause the cat to become more resistant to going to use a litter box in a dimly lit area. Sensory decline can also lead to increased anxiety which can impact where the cat chooses to go within the house.

For further information on house soiling issues, please see Chapter 6.

Summary

When evaluating the senior cat, there are multiple intersecting factors to consider. Medical illnesses and changes in behavior need to be viewed collectively to create complete diagnostic and treatment plans. A careful and detailed history, in addition to a thorough physical examination, is very important, as is the tracking of behavioral changes from visit to visit. Treatment plans need to address not only the specific medical aspects, but also incorporate any relevant behavioral treatment plan components to fully meet the needs of the senior cat.

Resources for the Companion Website

https://www.purinainstitute.com/science-of-nutrition/advancing-brain-health/cognitive-dysfunction-syndrome

References

1 Quimby J, Gowland S, Carney HC, DePorter T, Plummer P, Westropp J. 2021 AAHA/AAFP feline life stage guidelines. *J Am Anim Hosp Assoc.* 2021;57(2):51–72.
2 AVMA. *AVMA pet ownership and demographics sourcebook: 2017–2018 edition.* 2018.
3 Gunn-Moore DA. Cognitive dysfunction in cats: Clinical assessment and management. *Top Companion Anim Med.* 2011;26(1):17–24.
4 Bamberger M, Houpt KA. Signalment factors, comorbidity, and trends in behavior diagnoses in cats: 736 cases (1991–2001). *J Am Vet Med Assoc.* 2006;229(10):1602–1606.
5 Landsberg GM, DePorter T, Araujo JA. Clinical signs and management of anxiety, sleeplessness, and cognitive dysfunction in the senior pet. *Vet Clin: Small Anim Pract.* 2011;41(3):565–590. Seibert LM, Landsberg GM. Diagnosis and management of patients presenting with behavior problems. *Vet Clin North Am Small Anim Pract.* 2008;937–950. doi:10.1016/j.cvsm.2008.04.001
6 Seibert LM, Landsberg GM. Diagnosis and management of patients presenting with behavior problems. *Vet Clin North Am Small Anim Pract.* 2008;38(5):937–950.
7 American Association of Feline Practitioners. Feline focus–2008 AAFP senior care guidelines. *Compend Contin Educ Vet.* 2009;31(9):402–407.

8   Stelow E. Behavior as an Illness Indicator. *Vet Clin Small Anim Pract.* 2020;50(4):695–706.

9   Laflamme D, Gunn-Moore D. Veterinary clinics of North America: small animal practice. *Nut Aging Cats.* 2014;761–774. doi:10.1016/j.cvsm.2014.03.001.

10 Weese JS, Blondeau JM, Boothe D, Breitschwerdt EB, Guardabassi L, Hillier A, Lloyd DH, Papich MG, Rankin SC, Turnidge JD, Sykes JE. Antimicrobial use guidelines for treatment of urinary tract disease in dogs and cats: Antimicrobial guidelines working group of the international society for companion animal infectious diseases. *Vet Med Int.* 2011;2011:263768.

11 Weese JS, Blondeau J, Boothe D, Guardabassi LG, Gumley N, Papich M, Jessen LR, Lappin M, Rankin S, Westropp JL, Sykes J. International Society for Companion Animal Infectious Diseases (ISCAID) guidelines for the diagnosis and management of bacterial urinary tract infections in dogs and cats. *Vet J.* 2019;247:8–25.

12 Slingerland LI, Hazewinkel HAW, Meij BP, Picavet P, Voorhout G. Cross-sectional study of the prevalence and clinical features of osteoarthritis in 100 cats. *Vet J.* 2011;187(3):304–309.

13 Hardie EM, Roe SC, Martin FR. Radiographic evidence of degenerative joint disease in geriatric cats: 100 cases (1994–1997). *J Am Vet Med Assoc.* 2002;220(5):628–632.

14 Lascelles BDX. Feline degenerative joint disease. *Vet Surg.* 2010;39(1):2–13.

15 Clarke SP, Mellor D, Clements DN, Gemmill T, Farrell M, Carmichael S, Bennett D. Prevalence of radiographic signs of degenerative joint disease in a hospital population of cats. *Vet Rec.* 2005;157(25):793–799.

16 Bennett D., Morton C. A study of owner observed behavioural and lifestyle changes in cats with musculoskeletal disease before and after analgesic therapy. *J Feline Med Surg.* 2009;11(12):997–1004.

17 Klinck MP, Frank D, Guillot M, Troncy E. Owner-perceived signs and veterinary diagnosis in 50 cases of feline osteoarthritis. *Can Vet J.* 2012;53(11):1181.

18 Robertson SA. Moving forward with detecting osteoarthritis in cats. *Vet Rec.* 2019;185(24):754.

19 Hardie EM. Management of osteoarthritis in cats. *Vet Clin North Am: Small Anim Pract.* 1997;27(4):945–953.

20 Sordo L, Breheny C, Halls V, Cotter A, Tørnqvist-Johnsen C, Caney S, Gunn-Moore DA. Prevalence of disease and age-related behavioural changes in cats: Past and present. *Vet Sci.* 2020;7(3):85.

21 Stadig S, Lascelles BDX, Nyman G, Bergh A. Evaluation and comparison of pain questionnaires for clinical screening of osteoarthritis in cats. *Vet Rec.* 2019;185(24):757.

22 Bartlett PC, Van Buren JW, Neterer M, Zhou C. Disease surveillance and referral bias in the veterinary medical database. *Prev. Vet Med* 2010;94(3–4):264–271.

23 Marino CL, Lascelles BDX, Vaden SL, Gruen ME, Marks SL. Prevalence and classification of chronic kidney disease in cats randomly selected from four age groups and in cats recruited for degenerative joint disease studies. *J Feline Med Surg.* 2014;16(6):465–472.

24 Carney HC, Sadek TP, Curtis TM, Halls V, Heath S, Hutchison P, Mundschenk K, Westropp JL. AAFP and ISFM guidelines for diagnosing and solving house-soiling behavior in cats. *J Feline Med Surg.* 2018;20(6):NP2.

25 Landsberg GM, Denenberg S. Behavior problems of the senior cat. In: *Feline behavioral health and welfare: Prevention and treatment.* Rodan I, Heath S, Elsevier, St. Louis, Missouri, USA; 2015:344–356.

26 Gunn-Moore D, Moffat K, Christie LA, Head E. Cognitive dysfunction and the neurobiology of ageing in cats. *J Small Anim Pract.* 2007;48(10):546–553.

27 Denenberg S, Liebel FX, Rose J. Behavioural and medical differentials of cognitive decline and dementia in dogs and cats. In: Landsberg G, Maďari A, Žilka N, eds. *Canine and feline dementia.* Cham, Switzerland: Springer International Publishing; 2017:13–58.

28 Landsberg GM, Nichol J, Araujo JA. Cognitive dysfunction syndrome: A disease of canine and feline brain aging. *Vet Clin Small Anim Pract.* 2012;42(4):749–768.

29 Overall K. *Manual of clinical behavioral medicine for dogs and cats.* St. Louis, Missouri, USA: Elsevier Health Sciences; 2013:432–439.

30 Landsberg GM, Denenberg S, Araujo JA. Cognitive dysfunction in cats: A syndrome we used to dismiss as 'old age'. *J Feline Med Surg.* 2010;12(11):837–848.

31 Whyte A, Gracia A, Bonastre C, Tejedor MT, Whyte J, Monteagudo LV, Simón C. Oral disease and microbiota in free-roaming cats. *Top Companion Anim Med.* 2017;32(3):91–95.

32 Gengler W, Dubielzig R, Ramer J. Physical examination and radiographic analysis to detect dental and mandibular bone resorption in cats: A study of 81 cases from necropsy. *J Vet Dent.* 1995;12(3):97–100.

33 Little SE. Managing the senior cat. In: *The cat*. St. Louis, Missouri, USA: WB Saunders; 2012:1166–1175.

34 Ray M, Carney HC, Boynton B, Quimby J, Robertson S, St Denis K, Tuzio H, Wright B. 2021 AAFP feline senior care guidelines. *J Feline Med Surg.* 2021;23(7):613–638.

35 Clarke DE, Caiafa A. Oral examination in the cat: A systematic approach. *J Feline Med Surg.* 2014;16(11):873–886.

36 Norsworthy GD, Carney HC, Ward CR. 2016 AAFP guidelines for the management of feline hyperthyroidism. *J Feline Med Surg.* 2016;18(9):750-750.

37 Peterson M. Hyperthyroidism in cats: What's causing this epidemic of thyroid disease and can we prevent it? *J Feline Med Surg.* 2012;14(11):804–818.

38 Overall KL. Medical differentials with potential behavioral manifestations. *Clin Tech Small Anim Pract.* 2004;19(4):250–258.

39 Syme HM. Cardiovascular and renal manifestations of hyperthyroidism. *Vet Clin North Am Small Anim Pract.* 2007;37(4):723–743.

40 Vaske HH, Schermerhorn T, Armbrust L, Grauer GF. Diagnosis and management of feline hyperthyroidism: Current perspectives. *Vet Med Res Rep.* 2014;5:85.

41 Langston CE, Reine NJ. Hyperthyroidism and the kidney. *Clin Tech Small Anim Pract.* 2006;21(1):17–21.

42 Vaske HH, Schermerhorn T, Grauer GF. Effects of feline hyperthyroidism on kidney function: A review. *J Feline Med Surg* 2016;18(2):55–59.

43 Peterson ME, Broome MR. Thyroid scintigraphy findings in 2096 cats with hyperthyroidism. *Vet Radiol Ultrasound* 2015;56(1):84–95.

44 Norsworthy GD, Adams VJ, McElhaney MR, Milios JA. Relationship between semi-quantitative thyroid palpation and total thyroxine concentration in cats with and without hyperthyroidism. *J Feline Med Surg.* 2002;4(3):139–143.

45 Norsworthy GD, Adams VJ, McElhaney MR, Milios JA. Palpable thyroid and parathyroid nodules in asymptomatic cats. *J Feline Med Surg* 2002;4(3):145–151.

46 Boretti FS, Sieber-Ruckstuhl NS, Gerber B, Laluha P, Baumgartner C, Lutz H, Hofmann-Lehmann R, Reusch CE. Thyroid enlargement and its relationship to clinicopathological parameters and T4 status in suspected hyperthyroid cats. *J Feline Med Surg.* 2009;11(4):286–292.

47 Bellows J, Center S, Daristotle L, Estrada AH, Flickinger EA, Horwitz DF, Lascelles BDX, Lepine A, Perea S, Scherk M, Shoveller AK. Evaluating aging in cats: How to determine what is healthy and what is disease. *J Feline Med Surg.* 2016;18(7):551–570.

48 Feldman EC, Nelson RW. *Canine and feline endocrinology and reproduction*. St. Louis, Missouri, USA: Saunders; 2004.

49 Scott-Moncrieff JC.Feline hyperthyroidism. In: Feldman, E, Nelson, RW, Reusch, CE, Scott-Moncrieff, J, eds.*Canine and feline endocrinology,* 4th ed. St. Louis, Missouri, USA: Elsevier Health Sciences; 2014:136–195.

50 Sparkes AH, Cannon M, Church D, Fleeman L, Harvey A, Hoenig M, Peterson ME, Reusch CE, Taylor S, Rosenberg D. ISFM consensus guidelines on the practical management of diabetes mellitus in cats. *J Feline Med Surg.* 2015;17(3):235–250.

51 Bennett N. Monitoring techniques for diabetes mellitus in the dog and the cat. *Clin Tech Small Anim Pract.* 2002;17(2):65–69.

52 Bijsmans ES, Jepson RE, Chang YM, Syme HM, Elliott J. Changes in systolic blood pressure over time in healthy cats and cats with chronic kidney disease. *J Vet Int Med*. 2015;29(3):855–861.

53 Kobayashi DL, Peterson ME, Graves TK, Nichols CE, Lesser M. Hypertension in cats with chronic renal failure or hyperthyroidism. *J Vet Int Med*. 1990;4(2):58–62.

54 Belew AM, Barlett T, Brown SA. Evaluation of the white-coat effect in cats. *J Vet Int Med*. 1999;13(2):134–142.

55 Acierno MJ, Brown S, Coleman AE, Jepson RE, Papich M, Stepien RL, et al. ACVIM consensus statement: Guidelines for the identification, evaluation, and management of systemic hypertension in dogs and cats. *J Vet Int Med*. 2018;32:1803–1822.

56 Hanås S, Holst BS, Ljungvall I, Tidholm A, Olsson U, Häggström J, Höglund K. Influence of clinical setting and cat characteristics on indirectly measured blood pressure and pulse rate in healthy Birman, Norwegian Forest, and Domestic Shorthair cats. *J Vet Int Med*. 2021;35(2):801–811.

57 Geddes RF. Hypertension: Why is it critical? *Vet Clin Small Anim Pract*. 2020;50(5):1037–1052.

58 Fox SM. Painful decisions for senior pets. *Vet Clin Small Anim Pract*. 2012;42(4):727–748.

59 Jergens AE. Gastrointestinal disease and its management. *Vet Clin North Am Small Anim Pract*. 1997;27(6):1373–1402.

60 Marsilio S. Differentiating inflammatory bowel disease from alimentary lymphoma in cats: Does it matter? *Vet Clin Small Anim Pract*. 2021;51(1):93–109.

61 Paulin MV, Couronné L, Beguin J, Le Poder S, Delverdier M, Semin MO, Bruneau J, Cerf-Bensussan N, Malamut G, Cellier C, Benchekroun G. Feline low-grade alimentary lymphoma: An emerging entity and a potential animal model for human disease. *BMC Vet Res*. 2018;14(1):1–19.

62 Sato H, Fujino Y, Chino J, Takahashi M, Fukushima K, Goto-Koshino Y, Uchida K, Ohno K, Tsujimoto H. Prognostic analyses on anatomical and morphological classification of feline lymphoma. *J Vet Med Sci* 2014;76:807–811.

63 Saito R, Chambers JK, Kishimoto TE, Uchida K. Pathological and immunohistochemical features of 45 cases of feline meningioma. *J Vet Med Sci*. 2021;83:1219–1224.

64 Motta L, Mandara MT, Skerritt GC. Canine and feline intracranial meningiomas: An updated review. *Vet J*. 2012;192(2):153–165.

65 Tomek A, Cizinauskas S, Doherr M, Gandini G, Jaggy A. Intracranial neoplasia in 61 cats: Localisation, tumour types and seizure patterns. *J Feline Med Surg*. 2006;8(4):243–253.

66 Falzone C, Lowrie M. Blindness and behavioural changes in the cat: Common neurological causes. *J Feline Med Surg*. 2011;13(11):863–873.

67 Griffin MA, Culp WT, Giuffrida MA, Ellis P, Tuohy J, Perry JA, Gedney A, Lux CN, Milovancev M, Wallace ML, Hash J. Lower urinary tract transitional cell carcinoma in cats: Clinical findings, treatments, and outcomes in 118 cases. *J Vet Int Med*. 2020;34(1):274–282.

68 Landsberg GM, Hunthausen W, Ackerman L. Fears, phobias, and anxiety disorders. In: *Behavior problems of the dog and cat*. Edinburgh, London, New York, Oxford, Philadelphia, St Louis, Sydney, Toronto: Saunders Elsevier; 2013;182–183, 327–344.

69 Notari L. Stress in veterinary behavioural medicine. In: Horwitz DF, Mills DS, eds. *BSAVA manual of canine and feline behavioural medicine*. BSAVA Library; 2009:136–145.

70 Landsberg G. Feline behavior and welfare. *J Am Vet Med Assoc*. 1996;208:502–504.

71 Černá P, Gardiner H, Sordo L, Tørnqvist-Johnsen C, Gunn-Moore DA. Potential causes of increased vocalisation in elderly cats with cognitive dysfunction syndrome as assessed by their owners. *Animals* 2020;10(6):1092.

14

Cat Relationships in the Home

Sun-A Kim and Elizabeth Stelow

Introduction

As noted elsewhere, cats are very popular pets. And, while there are households in which one or more adult lives with a single cat, this is not the norm. Most live with other cats, kids, dogs, and/or other types of pets. So, consideration must be given to those relationships. Chapter 11 focuses on cats having challenging relationships with other cats in the household. But, how do we foster positive ones? How should cats get along with kids, dogs, and other pets?

This chapter focuses on four major aspects of the relationships of cats in the home:

- Cats and children, particularly the introduction of new cats or new children
- Cats and household dogs
- Cats and household pets of other species
- Introducing a new cat to a household with kids, other cats, dogs, or other pets

While each of these makes slightly different recommendations, a few common themes include: plan ahead, safety first, and move slowly.

Cats and Children

According to the 2017–2018 US Pet Ownership & Demographics Sourcebook, approximately 25.4% of households in the United States own cats, with an average of 1.8 cats per household. This translates to over 58 million cats living in households across the country. In America, "dogs may be considered man's best friend," but cats come in at a very close second, as cats are the second most owned pets in the US, just behind dogs.[1]

The Benefits and Risks of Cats and Kids Living Together

Perhaps Charles Dickens was ahead of his time when he said, "What greater gift than the love of a cat?" Evidence suggests that cats may be considered to be a child's greatest gift. Each year, the number of cats being adopted to homes has increased, but, more importantly, in homes with children. Studies have reported that virtually all children wanted a pet, and children lacking pets often desired one and sought out contact with their neighbors' pets.[2,3] Still, there are advantages and disadvantages to having kids and cats in the same household.

Benefits

Arguments can be made from both sides on the advantages and disadvantages of living with a cat. When looking at the evidence, it may surprise many how beneficial raising an animal can be to the overall health of humans, when assessing diseases, stress, and relationships.[4] "Zooeyia," a fairly recent term, was created to underline the importance of animals to human health. Zooeyia, defined as the "positive impact of animals on human health," is formed from two Greek root words, zoion (animal), and hygiea (health) after the Greek Goddess Hygiea, also the same root for hygiene.[4] Positive impacts of companion animals are numerous and seen in various circumstances, such as contributing to the social and behavioral development support and improved mental health and quality of life of children with Autistic Spectrum Disorder (ASD).[5] In a study of ASD children and their pets, researchers found that ASD children valued their relationship with their pet cat more than their dogs, where they displayed much more visual attention to their pet cat than to their pet dog.[6] Positive impacts of raising cats are not limited to ASD children's social–emotional and cognitive development[7,8] but also include impacts on the social–emotional support of typically-developing children as well. Raising cats provides all children the opportunity to learn about the responsibilities of caring for another being; experience the love, respect, affection, and companionship that come from caring for an animal;[9–11] and help to improve children's overall attentiveness and motivation.[12] The biggest advantage of raising cats is that the benefits are not limited to only a small group of cats or children, but can be experienced by all in a symbiotic relationship. Cats are dependent on humans for food, love, attention, and a warm home, and in return, children and adults alike enjoy the cute, furry, cuddly creatures that bring joy and love to our lives.

Risks

As cute and cuddly as cats may be, they are predatory animals that have sharp teeth and claws. Therefore, feline aggression can be a problem in households with children. Although not seen often, aggressive behavior against children of any age can be seen in cats of any breed, size, age, or sex. Aggressive behaviors can come from a variety of motives and causes including fear, defense, territoriality, redirection, play hyperstimulation, pain, and discomfort. Cats that are chased or picked up when they try to run away are likely to scratch or bite, either accidentally or defensively. To address a cat's aggression, working with a professional who can look at the context of the incident will be of utmost importance.

Cats can injure children during play, as well; in fact, one type of feline aggression is known as "inappropriate play" or "play-motivated" aggression.[13] Therefore, it is of paramount importance that owners prepare their environmental management strategies ahead of time, so cats are never in a situation encouraging inappropriate play behavior, but promote only acceptable play behavior.

Taking care of children is already a great responsibility for parents, and taking on the added responsibility of adopting a cat or cats would mean extra commitments, such as finding a sitter when on holiday, time and work involved in training/pet care, and cleaning up/dealing with the mess caused by the animal(s).[9]

Still, cats and kids can live comfortably together if certain steps are taken to provide everyone with the resources and protection they need.

Managing the Relationship between Cats and Kids

Many considerations must be met when pairing cats and children in a household. The safety of both the cats and the children will be most important. But goals should exceed the most basic safety measures: How can cats *thrive* with children? Whether the family is adding a cat or child – or just wants to make sure they're doing everything they can – the following questions can guide cat owners with children to provide the best situation:

- *Where should the cat's litter box, food, and water bowls be located?* They should be located in a safe and quiet place that young children cannot reach. If a litter box needs to be relocated, then it is recommended that it be moved little by little, and not far from the place where the cat usually spends the day. Food and water can be moved farther, as long as the cat is introduced to the new location.

- *Does the cat have space to get away?* Even the most social and tolerant cat may need a space that it can get away to when things around it become too noisy, chaotic, or otherwise stressful. Children can lack the impulse control to avoid the cat when it signals that it needs space. Giving the cat ample places to go where the children – especially young children – cannot follow allows it time to destress. The "safe space" may come in the form of vertical spaces, like cat trees, wall shelves, or bookcases. Or the house can be fitted with baby gates manufactured with cat doors in them, allowing the cat to move into rooms that the children cannot. If the cat has an enclosed outdoor space, like a "catio," that, too, can be a child-free zone. Figure 14.1 shows one example of a catio.

- *How does this cat like to play?* Some cats play rough, while others are perfectly gentle. Some may need to be enticed with a wand toy, while others may choose to explore whatever activity their humans are doing. Based on the personalities of all involved, decisions should be made about how children should be allowed to play with the household cats (no playing with hands, please!!) and guidelines set for the specific toys to be used. Wand toys keep teeth and claws away from hands. Soft catnip toys can be tossed for a game of fetch. Hide-and-seek can be rewarding for everyone.

- *Should cats and kids sleep together at night?* This is a decision that should be negotiated, in part, with the cat. Some cats want to cuddle with people and others like time exploring and "hunting" at night. Some children sleep better knowing they have a companion and others awaken too easily to have a cat prowling around them at night. So, again personalities of all involved will drive the decision about whether cats and kids should be expected or allowed to sleep together.

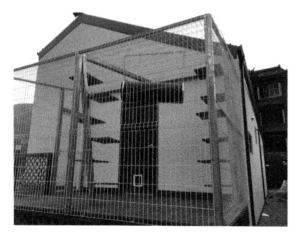

Figure 14.1 A "catio" with a cat door gives the resident cat enrichment and a space to call its own. Photo courtesy of Sun-A Kim.

- *How do the children interact with the cat?* Like adults, children approach cats in many different ways, sometimes in the same day. They may be gentle and patient one moment, rambunctious and loud the next. But, they can learn to be respectful of the cat's body, his sense of hearing, and his nature as a prey animal, as well as a predator. A child is never too young to learn how to interact with a cat respectfully.[14,15]
- *How does the cat interact with the children?* The majority of cats seem to integrate well with the children in a household. It's natural for a cat to choose to get away from child-induced chaos periodically. But, if a cat in a household with children rarely appears, seems particularly withdrawn, or becomes aggressive during interactions with the children, diagnosis and treatment should be sought. Some cats are not a good fit for households with children and would be happier with child-free owners.
- *Is the cat's environment sufficiently enriched?* Chapter 3 discusses feline enrichment in households; but it bears repeating here. Cats are highly sensitive creatures, especially to their environment. The slightest imbalances in their environment can be a source of stress. On the other hand, when provided with a livable environment, cats can better respond to stressful situations. Behavioral environmental enrichment is a therapy to proactively promote healthy behaviors and emotions.
- *Do the owners understand feline body language?* It is crucial that owners are able to tell when their cats are becoming stressed, fearful, frustrated, interested in pouncing, or otherwise potentially risky for a child to be around. In addition, children, even young ones, should learn to "read" their cats, as well.[15,16] Many online resources are available for owners and their children to learn more about feline body language. One such is the Maddie's fund website, https://www.maddiesfund.org/feline-communication-how-to-speak-cat.htm.

Behavioral environmental enrichment for resident cats

- Is enough vertical space provided (i.e. cat tree, shelves, etc.) for the cat? Are there enough safe spaces to escape to?
- Are enough toys provided for sufficient play behavior? And are they rotated to prevent boredom? Does the owner spend sufficient time playing with the cat?
- Are nutritionally balanced meals provided in appropriately sized portions at set mealtimes? Is clean water in a clean bowl or fountain provided always available?
- Is the litter box big enough and filled with the cat's preferred type of litter, and placed in the best location? Is litter-box hygiene maintained frequently, by scooping out the litter 1–2 times a day?
- Is the cat's favorite style of scratcher provided in a safe and desired location?

Introducing a Baby into a Home with a Cat

Managing the relationship between household cats and children in the family never stops. But one crucial period is the preparation for bringing a baby home. The household cat has a routine that will soon be disrupted. Its relationship with the adults in the family will change. The birth of a baby can create stress in both humans and companion animals. Thus, preparations should be made slowly and methodically to deal with the changes. Appropriate preparations that are made sooner than later would lead to the success of the changes.

These preparations include three distinct phases:

- Rearranging the cat's lifestyle to accommodate the changes that will come with a new baby
- Acclimating the cat to the baby's new belongings, as well as the sounds and smells of a baby
- Introducing the cat to the new baby

Each one is important and should be undertaken with care, so that the cat and the baby get started on the right foot.

Rearranging the Cat's Lifestyle

It is important that the home (therefore the spaces set aside for the cat) be prepared long before the baby makes its appearance.[15] These are some things for expectant parents to consider:

- **Do the cat's resources need to be moved?** If the current litter box is not located in a place that can continue to be used after the baby is born, then it must be relocated to the new location in advance. Similarly, the cat's food and water need to be out of reach of a baby, especially when it becomes a toddler.[14]
- **How will everyone keep up the cat's feeding schedule?** When the baby is born, days will seem longer and hours of sleep even shorter. Responsibilities will seem as if they've multiplied and managing the simplest chores may be the last thing anyone will want to do. There may also be times when you forget to feed the cat or accidently feed him twice because you forgot you had already fed the cat earlier. So, employing a checklist or calendar to keep track of feeding time(s) for your cat is a great idea. Also, cats like routine and regular feeding times; so even if a cat-sitter feeds the cat, maintaining the routine of a regular feeding time will make your cat very happy.

    If the cat is not meal fed, it is advisable to convert it to meal feedings. That way, feeding locations and times can be controlled and there will not be constant presence of food to be considered when the baby becomes mobile.[15]
- **Do resting spots need to be changed?** If the cat is currently spending much of its time in the baby's nursery room, prepare ahead of time and transition slowly to a new location in advance of the baby's arrival. Cats are better at adapting to slow changes than to sudden changes, so move your cat's bed/bedding in small increments until the new location is finally reached.
- **Are there safe spaces for the cat?** When unable to supervise the cat and baby together, provide a safe space for the cat to stay in comfortably and safely. A safe space can be a cat tree, window perch (Figure 14.2), a room behind a baby gate, wall shelves (Figure 14.3), or a tall bookcase. A variety should be available.[15]
- **How will play time with the cat be accommodated?** Just as daily walks are important for a dog, playtime is important for a cat. When a baby is born and is constantly the center of attention of everyone in the family, it may be easy for the cat and its needs to be neglected, especially its playtime. Cats need attention and daily exercise, otherwise, they may begin to display negative behavior changes. As such, maintaining a journal to keep track of how often and how much play time you can dedicate may go a long way in keeping your cat happy and feel loved.
- **Where will the cat sleep at night?** Perhaps a better question is, "Where will the baby sleep at night?" If the baby is to sleep in a nursery, it will be important to avoid unobserved interactions between the baby and the cat. A screen door or tall baby gate mounted on the nursery door frame (Figure 14.4) can prevent the cat from entering while allowing sounds to travel.[14] The cat will be able to sleep with the parents while the baby is asleep in the nursery. If the baby is to sleep in the parents' bedroom, keep the cat from entering the bedroom during sleep time.[14] The image of a cat and baby snuggled up together sleeping peacefully may be heartwarming and sweet; but in reality, there is a small possibility for the sleeping cat to encroach on the baby's nose and mouth, causing suffocation. Thus, it is important to keep the baby and cat separated at all times when unsupervised.[14]

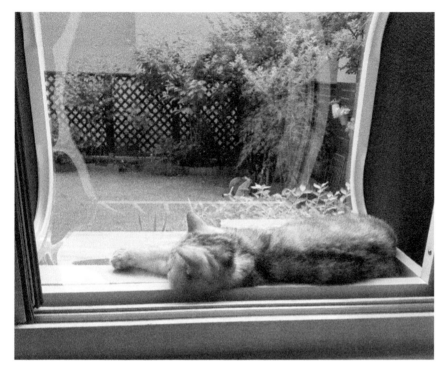

Figure 14.2   A cat-only zone. Photo courtesy of Hyunjin Yoo.

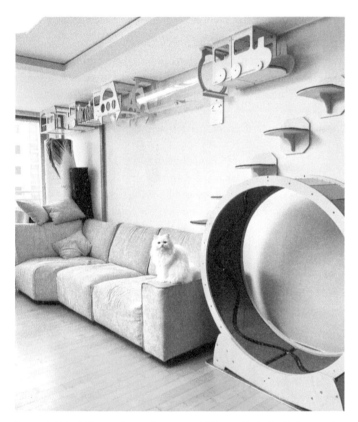

Figure 14.3   Cats needs a safe space, which may include shelves and cat walk. Photo courtesy of Wooyul Jung.

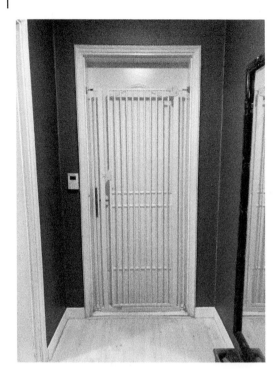

Figure 14.4 Keeping the door closed or adding a high baby gate will prevent cats from entering the baby's room without supervision. Photo courtesy of Sun-A Kim.

Preparing the Cat for Baby

The cat will need to become accustomed to new furniture, play things, and other of the countless new things acquired by expectant parents. The sooner this is done, the better.[15]

- **Treat any behavior issues that may exist:** In general, it is best to treat behavior problems as early as possible before they worsen. But, it's particularly important to address anything that might be worsened by – or be a threat to – a new baby. If the cat owner recognizes that there is a problem, they can fill out the Fe-BARQ (https://vetapps.vet.upenn.edu/febarq) questionnaire. Based on the results of Fe-BARQ, they can pursue consultation with their veterinarian or a veterinary behaviorist.[17]

- **Habituate the cat to baby items:** Cats are sensitive to new objects and babies tend to require many of them. With the birth of a new baby, unless planned carefully, the cat may feel that its home is suddenly bombarded with new and foreign objects and be a source of stress and anxiety for the cat. Therefore, it is important to organize a list and make a plan of what items (i.e. furniture, clothes, stroller, car seat, etc.) will be needed and how to incrementally introduce the new items to the house so that the cat will not be overwhelmed by the sudden influx of new items. It should be noted that cribs, car seats, and strollers are ideal places for cats to climb onto and use as a bed. So, making it difficult for the cat to get access to these areas by covering them up will be key to maintaining a safe home. Cats love fluffy blankets and lying on a comfortable bed. So, parents need to be wary and prevent the cat from entering the crib to sleep on the bed where the baby may be sleeping, as there is a risk of suffocation and must be prevented.

- **Habituate the cat to baby scents:** Cats are extremely sensitive to smells. A new baby in the home will mean a host of new smells (e.g. fragrances from baby products) that the cat is unused to and its senses may be a bit overwhelmed. It will be impossible to prepare all of the unborn baby's items (lotion, shampoo, cream, etc.) ahead of time, but there are some simple solutions that go a long way to help the transition be easy for the cat. For instance, the owners can apply some of the baby lotion or cream on themselves so that the cat can gradually adapt to the new scents. Once the baby is born, actual items from the baby (blankets, hats) can be brought home for the cat to smell.[15]

- **Habituate the cat to baby sounds:** Cats are also highly sensitive to sounds. A surprising fact that many may be unaware of is that cats are able to hear higher frequencies than humans and dogs! Just as a new baby brings a host of new smells, a whole new of sounds will be introduced into the home. These may include:
  - Babies crying, babble, babies screaming, babies laughing
  - Play sounds (tapping, clapping, banging)
  - Music for young children (often high-pitched, upbeat)
  - The sounds of common electronic baby toys

  Cats may not be ready to deal with these new and ear-piercingly loud sounds like that of a baby's crying. Therefore, introducing these sounds ahead of time will help to reduce stressing and overwhelming the cat's senses.

  These sounds can be downloaded from the internet or recorded by an acquaintance who also has a baby. One of these sounds can be turned on the sound at the lowest volume while the cat is doing something it enjoys (e.g., playing, eating snacks, etc.). If the cat doesn't show any signs of stress or anxiousness, then the volume can be increased over time.
- **Find a cat-sitter for the future:** Raising a newborn baby will result in unpredictable situations that will lead to needing to leave the house suddenly and unexpectedly. Therefore, it will be important have a reliable person, who will already be aware of the cat's needs and routines, to take care of the cat with just a phone call. As such, a cat-sitter should be met with in in advance to meet the cat and be informed of all the pertinent information about the cat.

Introducing the Baby to the Cat

The initial meeting of the baby and cat can go smoothly without any drama – that is, if the parents-to-be have successfully prepared all the tips provided so far. On meeting day, after all the anticipation and build-up preparing for the big day, a successful day should begin with greeting the cat in the same manner as usual, like any other ordinary day. Rather than making a big fuss about the arrival of the baby, the day should feel almost anticlimactic because "no drama" equals a successful beginning to a peaceful transition!

The new parents should enlist the help of a friend or family member for the initial introduction. The parents should enter the home first without the baby so that they can greet the cat.[14] Then the friend/family member can bring in the baby. If the cat is interested or insistent on checking out the baby, then one parent should hold the baby covered with a blanket, and let the cat sniff the baby blanket. Keep in mind, it is not necessary to deliberately introduce the baby to the cat.

From that moment on, the new parents should be sure to give the cat attention only when the baby is present. This seems counterintuitive; after all, the parents will have more time to pet and play when the baby is asleep in its crib. But, giving the cat attention only in the baby's presence will help the cat to look forward to the baby being present. Conversely, attention only in the baby's absence will have the cat looking forward to the baby going away.[15]

Introducing a New Cat into a Home with Children

The considerations discussed earlier in the chapter are relevant when introducing a cat into a home with children. A plan must be made about where resources will go, who in the household is primarily responsible for care (ideally an adult), and expectation set about respect and kind treatment.

If the cat is an adult, it is best to assess its history of living with children. In fact, it is ideal to adopt adult cats into families with children only if they are shown to be tolerant of children. If the history is unknown, designating the new home as a "foster" home will allow the cat to be easily returned if it turns out that it is a bad fit.

If the new cat is a kitten, there is less history to worry about – but there are more rules to set in place with the children. Kittens are open to being taught to play roughly (especially with hands) and can easily be encouraged to climb things they should not (peoples' pant legs, draperies, etc.) It is also tempting to dress or put them in something potentially harmful because they are less likely to struggle. Therefore, younger children should have clear ground rules for what the kitten is and is not allowed to do; and their time together should be carefully supervised. Older children can be called on for input into the rules as a way to encourage them to think about the value of the rules (therefore get buy-in).

Cats Living with a Baby or Children

The cat should never be punished around the baby because cats should never associate punishment with the children, which will only cause fear or discomfort toward them. Rather, only good and positive events should occur for the cat when the baby is around (i.e. playing, treats, etc.) To note, a crawling baby can easily surprise or frighten a cat, so, as a rule, the baby and cat should never be left alone unattended.

A baby gate with a cat door should be installed around the cat's safe space to prevent the baby from accessing it. An example of this is included as Figure 14.5 and 14.6. A shelf or catwalk along the wall can be installed so that the cat can move to a safe space without having to step on the floor at any point in the house. Cats are animals that tend to avoid and run away from uncomfortable or fearful situations. A cat's avoidant behaviors are necessary not only for its safety, but more importantly, for the baby's safety as well.

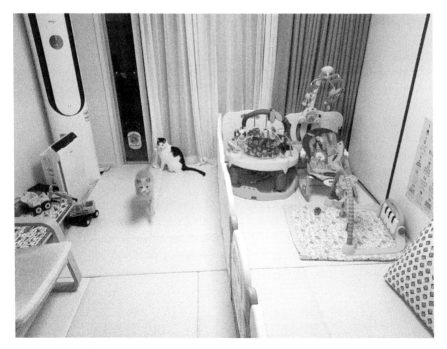

Figure 14.5   A baby gate system allows for babies and cats to keep separate spaces. Photo courtesy of Sun-A Kim.

Figure 14.6 Baby gates also allow cats and babies safe exposure to each other. Photo courtesy of Sun-A Kim.

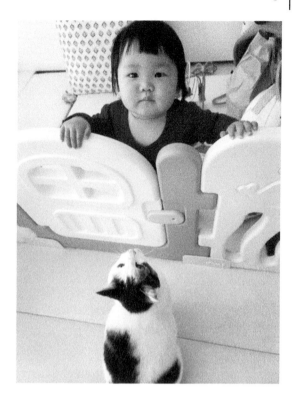

Cats and Dogs

Can cats and dogs be best friends – or are they doomed to play their cartoon roles as adversaries? While it certainly depends on the cat and dog in question, there is ample evidence that cat and dog owners can be optimistic.

> "Aspiring owners should not blindly believe popular assumptions, but both knowledge and respect for species-specific pet behaviours are essential to establish a balance in the household."
>
> *– Menchetti, et al.*[18]

In the Menchetti study, 62.4% of the 1270 owners surveyed reported that their cats and dogs living in the same households played together.[18] Other responses suggested that 58.1% of the dog–cat pairs chased each other, 40.9% fought, 43.9% of cats played with the dog's tail, and 63.8% made ambushes of some type (respondents could choose more than one selection). Many dog–cat pairs reportedly groomed each other, slept nearby each other, and tolerated each other near their food at mealtimes. An example of a positive relationship is seen in Figure 14.7.

A study by Thompson found that the cat in a cat–dog pair appeared to be the primary controller in deciding the friendliness of their relationship; this was deduced because owners weighed "cat factors" higher than "dog factors" when assessing the friendliness of the relationship. In addition, the comfort of the cat in the dog's presence was a stronger predictor of friendliness than the comfort of the dog.[19]

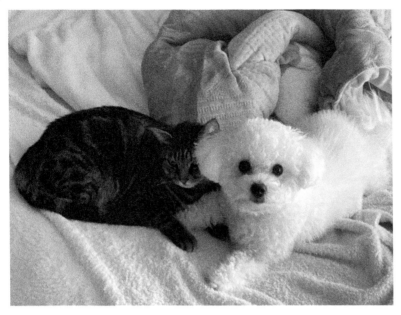

Figure 14.7 It is possible for cats and dogs to get along very well. Photo courtesy of Krista Mangulsone / Pexels and Sun A Kim.

Dogs and cats are vastly different, so raising them together can double the cuteness; or, on the flip side, the problems can be doubled. Problems between animals can become more difficult when they are not properly socialized when they are young.[20,21] The socialization window is around 3–14 weeks for dogs and 3–8 weeks for cats. Cats that meet dogs when the cats are young are likely to be much more accepting of living with dogs in the future.[21] In addition, they seem to get along best when the cat was brought into the household first.[20]

If a dog owner wishes to adopt a cat, or vice versa, it is important to be able to answer the following questions:

- Has your dog (cat) ever met a cat (dog) before?
- How did the interaction go?
- Did they get along or was one afraid of the other?

If the pet's experience was positive, the chances of living harmonious with another cat/dog will have increased drastically.

That being said, however, just because your cat met a dog and had successful meetings with other dog(s) does not necessarily guarantee a seamless adoption of a new dog in the home. Therefore, owners may wish to first try fostering a dog, living with the dog for a few weeks or months to see how their cat interacts and deals with a new family member. The last thing any family wants is to welcome home a new dog, only to live in constant chaos and stress because the two animals can't seem to get along. However, while fostering a dog, if the family dynamic remains calm and peaceful, the chances for a smooth transition of a new member would almost be certain! Hence, it is highly recommended have foster dog to have a trial period or a test run to see how your cat will react to a new member and be able to adjust.

When a Cat and a Dog First Meet

When welcoming a new animal to the home, the two animals should initially be kept separate with a safety door/gate between them, so that when the two animals are ready to meet, they are able to do so through the safety of the gate, figure 14.8 shows an example of such an arrangement. Before meeting for the first time, and if the owners have not yet set up a gate, the dog should be in a harness and leash for a safe meeting. It is always ideal and helpful to give delicious treats to both animals when they meet so that they are able to experience a create and reinforce a positive association with meeting each other. However, even if the meeting is positive and peaceful, it is of utmost importance to maintain a safe path and place for your cat to run away to, for any time it may need to get away.

Arranging the Environment

Even if the dog and cat are able to live together peacefully, the most important factor in maintaining peace and harmony in the home is for everyone to feel safe in the home environment. First, let's check the current environment and remember dogs are considered to live in 2D spaces, but cats are 3D animals. Understanding the current situation is the key to a successful preparation.

Checking the current situation

- Is there a safe space for a cat (cat-only zone)?
- Where is the cat's litter box located? Or where would you like to put the cat's litter box?
- Where are the food and water bowls located? Or where would you like to put the food and water bowls?

Do you have a safe space for the cat (cat-only zone)? An important factor when dogs and cats live together is maintaining the "cat-only zone." Often times, when cats and dogs live together, the dog becomes the "chaser" and the cat the "chasee," so providing multiple levels of vertical space in every corner of the house is crucial, where the cat can retreat to if in danger. Catwalks are ideal, but if they are not feasible, shelves or cat trees are fine alternatives.

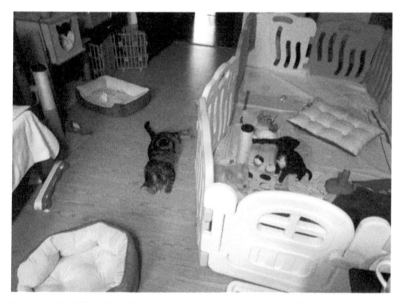

Figure 14.8   When introducing a new puppy to a home that has a cat, a puppy pen is recommended to help the animals adjust to each other. A cat can see, hear, and smell a puppy, and can choose to approach the pen or not. Photo courtesy of Dr. Sun-A Kim.

Where would you like to put the cat's litter box? Although many first-time owners may be shocked the first time they see their dog eating cat feces, it is common canine behavior and a common complaint from owners. To prevent the dog from feasting on feces, the cat's litter box should be located in a safe and quiet place that the dog cannot disturb. If the litter box needs to be relocated, then it is recommended that the litter box be moved little by little, and not too far from where the cat usually spends its day.

Where would you like to put the food and water bowls? Usually, dogs are voracious eaters and eat immediately as soon as they are fed. Conversely, most cats are more finicky and tend to eat little by little throughout the day. So, if your cat's food bowl is in a place that dogs can easily reach, then you may have a constantly hungry cat. As such, the cat's food and water bowls should be placed on a higher vertical plane than the dog can reach, but not too far from where the cat normally rests. If the bowls need to be relocated, move them little by little every day to a place where the cat can eat safely and undisturbed.

Cats and Other Pets

Aside from the studies of cats and dogs living in the same home, little has been studied about cats sharing living spaces with other non-human species.[22] Therefore, we turn to the natural history of the cat for guidance.

As has been said many times in this volume, cats are widely accepted as both predator and prey;[23] this dichotomy guides their interactions with other species. From the first perspective, dogs are the only house pet likely to see a cat as prey.[23] But, from a predator perspective, many popular pets are potentially at risk of being attacked by the family's cat.

In 2016, the AVMA reported that, of the 25% of all US households that owned a cat, 4.1% also had at least one bird. That same year, 14% of US families owned a total of over 100 million exotics, including more than 2 million rabbits (in 1.2% of US households), 3.5 million small mammals, 6 million reptiles, and 76 million fish (in 8.3% of households). Figure 14.9 and 14.10 show cats living closely with small mammals. The report does not say how many of those homes with exotic pets also had cats. But, it does note that, among the 71 million households (57% of all US households) who owned a pet, only 20.4% had only cats, whereas 25% had various combinations of different pet species.[1] So, odds are good that many households with cats also have small mammals, fish, birds, or reptiles. Many species within those broad groups are considered viable prey for free-ranging housecats.[24]

Despite being reported by their owners to be well fed and to have access to wet or dry food ad libitum, at least some domestic cats clearly hunt live prey and appear to show distinct differences in the types of prey that they hunt.

Because it is not possible to ask housecats not to hunt the captive prey species that may be living alongside them in the home, consideration should be given to the safety of those prey species living in the same home as cats. Safety comes in the form of secure housing (Figure 14.11) and sequestering the cat/s during prey species play times.

Secure housing includes (but is not limited to) a housing structure that cannot be breached by any part of a curious cat. In addition, the housing should be placed in a location that prevents a cat from stalking, staring at, or otherwise threatening a sensitive species (like rabbits, small mammals, and birds). Finally, the housing should not be able to be moved or knocked over by a cat trying to test the security of said housing.

Play or exercise time for birds, rabbits, or small animals should be limited to areas of the home from which cats have been temporarily or permanently barred.

Figure 14.9 Cats and rabbits can be tolerant of each other, or even close companions, but should always be supervised together. Photo courtesy of Liz Stelow.

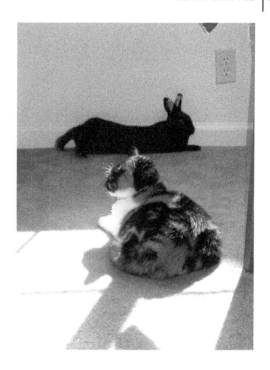

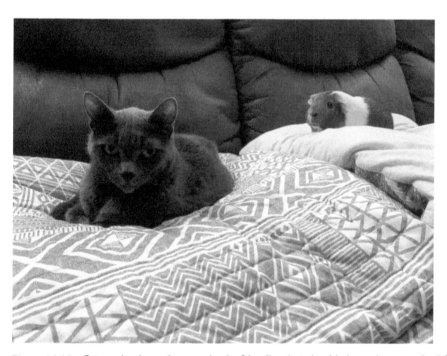

Figure 14.10 Cats and guinea pigs can also be friendly – but should always be supervised. Photo courtesy of Amanda Aguilera.

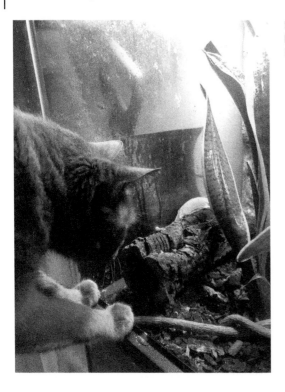

Figure 14.11 It is important that small animals be kept in secure housing when curious cats are in residence. Photo courtesy of Amanda Aguilera.

Introducing a New Cat to a Household

Whether this new cat will be sharing space with children, other cats, dogs, or other animals, careful plans must be made to ensure everyone's comfort. There are some basic preparations to be considered, regardless of the other species in the home; additionally, there are some species-specific factors to be addressed.

Deciding to Add a Cat

When it comes to the decision to add a cat to a household, there are many considerations, including:

- How do all the human residents feel about having a cat (or a specific cat, if there is one)?
- How will it fit in with any other household pets?
- Is the size and layout of the house suitable for a cat? Will there be adequate space for resting, feeding, and enrichment opportunities?
- Does the family have a plan for the everyday care, feeding, and health maintenance of the cat?
- Is the family prepared for the possibility that the cat will not, in fact, get along well with the other animals or humans in the household? Are there contingency plans?[25]

These considerations become irrelevant if the family acquires a cat without setting out to do so. According to a 2012 study by Bayer, more than 50% of clients report that they did not seek out cat ownership, but rather, that their cat "found them." [26]

However the decision is made, it is crucial that the cat be brought into the house with successful acclimation in mind.

Preparations for the New Addition

A new cat will need all the comforts of home: litter, food, water, perches, play time, affection, and a safe place to hide away when necessary.

Providing for the cat's needs – particularly the feeding, litter, and safe spaces – will likely require keeping children and dogs (and perhaps other species) away from those resources. Therefore, baby gates, tall cat trees or wall shelves, and other adjustments to the home may need to be made. Because the cat's retreat should be a quiet space, it should not be a high-traffic room; owners may need to remove frequently used items from it ahead of the cat's arrival.

Other pets may need to have their routines adjusted beforehand, as well. If a dog will be crated or otherwise sequestered during certain times of the day, training for that should happen before the cat arrives. This is particularly true if the dog is accustomed to having free run of the home. Crate training and the willingness to remain in a room away from the family may take time and patience and should not be rushed. The changes should be positively reinforced and done at the pace the dog feels comfortable.

If there are house rabbits, ferrets, birds, or other small animals that are accustomed to ample time loose in the home, their schedules and access to certain spaces may need to be adjusted, as well.

To minimize any competition over food resources, all free-ranging pets should be meal fed rather than free fed. In this way, the pets that need to eat alone, in a separate room or on a perch, can be given a discrete time to do so. This ensures that all pets and their humans can be respectful of each other.

The Introduction

There is no one "right way" to add a new cat to the household. But, there are steps to be taken that may maximize the odds of a smooth transition. These are as follows:[15]

1) Maintain Separation. Keep the newcomer separated from the resident animals – at first. They should be separated by a door. Articles of bedding can be traded back and forth to allow for acclimation. Or the resident animals and the newcomer can trade spaces for certain periods each day. Once the newcomer has adjusted and there does not appear to be excessive curiosity or overt aggression at the door, move cautiously to Step 2.

2) Feed in Adjacent Spaces. Feed the newcomer and one of the resident animals on opposite sides of the closed door. If there are multiple resident animals to consider, rotate them through this process. The act of feeding together this way creates positive associations between the newcomer and the resident animals. If everyone is willing to eat meals this way, move to Step 3.

3) Offer Visual Access. Use a baby gate, screen door, carriers, or a door left ajar to allow the resident animals visual access to the newcomer. Safety for all involved must be maintained; the animals should not be allowed to interact physically until it's clear that they can do so without aggression. Once this is the case, move to Step 4.

4) Offer Physical Access. Allow the newcomer to interact with the resident animals with direct supervision to avoid injury (Figure 14.12). Watch carefully for signs of excessive arousal or aggression. Allow these encounters to take place in large spaces with ample opportunities to retreat. Keep sessions brief at first and lengthen them over time. Continue to build on the success of these encounters until the newcomer is integrated into the household.

Throughout this process, it's best to keep all cats indoors, since fighting is most likely to occur after a cat returns from outdoors or in response to new odors.

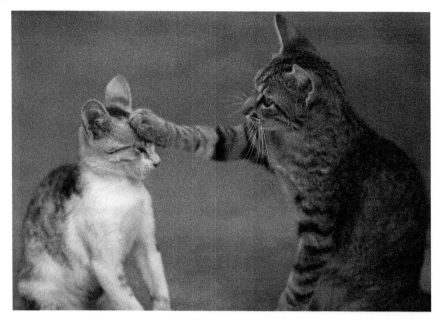

Figure 14.12 When introducing a new cat or kitten, supervise interactions with resident animals. Photo courtesy of pixabay.

While gradual introduction is recommended, it is no guarantee of future acceptance of the new cat. Studies have shown that future aggression between the newcomer and resident cats was best predicted by the newcomer having bit or scratched one of the resident cats during the first meeting. Factors that do not appear to influence the likelihood of future aggression are the number of cats in the household, the age or sex of the cats, the size of the house, or the method of introduction of the newcomer.

Conclusion

Cats can – and do – live happily in human homes with children, other cats, and other types of pets. That is not to say that every cat would flourish in every type of household. But, with proper planning, thorough understanding of the cat and proposed family life, and adequate access to experts who can assist in any necessary problem solving, cat-loving families can be hopeful of harmony within their feline-friendly homes.

References

1 AVMA. *AVMA pet ownership and demographics sourcebook: 2017–2018 edition.* 2018.
2 Kidd AH, Kidd RM. Children's attitudes toward their pets. *Psychol Rep.* 1985;57(1):15–31. https://doi.org/10.2466/pr0.1985.57.1.15.
3 Kidd AH, Kidd RM. Social and environmental influences on children's attitudes toward pets. *Psychol Rep.* 1990;67(3I):807–818. https://doi.org/10.2466/pr0.67.7.807-818.
4 Hodgson K, Darling M. Zooeyia: An essential component of "One Health." *Can Vet J.* 2011;52(2):158–161. http://www.statcan.gc.ca/pub/82-230-x/82-230
5 Byström KM, Lundqvist Perssontt CA. The meaning of companion animals for children and adolescents with autism: The parents' perspective. *Anthrozoos.* 2015;28(2):263–275. https://doi.org/10.1080/08927936.2015.11435401

6 Grandgeorge M, Gautier Y, Bourreau Y, Mossu H, Hausberger M. Visual attention patterns differ in dog vs. cat interactions with children with typical development or autism spectrum disorders. *Front Psychol*. 2020;11:2047. https://doi.org/10.3389/fpsyg.2020.02047

7 Endenburg N, Van Lith HA, Kirpensteijn J. Longitudinal study of Dutch children's attachment to companion animals. *Soc Anim*. 2014;22(4):390–414. https://doi.org/10.1163/15685306-12341344

8 Hart LA, Thigpen AP, Willits NH, Lyons LA, Hertz-Picciotto I, Hart BL. Affectionate interactions of cats with children having autism spectrum disorder. *Front Vet Sci*. 2018;5(Mar). https://doi.org/10.3389/fvets.2018.00039

9 Fifield SJ, Forsyth DK. A pet for the children: Factors related to family pet ownership. *Anthrozoos*. 1999;12(1):24–32. https://doi.org/10.2752/089279399787000426.

10 Kidd AH, Kidd RM. Children's drawings and attachment to pets. *Psychol Rep*. 1995;77(1):235–241. https://doi.org/10.2466/pr0.1995.77.1.235

11 Triebenbacher SL. Pets as transitional objects: Their role in children's emotional development. *Psychol Rep*. 1998;82(1):191. https://doi.org/10.2466/pr0.82.1.191-200

12 Borgi M, Cirulli F. Children's preferences for infantile features in dogs and cats. In: *Human-animal interaction bulletin* (Vol. 1, Issue 2). 2013.

13 Curtis TM. Human-directed aggression in the cat. *Vet Clin North Am Small Anim Pract*. 2008;38(5):1131–1143.

14 Bergman L. Ensuring a behaviorally healthy pet-child relationship. *Vet Med*. 2006;101:670–682.

15 Bergman L. Expanding families: Preparing for and introducing dogs and cats to infants, children, and new pets. *Vet Clin North Am Small Anim Pract*. 2008;5(38):1043–1063.

16 Heath S. Feline aggression. In: Horwitz D, Mills D, Heath S, eds. *BSAVA manual of canine and feline behavioural medicine*. Gloucester, UK: BSAVA; 2002:216–228.

17 Duffy DL, de Moura RTD, Serpell JA. Development and evaluation of the Fe-BARQ: A new survey instrument for measuring behavior in domestic cats (Felis s. catus). *Behav Processes* 2017;141:329–341. https://doi.org/10.1016/j.beproc.2017.02.010

18 Menchetti L, Calipari S, Mariti C, Gazzano A, Diverio S. Cats and dogs: Best friends or deadly enemies? What the owners of cats and dogs living in the same household think about their relationship with people and other pets. *PLoS One*. 2020;15(8):e0237822.

19 Thomson JE, Hall SS, Mills DS. Evaluation of the relationship between cats and dogs living in the same home. *J Vet Behav*. 2018;27:35–40.

20 Fawcett A. Cats and dogs compatibility. *Anthrozoology Research Group*. 2008. www.petnet.com.au/welfare.asp (accessed July 26, 2021).

21 Feuerstein N, Terkel J. Interrelationships of dogs (Canis familiaris) and cats (Felis catus L.) living under the same roof. *Appl Anim Behav Sci*. 2008;113(1–3):150–165. https://doi.org/10.1016/j.applanim.2007.10.010

22 Bernstein PL, Friedmann E. Social behaviour of domestic cats in the human home. In: Turner DC, Bateson P, eds. *The domestic cat: The biology of its behavior*, 3rd ed. Cambridge, UK: Cambridge University Press; 2014:71–80.

23 Landsberg G, Hunthausen W, Ackerman L. *Behavior problems of the dog and cat*, 3rd ed. Edinburgh, UK: Elsevier Health Sciences; 2012.

24 Dickman CR, Newsome TM. Individual hunting behaviour and prey specialisation in the house cat Felis catus: Implications for conservation and management. *Appl Anim Behav Sci*. 2015;173:76–87.

25 Rodan I. *Importance of feline behavior in veterinary practice. Feline behavioral health and welfare*. 2015;2.

26 Volk JO, Thomas JG, Colleran EJ, Siren CW. Executive summary of phase 3 of the Bayer veterinary care usage study. *J Am Vet Med Assoc*. 2014;244(7): 799–802.

15

Cats in the Clinic
Margie Scherk

Introduction

As veterinarians, we believe in, and promote, preventive healthcare. When it comes to bringing our own cats in to the clinic, we may feel trepidation, just as our clients do,[1] yet they do so without the benefit of years of scientific training. That clients even bring their cats to the clinic, is a tribute to both their love of their companion and their trust in veterinarians.

What is a cat's experience in the veterinary clinic? What is their mental and emotional state? How do these affect their physiologic state in the short term? In the long term? How much of their experience do they remember and do they (or what might they), anticipate about subsequent visits? The goal of this chapter is to examine these ideas from the basis of science, where available, anecdote/observation, and a few unabashedly anthropomorphic imaginings by the author.

Imagine the scenario from the cat's point of view: *The carrier comes out, your caregiver is nervous, she chases you around and tries to force you into the carrier. You resist and may resort to self-defense. There are smells of human sweat, fear, maybe even blood. You may feel so anxious that you soil yourself! Eventually you are in the carrier. Everyone is exhausted. Then you are moved into a "car" that moves without you moving. You may be a bit nauseated; certainly you are scared. You cry out repeatedly. You may vomit or soil yourself. Then the "car" stops and you get carried on a noisy and unfamiliar street and into a place with overwhelming smells and sounds! Help! And you are already aroused and anxious ... look out!*

Why is this the default scenario? It's a combination of feline physiology and, frankly, human failing that makes veterinary visit so stressful for the cats.

First, cats are programmed to respond to new situations with concern. They are innately cautious because their amygdala is "preadapted" to respond to perceived threats.[2,3] This means that anything out of the ordinary, like a car ride in a seldom-used carrier, can set them up for disaster.

Second, to add insult to injury, humans (caregivers, their family, veterinary staff, veterinarians) don't always do the things that would make veterinary visits less scary. It's not through lack of desire to do a better job of caring for feline emotions; rather, it's often lack of knowledge and a solid plan.[4,5]

Animal welfare, with a focus on the emotional needs of animals, is a relatively new discipline. Presently, beliefs and practices around animal welfare go beyond the "five freedoms." It is no longer enough merely to provide for physical needs, instead we now look to the type and quality of experiences the individual has.[6] These can have both short- as well as long-term effects on physiological health and emotional suffering.[7]

Clinical Handbook of Feline Behavior Medicine, First Edition. Edited by Elizabeth Stelow.
© 2023 John Wiley & Sons, Inc. Published 2023 by John Wiley & Sons, Inc.
Companion Website: www.wiley.com/go/stelow/behavior

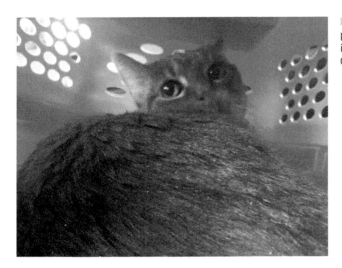

Figure 15.1   This cat is showing body posture and facial expressions indicating fear. Photo credit: Fish Griwkowsky.

McMillan describes the neurobiological mechanisms that are associated with stress and distress; indeed, there is evidence that emotional pain may induce greater suffering than physical pain. Individuals of many species (including cats) will knowingly put themselves at repeated risk for harm and pain when the emotional stakes are high.[8] (https://web.archive.org/web/20150320220111/http://www.animalleague.org/events-news/press-center/scarlett-passes-away.html) A desire to be taken to the veterinarian when ill or healthy doesn't seem to fall in this category, however. Repeated veterinary visits and longer-term hospitalization can have profound negative effects on the well-being of cats.[7,9,10]

The Goal of the Feline Practitioner Must Be to Put Feline Welfare First

There are several reasons that a stressful feline veterinary visit does lasting harm, and therefore should be avoided:

- Caregivers are more stressed when their cats are stressed
- They may choose to change clinics or avoid veterinary visits altogether
- Stressful visits are difficult for staff and may lead to injury
- The visit may yield less useful diagnostic data due to stress
- Stressful visits take a toll on our feline patients.

Let's look a little closer at these issues.

Caregivers Get Stressed When Their Cats Are Stressed

Susan, Kitty's person, hates bringing Kitty in: *Kitty hates going to the vet so much, I only take her when she absolutely has to go in. I believe in preventive health care but it is so stressful for me and for Kitty that I just can't justify it. She struggles when I put her in the carrier; she cries the whole way to the clinic; she hides and then tries to bite people when they handle her. I feel badly for the staff, but I hate seeing her so upset. And I don't like seeing how they handle her! All of it makes me feel guilty. Plus, I hate having to give her medication. I want her to love me and have a good life at home.*

Caregivers "don't care how much we know, until they know how much we care." A survey of 1,111 cat guardians in Italy was performed to assess the cat guardian's perception of cat welfare and behavior at the cat's veterinary clinic.[11] Caregivers assessed poor welfare starting on the trip to the clinic, in all locations and at all stages in the clinic and once the cat returned home. Repeated visits resulted in worsening stress and spilled over to other travel and handling at home. Restraint was viewed as playing a major role in aggression.

A major reason for changing veterinarians was the perception of poor welfare.[11] Another web-based survey of over 3,000 respondents, showed that *one* of the factors influencing the cat's current vaccination status was the caregiver's perception of the importance of stress on their cat.[12] As the relationship between cats and their people has evolved, pet parents expect a more considerate approach to handling their companion.[13]

The Veterinary Team Suffers When Our Patients Are Stressed

Working with stressed and unhappy patients is emotionally draining and can result in physical harm to veterinary team members. Cat bites and scratches have been reported among the most frequent injuries at veterinary clinics.[14]

Let's look at it from the perspective of the veterinary team member: *Kitty has an appointment at 3 p.m. tomorrow. Kitty is never happy in the clinic and everyone is a little anxious in the morning, seeing her name on the day sheet. In fact, until her appointment, this manifests as team members being a little short tempered and worried. Once the appointment is over, everyone breathes a collective sigh of relief and harmony within the team is restored.*

But it goes beyond fear of or actual physical harm. Feline distress causes human distress. Many people working in veterinary clinics feel less comfortable working with cats because they perceive them as being "harder to read."[4] Humans are also physiologically hardwired to respond to threats but allowing our natural reactions (becoming tense, wanting to avoid risk by increasing restraint or restrainers) exacerbates the cat's response. Subconsciously, we may recommend pre-visit sedation (e.g., gabapentin) or take steps to see Kitty less frequently in order to limit *our* distress but justify it as a means of reducing *Kitty's* distress. By becoming aware of our response, we can reduce our reactive, instinctual self-defensiveness and prevent this upward spiral.

We Struggle to Get Appropriate Diagnostic Results Due to the Physiologic Effects of Fear and Stress

During veterinary visits, not only do we have unmeasurable effects of fear, stress, or arousal, we also have those that affect the physical examination and confound diagnostics and behavioral means of assessing our patients.[15] When compared to measurements taken at home, blood pressure, rectal temperature, heart and respiratory rates (HR, RR) were higher in the clinic.[16] Increased epinephrine and cortisol levels result in stress hyperglycemia ($\pm$ glucosuria), increased serum lactate concentration, and a physiologic or a stress leukogram, hypokalemia,[17] and alkaluria. Importantly, stress hyperglycemia generally resolves within 90 minutes of struggling,[18] supporting the ALIVE guidelines that a diagnosis of diabetes may be made either through measuring fructosamine or by finding glucosuria on more than one occasion on a naturally voided sample acquired in a home environment at least two days after any stressful events.[19]

Urine corticoid: creatinine ratio values (using extracted corticoid results) increase between samples collected at home and then in the clinic.[20] When hospitalized over a three-week experimental period, cats experiencing an irregular and unpredictable cleaning/feeding schedule, social interactions, and manipulations were found to have consistently elevated urine-cortisol increased ACTH sensitivity and decreased pituitary sensitivity to luteinizing hormone-releasing hormone. More relevant, perhaps, for practitioners and care providers was that exploratory and play behaviors decreased and the stressed cats spent more time being watchful and trying to hide. Cats able to hide had lower cortisol levels, implying that hiding/evading/controlling exposure to fear-inducing stimuli is critical for the welfare of cats in our care.[21] Neurochemically, elevated cortisol levels interfere with learning to adapt while being frightened[2] and inappropriate learning may occur when repeated negative responses are given to the cat attempting to protect themself.[5]

Stress Takes a Toll on the Cat

Without addressing or thinking also about emotional pain, we risk medicalizing our patients. Emotional pain may be as, or more, debilitating as physical pain. In fact, to separate these two is artificial. Both affect each other: physical health is compromised through stress, anxiety, and fear in many species. Idiopathic cystitis is just one of a lengthy list of illnesses associated with stress in cats.[22,23] McMillan states that: "efforts to promote and maintain optimal health are incomplete and less effective without proper attention to emotional health and well-being."[24]

Over repeated visits, or when a cat has to be hospitalized for a longer period (more than a few hours or days), the physiologic and neurochemical responses to prolonged perceived threat and the inability to cope, can result in illness. In a study of healthy caged cats, after only five days of an altered and unpredictable schedule, "sickness behaviors" including vomiting, diarrhea, anorexia, or decreased food and water intake, lethargy, decreased overall activity levels, grooming, social interactions, somnolence, enhanced pain-like behaviors, and even fever were seen.[25] A study to evaluate behavioral changes over hospitalization was performed using healthy cats being hospitalized (post neutering), for 3–5 days showed that regardless of initial behavioral category ("friendly" through overtly "aggressive"), after two days, their demeanor improved.[26] This may reflect boarding or other minimal handling situation in which cleaning and feeding schedules are maintained.

Anxiety and frustration have been shown to reduce local immunity but that behavioral interventions reducing these emotional states to contentment through gentling, cognitive enrichment, and positive human interaction resulted in enhance IgA-mediated immunity and reduce incidence of URD in shelter cats.[27]

Using radiotelemetry implants to measure BP and HR, Belew et al. showed that a "white-coat effect"/situational hypertension was observed in research colony cats when they were exposed to a simulated clinic visit.[28] Over the period of the office visit, the magnitude of the increases tended to decrease, but not disappear. They concluded that cats should be given time to acclimate to the clinic in an undisturbed, quiet environment.

Interestingly, when stress was compared between examinations performed at home compared to clinic, there was little difference. It must be noted, however, that in this cross-over study, low stress handling techniques were used in both locations. Stress was assessed through serum cortisol and glucose concentrations, temperature, HR, RR, blood pressure, and behavioral parameters. Serum glucose levels and hiding were higher in the clinic. Familiarity with the procedure and the veterinarian appeared to play a role in lower cortisol seen at the second visit, regardless of where it was performed.[29]

Making Feline Veterinary Visits Better

Veterinarians strive to excel at providing top quality medicine for patients. Over the past 30 years, awareness of pain and the importance of preventing, recognizing, and alleviating pain is as much a part of veterinary care as the previous focus of treating physiologic ailments. Herron states it most succinctly: "The commitment to ensuring the emotional well-being of the patient should be equal to that shown toward the physical well-being of the animals under a veterinarian's care."[30] Too many of us struggle with moral distress when caregiver wishes "prevent" us from providing that care.[31] But within the parameters of emotional well-being there is a lot we CAN do.

Reducing fear and anxiety within the clinic itself requires an awareness of how we interact with patients and being thoughtful of the effects of the physical – and social – environment on our patients. This must not be simply replaced by use of anxiolytics or sedatives, although these may be necessary in some cases. The goal has to be providing a more positive, low-stress experience or one in which they feel that they can cope.[32] Being solitary survivors, they anticipate threats in new surroundings. Cats deal with fear or conflict through avoidance or flight. When we can't give them reasons to not be afraid of us or the strange environment, we need to provide them with opportunities to continue to respond to the challenging situation in a species-appropriate manner (hiding/withdrawing, still able to collect sensory information) while we safely perform diagnostics and provide care.[33]

Rochlitz summarized the appropriate goal succinctly by saying that: "Provided extremes are avoided, if the cat has a variety of behavioural choices and is able to exert some control over its physical and social environment, it will develop more flexible and effective strategies for coping with stimuli."[34]

How can the scenario be improved for the cat, for the caregiver, and for the veterinary team? The frightening experience begins at home and continues in the clinic, with recovery taking some time once back at home. Therefore, the path to more comfortable feline veterinary visits includes these four steps:

1) Teach caregivers how to teach their cats to be more comfortable with veterinary care.
2) Arrange our clinics in a way that welcomes cats, by using cat-friendly lighting, reduced noise, pheromones, substrates, furniture, etc.
3) Learn and use handling and diagnostic techniques that minimize fear and stress in our patients.
4) Use medications where necessary, if all of the above fail to achieve sufficient relaxation (or early in the work the pet parent is doing).

1. Teach caregivers how to teach their cats to be more comfortable with veterinary visits

As a first step, veterinarians can provide information on things that caregivers can teach their cats, ideally starting in kittenhood. These include helping the cat feel safe and comfortable with:

- Handling that mimics a physical exam
- Being in the carrier
- Riding in the carrier in the car
- The administration of medications (especially injectables and fluids), nail trims, combing to prevent matts, tooth brushing, and other elements of cat care that can avoid unnecessary visits to the vet clinic.

Handling that Mimics Physical Exams

Starting with kittens (but it is never too late!), teaching cat parents to handle their cats in a way that feels like a physical exam may translate into a less stressful experience for the cat in the clinic. Caregivers can learn from the veterinarian how to pick up their cat, handle their toes, rub inside their ears, lift their tail, "feel around" the abdomen, and open the mouth (gently). This type of training can be rewarded with treats and stroking and can be part of human–animal bonding time.

Being in the Carrier

Ensuring that the cat sees the carrier as a safe space that they choose for sleep and comfort at home is an important part of reducing clinic visit anxiety. The firm-sided, easily cleanable carrier should be easy to disassemble so that the cat can sleep in the bottom, with the lid being added for travel and removed again in the clinic. This way the cat can explore or hide, depending on their state of anxiety.

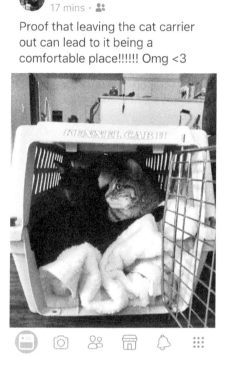

Figure 15.2 Carrier training makes the trip and experience less stressful for the cat.

Riding in the Carrier in the Car

Teaching the cat that travel isn't necessarily a bad thing and isn't always associated with a trip to the veterinary clinic is extremely valuable. Useful tips on this can be found in a caregiver article entitled: Have Cat, Will Travel: https://www.fundamentallyfeline.com/have-cat-will-travel along with accompanying video showing carrier training: https://www.fundamentallyfeline.com/getting-your-cat-in-the-cat-carrier. Another video may be found here: https://www.youtube.com/watch?v=V5a19du2BjA&feature=emb_rel_pause and one showing car travel is here: http://catalystcouncil.org/resources/health_welfare/cat_carrier_video.

Crash-test trials have been performed, showing that placing the carrier in the footwell of the back seats of the car is the safest location. In an accident, even with a safety belt through the top of the carrier (e.g., handle), the seatbelt will stay put but the carrier shell will break and the cat will be flung forward. (time points 1:15-1:50 in this video: https://www.youtube.com/watch?v=fZaQJfHwEN8&t=4s)

Training steps: once kitty enjoys the carrier, cat parents take the carrier into the car, place it in the footwell, start the car and turn it off again, retracing steps to the home. Treats should be given at multiple points to reinforce the positive nature of the experience. Subsequent training sessions expand on this by driving around the block, driving to a destination and taking the carrier out of the car, driving to the veterinary clinic and going in to the clinic without any handling or evaluation by veterinary team members, with each step reinforced by a reward.

Administering Medications and Other Treatments so that We Hospitalize Cats Less

Caregivers can learn lower-stress methods of giving oral medications, delivering subcutaneous fluids, doing at-home nail trims, and other maintenance activities that they occasionally rely on veterinary staff to do. The Fundamentally Feline website has lots of excellent videos about how to give subcutaneous fluids, how to administer medications, and how to truly have this be better accepted. (https://www.fundamentallyfeline.com/how-to-videos)

2. Arrange Our Clinic in a Way that Welcomes Cats

Assuming the cat has found the ride to the clinic to be acceptable, it's important that its time in the clinic is not traumatizing. As discussed previously, we can consider how best to support the cat in the layout and ambience of the clinic and the behavior of the staff. This section discusses how to adapt a clinic's physical space to become a cat-friendly facility.

In the Lobby/Seating Area

The lobby/seating area poses a visual challenge. To prevent the cat from seeing other cats or being sniffed by dogs, the carrier should be placed on a chair or shelf adjacent to the caregiver, or on their lap. Covering the carrier with a towel may help; hospitals may supply a stack of towels for this purpose. Office staff should keep the volume of their voices low and ensure that no other cats or dogs or new people are visible. Make the environment safe for the cat.

The caregiver and cat should be invited into an examination/consultation room as quickly as possible. If all rooms are busy, it may be better for the caregiver to wait in the car with the cat until the examination room is ready for them. The examination room should be as scent free as possible, both from another animal perspective as well as fragrances. Feline facial pheromone F3 plug-in diffusers may be helpful.[35,36]

In the Examination/Consultation Room

For an examination room to be most comfortable for a cat, it requires a few basics: It should:

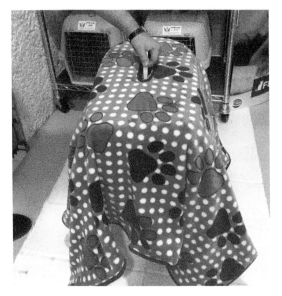

- Provide hiding places for the patient; height-seeking cats may like a tree or tower.
- Be free of noisy equipment, running water, or the sounds of other patients. Calm music may be soothing.
- Smell neutral or pleasant (to the cat); pheromones may be soothing.
- Have lowered light levels.
- Have surfaces covered with towels or mats.

Once in the room, staff can encourage the cat to exit the carrier on their own. If the cat is reluctant to exit, it's best disassemble the carrier rather than dump the cat out or

Figure 15.3   A cat carrier cover. Photo credit: Tamara Iturbe.

reach in to pull them out. Cats should have the opportunity to explore their environment and find a spot they feel comfortable in, whether that is in the bottom of the carrier, on the weigh scale, under the seating, in the examination room sink, or on their person's lap. They can explore or observe while the history is being taken and familiarize themselves with the sensory stimuli and, hopefully, learn to feel safe.

Throughout the appointment, it is good to move gently, speak quietly, reinforce relaxed behaviors, remain calm and attempt to provide reassurance when the cat is anxious.[30] Staff should avoid direct eye contact; sideways glances with hooded eyelids may be somewhat appeasing to cats. Encourage the cat to approach staff: trill, slow blink and offer a hand for them to sniff. If accepted, stroke only the top of the head or chin until the cat indicates that they feel comfortable with further intimacy. Don't pet the cat caudal to the waist.[37]

Plan for the cat to remain in the examination/consultation room for the entire visit. One randomized crossover study evaluated whether cats experienced more stress in the examination room with the caregiver present or in the treatment area without the caregiver. Using HR and Fear Anxiety and Stress (FAS) scores, separation from the pet parent along with being in the treatment area resulted in higher values for all parameters, indicating a higher level of stress.[38] This means that all materials needed for the diagnostics and treatments during this visit should be gathered and prepared ahead of time or brought into the consultation room ready for use.

It is important that everyone understand that the cat's negative emotional state in the examination room doesn't have to be eradicated, rather, that by recognizing its presence, adaptations can be made so that the cat is able to cope.

Please see Box 15.1 for information on feline senses and how to make the examination room a more suitable place for cats. A summary of these concepts is found in Table 15.1.

3. Learn and Use Handling and Diagnostic Techniques that Minimize Fear and Stress in Our Patients

It is crucial that all staff working with feline patients read, check, and recheck the signals the cat is providing. The FAS scale is a very valuable tool to help assess a patient's emotional/mental state. It defines which physical and behavioral signs a cat shows at a certain state of fear, anxiety, stress, or frustration and how to approach that individual. This helps to inform us how we need to change

---

Box 15.1   The physical and social environment: from a feline perspective

What role does the physical environment with human-centric design have on the state and response of the cat? Aroused already from being taken from their safe home, they enter a foreign environment that is filled with olfactory, visual, auditory, tactile and, possibly, taste inputs that are strange.

1. Olfactory Sensations:

While we are primarily a visual species, the most informative sense in cats is their sense of smell. Mills et al. have suggested however, that sensory preference is an individual trait.[39] The surface area of the olfactory epithelium of a cat is 20 cm^2 compared to that of a human at a mere 2–4 cm^2.[40] Additionally, like many other species, but different from us, they have a vomeronasal

(Continued)

Box 15.1   (Continued)

system that detects sensiochemicals (including pheromones) designed for intraspecies communication.[3] Together, the "smells" of an environment provide essential survival information, that we cannot comprehend, upon which they base their behaviors.[3] On entering the clinic, they are greeted with a cacophony of smells: cleaning and disinfecting products, urine, feces, anal glands, which we try to mask through cleaning and by using deodorizers or aromas we find pleasant. They likely are overwhelmed by the "pleasant" fragrance but still smell the confusing mixture of bodily excretions along with scented cat litters, human odors, isopropyl alcohol, and fear pheromones. When boarding or hospitalized, cats are comforted by the scent of themselves or their affiliates.[41] When a cat returns home from the veterinary clinic having lost their characteristic odor, other cats may attack them.[3] As cats investigate a space and become comfortable with it, they will incorporate the smells in their safe repertoire ... but should the experience have negative associations, then the smell will trigger fear, anxiety, or stress.[41]

Olfactory Recommendations: Recognizing that we can't smell many of the odors that cats do, and most certainly not as strongly as they do, we should try to find the least odorous disinfectants and avoid using them near cats (let surfaces dry thoroughly), use isopropyl alcohol sparingly, minimize exposure to the smells and pheromones from other animals, have good ventilation, not share towels, be aware of the myriad smells and pheromones on protective gloves and masks, and consider the use of pheromones throughout the clinic as well as on clothing/hands. Volatile/essential oils should be avoided around cats because they could end up on their coat and be ingested through grooming. Washing their scent away in the kennel or using cleaning products removes their ability to feel secure. By placing two blankets or towels in a cage and replacing only one every day, scent may be preserved.

Catnip, silvervine (*Actinidia polygama*), honeysuckle (*Lonicera tatarica*) and valerian root (*Valeriana officinalis*) may provide olfactory enrichment for cats in the clinic.[42] Outpatients should not be given catnip before examination without knowing whether they become aroused or relaxed from it.

2. Visual Sensations:

Feline vision is geared to hunting. They have a wider visual field than we do (200 degrees, vs our 180 degrees), and by having a larger proportion of rods to cones, they are able to detect movement in dim lighting – dawn and dusk – when they are most active. The large eye that focuses light through a larger (i.e., longer) pupil onto a tapetum lucidum allows them an advantage in poor lighting. While controversial, they appear to see color similar to that of someone with red–green color blindness: they see blue, yellow, and some hues of green.[43] And they do not see color with the same intensity that we do. A color palette that takes what cats see into consideration has been hypothesized.[32,44] Cats are also near sighted: their acuity is 20/100–20/200 meaning that they can only focus up to about 25 cm. Close-range manipulation of prey depends on their vibrissae.[40,45] They see rapid movement more readily than slow movement. The cat's large lens is less flexible making their ability to accommodate and see detail poor, whether near or far, so movement is a key stimulus. Interestingly, adult indoor-raised cats have stiffer lenses and poorer acuity.[40] Artistic interpretation of this can be found at: https://www.livescience.com/40460-images-cat-versus-human-vision.html. Bright lights, rapid movements, anything coming toward their faces will all be stressful and risk initiating a fear response.

Box 15.1	(Continued)

Visual Recommendations: Consider reducing the wattage and install dimmer switches in exam and treatment areas. Be aware of how you move: minimize sudden, quick movement. Allow the cat to reduce visual stimuli under a towel during handling or behind a partly covered door in their kennel. Ensure that while in the clinic proper, they aren't exposed to seeing other cats or dogs. Perform exams and treatments from behind the patient in order to avoid direct eye contact.

3. Auditory Sensations:

With ears that can swivel independently, sideways and backwards, cats have the auditory acuity needed to locate prey before they can see it. The range of frequencies they perceive is between 48 Hz to 85 kHz with the upper ultrasonic range being about an octave higher than we perceive. They developed high-frequency hearing to hear rodents without losing lower frequency range.[46] Yet they also hear low-pitched sounds, including male voices and, very low frequency sounds may be perceived through their pads.[3] The result is that our volume is too loud and they hear things that we don't, such as compact fluorescent light bulbs, light dimmers, some computer and television displays, etc. In the safety of a familiar place, they will blank out stimuli, however in unfamiliar surroundings, these sounds (or smells, or movements) may result in stress.

Auditory Recommendations: In a clinic, there are many strange voices, often loud or abrupt, sudden noises, hissing (spray bottles), shushing, beeps, pings, rings, etc. Speak quietly and gently and baffle ambient noises through use of towels – over the carrier, around the cat, over part of the kennel door, on the floor of the kennel, etc. Open syringe cases or paper wrapping slowly or in another room. Close cage doors quietly. White noise may help dampen disruptive background noise.[30]

Avoid using music that may invoke fear: this includes heavy metal and rock, but even classical music may be problematic.[47] Snowden et al. report that auditory enrichment/mood evocation needs to be species specific.[48] In independent studies, Hampton and Paz have shown that cat-specific music appears to be beneficial, however classical music had no greater effect than silence in the first, whereas it was helpful in the second report.[49,50] To calm an aroused or frightened cat, tones based on affiliative vocalizations (purring, trilling, chirruping) and rewarding sounds will be most effective. Noisy calls, dissonance, short staccato-like sounds may contribute to fear and defensive behavior.[48]

4. Tactile Sensations:

Touch is very important to cats. Cats prefer to be stroked in the temporal region showing fewer negative responses when compared to being stroked over their tail base. Response to being stroked along perioral and non-gland areas was intermediate to the other areas assessed.[51]

Restraint is truly a "less is more" phenomenon in cats. Moody et al. evaluated the negative responses of cats to passive vs. full-body restraint during a physical examination. Behavioral and physiological responses (licks/minute, ears position, pupil diameter, RR, staying on table after being released) were assessed during placement into restraint, restraint and

(Continued)

Box 15.1   (Continued)

following restraint. In passive restraint the cat was able to stand, sit, or lie as they chose and had full movement of their limbs. In full-body restraint (FBR), the cat was held on their side with their back against the handler, while the handler grasps the front and back legs, with a forearm across the cat's neck. The cat was allowed little to no movement of its head, body or limbs. While being placed into FBR, struggling increased; during restraint, lip licking, RR and pupil diameter size increased with ears being positioned down to the side or back; following release from FBR, more cats jumped off the examination table.[52]

Scruffing or using calming clips results in some cats becoming "calm," and semi-immobile.[30] While convenient as clips allow for hands-free restraint, "clipnosis" and scruffing remain controversial due to the ethical concerns around controlling behavior through inhibition resulting in freezing, a negative emotional state, rather than relaxation. The ISFM/FAB feline expert panel strongly support the view that scruffing should never be used as a routine method of restraint, and should only be used where there is no alternative.[53] With time, scruffing, along with pinning and intense or rough restraint has been delegated to be an inappropriate handling technique.[33] Massaging or petting the cat over the perioral and temporal gland sites helps to prevent fear and is recommended to replace scruffing.[54]

Cheek vibrissae are critical for guiding prey to the mouth, so that a fatal neck bite can be delivered.[55] But these exquisitely sensitive structures are also responsible to detecting air movements that could reflect a predator (including human caregivers) or prey. In addition to those found on a cat's cheeks, there are whiskers on chin, in the preauricular area and on the caudal aspect of the carpus and, in some cats, tarsus. Cats dislike being wet or cold and they are uncomfortable with slippery surfaces. The "Physical exam" section below discusses whisker position as a way to understand a cat's emotional state.

Tactile Recommendations: Cover surfaces (tables, cage floor, floor) with towels or soft fleece pads. Administer subcutaneous fluids warmed to body temperature. Don't shave whiskers!

5. Taste Sensations:

Cats appear to lack the ability to taste sweet but are able to taste salty, sour, bitter, and umami (meaty/amino acids) flavors. Additionally, they taste water.[55] They have fewer taste buds than do humans or dogs. Their food preferences are strongly affected by early experience however, they may modify their choices under favorable emotional circumstances.[56]

Taste Recommendations: Offering palatable food or treat (e.g., Churo, Catit Creamy, a syringable recovery diet, Temptations, SmartBites, etc.) may change the emotional state to one of pleasure and can be used for counterconditioning.[30] Bitter-tasting medications can be disguised in a pill-pocket/pilling dough or placed into a size 4 gelatin capsule before administration. Follow pilling with a palatable treat to ensure passage through the esophagus.

Performing a clinic inventory, such as in Table 15.1, is a useful exercise to try to imagine, based on the science, what elements of our surroundings appear threatening to a cat. With this information in hand, the clinic team can take steps to reduce the impact of those threats or remove them completely.

Table 15.1   Sensory threats and management techniques.

Sense	Threats	Reduce threat by?
Smells	Dogs, other cats, people, urine, feces, anal gland secretion, vomit, blood, disinfectants, isopropyl alcohol, medication, deodorizer candles, aromatherapy, perfumes, laundry detergent (Feliway?)	Avoid strong disinfectants, let surfaces dry thoroughly; use isopropyl alcohol sparingly; have good ventilation; don't share towels; use feline pheromones in rooms, on clothing/hands. Exchange one of two towels to preserve own smell. Avoid volatile/essential oils
Sounds	Dogs, other cats, strange voices, phones, faxes, computer printers, doors, water, centrifuge, dishwasher, music, traffic, spritzers/spray bottles, shushing	Speak quietly, gently; quiet noises through towels – over the carrier, around the cat, over the kennel door, on the floor of the kennel, etc. Open products and close cage doors quietly. Use white noise. Avoid loud music. Use purring, trilling, chirruping to calm patient
Sights	Dogs, other cats, strange people, reflections, things approaching face, bright lights, strange clothing (lab coats), masks, gloves, dark silhouettes, sudden movement	Lower the lights. Minimize sudden, quick movement. Reduce visual stimuli with a towel during handling or behind a partly covered carrier door. Prevent seeing other cats or dogs. Wear street clothing (not lab coat) as uniform
Sensations	Cold, wet, slippery, restraint, blood pressure cuff inflating, needles, being syringe fed, cold SQ fluids/injections, stinging injections	Cover surfaces with towels or soft fleece pads. Use minimal but gentle restraint. Warm subcutaneous fluids to body temperature. Don't shave whiskers!
Tastes	Strange diets, medication	Offer palatable foods and treats; disguise bitter medications; follow medications with a treat

how we are approaching and working with a patient at this and subsequent visits. Please see Chapter 8 for more information.

The programs and materials offered by Fear Free Pets are of huge value and all staff should be comfortable using them routinely. https://fearfreepets.com. The program recommends the following tools to help reduce the stress experienced by the cat:

Before the visit
- Medicating for motion sickness [dimenhydrinate 12.4 mg/cat PO lasts 8 h; maropitant 1 mg/kg PO lasts 24 h]
- Pre-visit anxiolysis with gabapentin [5–10 mg/kg PO, given 90–120 minutes before visit, lasts 12 h], a benzodiazepine that allows learning [alprazolam, lorazepam], or trazadone [50 mg PO 90–120 minutes before visit, unknown half-life[57,58]
- Compression garments

During the visit
- In-hospital sedation
- Whether the caregiver and cat have a preferred healthcare provider, a preferred entrance, specific known triggers, favorite/most effective distraction techniques, a preferred exam location, or a most favorite positioning for sample collection.[13,59]

Please note that this author considers the use of anxiolytics before the visit or sedation during the visit as a last resort. Routine use is an admission that not enough attention is being paid to accommodating the patient's emotional needs. Staff should assess the caregiver's body language and try

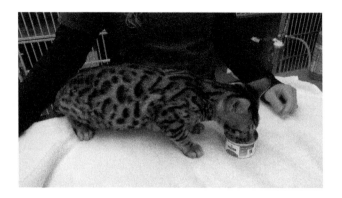

Figure 15.4   Positive conditioning in the clinic for vaccination or for sample collection.

to help them relax. Listen to the words and tone they use regarding the cat (derogatory or tense) and reassure them. Human body language of veterinary team and caregiver can convey unintended messages to a hyperalert patient; helping the caregiver to be relaxed assists with calming the cat.

In emotionally naïve patients (e.g., those who have never been to a veterinary clinic before regardless of age), we have a chance to lay the foundation of positive emotional experience. In these cats, we can offer food treats (by passive delivery on the table top, not by hand) while performing examination, vaccinations, etc. (Figure 15.4) We can reassure them that their fearful behaviors will not be prevented, chastised, or corrected; rather, an option to control their level of exposure to the perceived threats (using towels, blankets) will be provided.

But in cats with established fear/anxious bias toward clinic visits, using food or toys to trigger desire-seeking risks creating a conflicted and confused emotional state that might lead to greater self-defensiveness. In this situation, using anxiolytics can help to shape a less fearful experience so that subsequent visits do not need chemical assistance.

The Physical Exam

Staff body language should be appropriate for interacting with cats. While we smile and show our teeth to convey joy or a desire to engage, cats show their teeth under very different circumstances. Similarly, a steady gaze directly into another person's eyes implies honesty and sincerity, yet for cats this same implies threat and imminent attack.

Examinations should be performed from behind the cat, as looking into the cat's face is threatening. Making oneself as small as possible to avoid looming over the cat also reduces threats. Exams can be done in the bottom of the carrier with the cat covered by a towel.

It takes a conscious decision on part of the entire veterinary team to learn to "speak" cat language. Most clinics have a natural cat advocate; if not, the person who relates best to cats should be appointed. Their role, as through the AAFP Cat Friendly Practice Program (https://catvets.com/cfp/veterinary-professionals) or the ISFM Cat Friendly Clinic Program (https://icatcare.org/veterinary/cat-friendly-clinic) will be to address the physical aspects of "felinizing the facility." Equally, or perhaps more, important will be teaching people to slow down, to move calmly and using a light voice, rather than harsh tones. Practicing towel wrapping and unlearning scruffing (Photo 15.5). Learning how to assess facial expressions (reflecting most rapid changes in emotional state) and whole-body posture and movements. Learning to look at whisker position to assess emotional state.[27] The better everyone is able to read body/facial language, the more appropriately the team can adjust their behavior to help the cat relax or, at very least, not escalate. Regardless of how defensive ("aggressive") cats are, they are more frightened than you are. Also, the manifestations of stress/fear and pain look similar; many cats are both in pain and fearful. (https://www.felinegrimacescale.com)

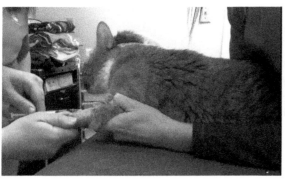
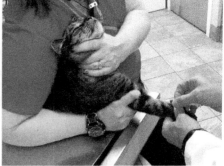

Figure 15.5   a) Scruffing is unnecessary and counterproductive in a feline friendly practice. b) This image illustrates less harsh restraint for purposes of administering a cephalic injection.

One key aspect of "reading a cat" that all staff should know is the common whisker positions that signal different states of emotion in the cat. For example:

- Relaxed, content – whiskers are neutral, slightly sideways
- Interested, engaged – whiskers are fanned forward, with closed mouth, relaxed lips, and plump muzzle
- Hunting – whiskers are fanned out, moving forward to detect prey's neck
- Fearful, anxious, stressed – whiskers are pulled back, often with ears dropping sideway or backwards, +/− open mouth vocalizing
- Self-defensive – whiskers are pointing forward, with ears upright and turned laterally
- Painful – whiskers are spreading forward, but with a flattened and tense muzzle

Facial Expressions

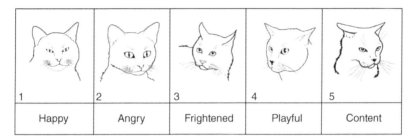

1	2	3	4	5
Happy	Angry	Frightened	Playful	Content

Handling for Specimen Collection

Similar to examination, sample collection should be done away from the cat's face, using as quiet a clipper as possible (or not shaving), very little or no isopropyl alcohol, with minimal restraint on a soft, non-slippery surface. Gentle handling with calm voices by relaxed personnel is extremely important. Having prepared all necessary materials (syringes, labelled tubes, slides, etc.) ahead of time, nursing staff can come into the room moving slowly and calmly. Avoid moving the cat to another room (e.g., treatment area) for procedures as the cat has become acclimated to the consultation room. As sample collection is best performed in this room, the caregiver will be with the cat in most cases.[60] Being calm will help the caregiver be calm. If this isn't possible, the caregiver should be asked to briefly leave the room.

Allow the cat to retain a sense of control over their body. The medial saphenous vein (Figure 15.6) is the author's first choice for blood collection as the cat's front end can remain sternal while the back end is rotated. In this position, without needing to reposition the cat, a cystocentesis can be performed to collect a urine sample and, if it hasn't already been done, blood pressure can be readily collected (prior to other sampling) in this position as well (Figure 15.7). Should this vein not provide the desired sample, then the cat's front end can be laid laterally for a jugular collection. Alternately, a jugular sample can be collected with the cat resting in sternal position (Figure 15.8) rather than moving the cat's forelimbs over the edge of the table – much like hanging someone over a cliff or out of a window, being directly in their visual field (threat) then approaching them with noisy clippers and smelly, cold isopropyl alcohol, topped off with a needle prick.

Blood pressure cuffs should be placed on the limb or tail at the same horizontal level as the heart (Figure 15.9). Tail measurements have been shown to be less affected by muscle condition and age and have the advantage of being away from the cat's face.[61] When using a Doppler, it is very helpful to use an ear covering headset to prevent the cat from hearing the noise of the probe on the fur while locating the artery. If this isn't possible, turn the volume of the machine as low as possible.

If a cat becomes extremely upset during handling, persisting with attempts to handle the patient risks creating long-term aversion/negative associations with the clinic. In this case, the clinician has two options: use chemical restraint or take a break from the procedure, allowing the cat to relax in a safe, quiet space (e.g., their carrier inside a kennel). Breaking the exam into portions, interspersed with rest periods, may allow them to relax and learn that the procedures are safe.

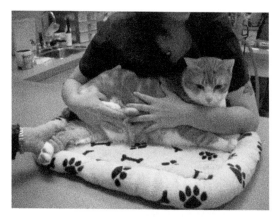

Figure 15.6 Positioning for medial saphenous blood collection.

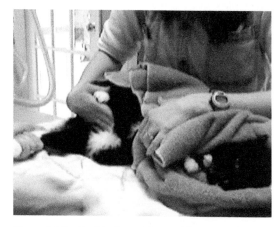

Figure 15.7 Positioning with towel for protection of holder for medial saphenous blood collection and for cystocentesis urine collection.

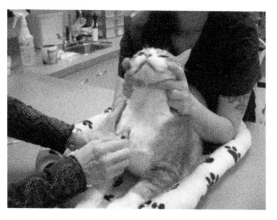

Figure 15.8 Positioning for jugular venipuncture.

Distraction using toys or food may work as long as the cat isn't too aroused. Sometimes having the caregiver leave may be preferable to having the caregiver stay with them. Counter-intuitively, a study evaluating blood pressure using continuous direct measurement via pressure transducer in healthy conscious cats found that mean blood pressures were higher (whether active or not) when they were stroked by a familiar person than when being stroked by an unfamiliar person.[62]

Hospitalization

Should a cat need to be hospitalized, it is important to not only keep the husbandry schedule constant, but also to understand the social needs of the individual cat. Despite being solitary survivors, they need some degree of interaction. For some cats, being spoken to multiple times a day suffices, while others want to be stroked. Cats have, as already noted, stroking preferences. While some cats will warm into allowing a full-body pet, it shouldn't be assumed. Many cats prefer top of head only.

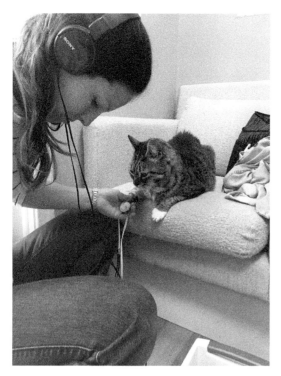

Figure 15.9 Placement of blood pressure cuff is in line with the heart and headset reducing noise heard by patient.

Because cats do not appear to be able to anticipate future events, much like us when we are frightened or in pain, the only reality is the present experience. Depending on the needs of both the patient and the caregiver provisions for regular visiting should be considered.

Social interactions with other cats and other species in the veterinary clinic should be restricted, especially when the cat needs to be hospitalized. Cages should not face other cages; cats should not be able to see the treatment table. Olfactory, auditory, and visual communication should be kept to a minimum. Towels used for other patients should be removed from the olfactory space (e.g., taken to the laundry promptly) to eliminate fear/alarm pheromone from the area. Cats should be kept away from noisy cats and dogs.

Providing multiple and separated resources in a kennel is difficult but should be considered.[63] Use of vertical space can help. Using the top of the cat's carrier as a perch and as a place to hide can move the cat away from the litter box. Water and food should be as far from the litter as possible. The bedding should be soft and the kennel as quiet and non-reflective as possible. Hanging a towel over the half of the door/gate that has the bed and food will provide additional privacy without completely eliminating light or the ability to observe. If possible, have the litter box in an adjacent compartment. Opportunity to play and puzzle solve should be provided to cats who aren't too ill. This may include a play box, as shown in Figure 15.10. Rather than disinfect and reuse them, the author sends these home with the caregiver, where they can be used for toys or as a modified puzzle feeder. This inexpensive tool has provided the additional benefit of caregivers telling friends about it resulting in referrals.

Stainless steel poses a lot of sensory difficulties to cats. It is reflective, cold, and loud. The floor of the kennel should be covered with a towel or fleece, rather than newspaper so it is warm and soft. As already mentioned, covering half of the cage door with a towel will reduce the reflections inside the cage that might scare the cat. Dimming the lights and/or rotating track lighting to face away from the patients will help cats relax. The latches of the cage door are very loud when the door is closed: applying tape or being extremely cautious when closing the door will help reduce that source of noise. A useful exercise for all personnel is to spend five minutes inside a cage looking out in order to see what their patients experience.

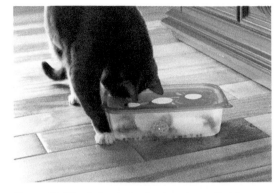

Figure 15.10 A simple toy box can be crafted from a plastic container containing kibble or soft toys or catnip.

When approaching the cat in their kennel, it is important to not block the entire opening. Blocking out all of the light and trapping the cat may make them feel threatened. Allow them the choice to come forward to even to try to leave. A happy cat has the sense of control.

Heading Home

Once the visit is over, the cat will most often willingly enter their carrier. If more than one cat came in one carrier, providing a loaner carrier, clean and free of previous cat smells, can be offered to help reduce the fear-induced aggression between housemates. The visit isn't over until the cats have adjusted to their home environment and family members. The cat returning home is at a disadvantage. The veterinary visit may have been for preventive care, may have included shaving (disfigurement), or the cat may be convalescing after anesthesia or illness. They may have a feeding tube or need repeated medication. They no longer belong to the previously harmonious group.

Upon returning home, place the cat in their carrier in a room and, with the door to the room closed, open the carrier. Let the cat groom themselves to remove clinic smells and re-establish the smell the other cats are familiar with before letting the cat into the rest of the home. One can also apply some talcum/baby powder to the bib (chest) of all of the cats so they all smell the same.

Most caregivers dread giving treatments; they may be leery of being hurt, feel guilt toward their cat, not have the skills to follow the recommendation, all of which can end up with a course of therapy being cut short. When oral medications are prescribed, pills are generally easier to give than liquids and subcutaneous injections easier still. (Which would you rather do?) Pre-drawn injections of once or twice daily medications can be sent home, depending on clinic policy. Pills may be administered in pill pockets or pilling dough, be ground up (depending on the medication) and mixed into an appetizer or Churo or Catit Creamy. If the medication is bitter, placing it inside a size 4 gelatin capsule will hide the flavor as well as allow multiple medications to be given at once. All pills and capsules should be chased with water or food to reduce the possibility of esophageal stricture formation.

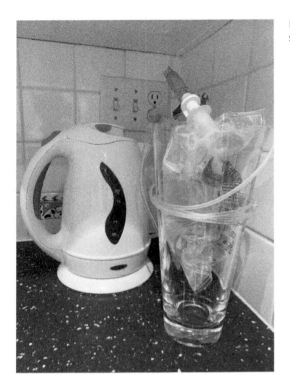

Figure 15.11 Set-up for warming fluids for subcutaneous administration.

Subcutaneous fluids (in clinic or at home) are more readily accepted when they are warmed to cat body temperature (Figure 15.11). **(See Appendix for Client Handout)** Pairing the fluids or any medication with a food or other reward will make the cat more accepting of the treatment.

Provide a web resource for how to perform treatments. (See Box 15.2). While we may gravitate toward the more professionally crafted videos, a YouTube home video posted by another cat parent may be more meaningful and reassuring to a caregiver than a perfectly staged one.

Caregiver stress and clinic team energy, speech and body language play a role in the emotional experience for the patient. Educating the caregiver as already mentioned toward creating a

---

Box 15.2

Having a library of YouTube links or making your own clinic "how-to" videos is extremely helpful. YouTube videos made by lay people may have the advantage of being more convincing rather than those by healthcare professionals. Find ones that your staff and you as well as a caregiver think are best. There are many good links. Examples of useful illustrative clips to have on hand include how to:

- Give your cat a pill (see below)
- Give subcutaneous fluids: www.youtube.com/watch?v=OLOVw35w4Ns
- Administer insulin: http://www.youtube.com/watch?v=XeZgKLflJn4
- Measure blood glucose: www.veterinarypartner.com/Content.plx?A=605

(Continued)

Box 15.2 (Continued)

- Use an inhaler for asthma medications: www.youtube.com/watch?v=INF1W8uaPEA
- Change a KittyKollar (video) and Living with an E-tube (handout): www.kittykollar.com

Syringe feeding, brushing teeth, etc. are also available. Cat caregivers like to show their skills and help others.

Similarly, having a selection of web resources that you have vetted and feel comfortable with guides caregivers to reading materials when they want to learn more about their companion's medical condition.

Cornell University has a series of videos on a number of procedures and diseases at www.partnersah.vet.cornell.edu. They include: Brushing your cat's teeth, Giving your cat a pill or capsule, Giving your cat liquid medication, Taking your cat's temperature, trimming your cat's nails. Other free videos include: Caring for your diabetic cat, Gastrointestinal diseases in cats, Cat owner's guide to kidney disease, Managing destructive scratching behavior in cats, and A pet owner's guide to cancer.

Everything on the icatcare website has been created by the ISFM and is excellent: http://icatcare.org/advice/general-care. They have an extensive library of handouts on medical conditions as well as general cat care, including several videos.

Feline Chronic Kidney Disease: www.felinecrf.org

Feline Diabetes: www.felinediabetes.com, www.petdiabetes.com.

---

relaxing transition from home to car to clinic will benefit the human as well. Making the clinic comfortable, homey, less clinical may also reduce the white coat response on the part of the caregiver.

4. Use Experience-altering Medications ("Chemical Restraint") When Necessary

This author believes that sedation should *not* be used *routinely* for bringing cats to the clinic or for the fearful cat during veterinary visits. It is too easy to believe the excuse that it is more humane for the patient and that it allows the team to get procedures done quickly, allowing the cat a shorter visit. For truly respectful and compassionate handling, time and effort put into making changes to the sensory milieu of the clinic and manner of handling allows the cat to learn that they can cope. Ask yourself who you are doing this for.

When all attempts to provide low stress handling have been employed, Sophia Yin recommended that: "If it is thought that the measures already taken will not be sufficient to keep the cat calm and cooperative through the visit, injectable sedatives should be considered before the cat has a chance to become highly aroused or reactive, since they have a more consistent effect when used at an early stage."

Reversible agents should be used to leave the cat with as little confusion as possible. A recommended protocol is 20–30 mcg/kg dexmedetomidine with 0.2–0.4 mg/kg butorphanol administered IM, to be reversed with ½ volume (dexmedetomidine volume) atipamezole IM. Geriatric, sick or cats with cardiac disease should not receive dexmedetomidine. Buprenorphine may be used in lieu of butorphanol at 0.02 mg/kg IM or via the transmucosal route. The cat needs to be monitored throughout the entire sedation and recovery period.[59] Put cotton into the cats ears and cover the cats eyes during sedation to reduce the level of external stimulation. Muscle tension, HR, RR, and blood pressure should be monitored.

Summary

As stated succinctly by Heath: "due to complex interconnections ... physical health cannot be optimised unless emotional and cognitive health are also considered."[33] Key to this is allowing the cat to perceive that they have control and choice in their experience. By making some environmental changes by continuously assessing the emotional response of the patient and adjusting our responses, we improve the clinic experience for our feline patients.

Appendix

How to Give Subcutaneous Fluids

To Warm the Fluids to Body Temperature:

1) Using an unopened bag:
   a) Remove the outside protective bag
   b) Microwave the bag for 2–3 minutes (depending on microwave)
   c) Massage the warmed bag to distribute the heat evenly
   d) Test the bag on your wrist. It should feel comfortably warm, just about body temperature.
2) If the bag has already been used and has the line attached, do not microwave it as the line will melt and seal shut.
   a) Boil water in a kettle or pot
   b) Put the bag into a vase or tall upright container with the bulb portion up so it will remain above the water
   c) Pour the hot water into the vase taking care to not reach the bulb
   d) Set the timer for about five minutes (depends on how much is remaining in the used bag)
   e) Massage the warmed bag to distribute the heat evenly
   f) Test the bag on your wrist. It should feel comfortably warm, just about body temperature

To Connect a New Line to a Bag

1) Prepare the line by rolling the wheel to a closed position
2) Take the cap off the line being careful not to touch the end of the line
3) Remove the end from the port on the bag
4) Insert the pointed end of the IV line into the port
5) Squeeze the bulb of the IV line to fill the bulb half full
6) Open the line by rolling the wheel to the open position and fill the line with fluids

To Give Your Kitty Fluids

1) Hang the bag of fluids on a curtain rod or shower rod with the still-capped line hanging down
2) Place an unused, covered needle on the line and place the sterile cap (from the end of the line) close by

3) Sit somewhere comfortable. I prefer the floor so that kitty feels secure
4) If you want, you can wrap your kitty in a towel leaving head and shoulders exposed and cradle him/her
5) Remove the cover on the needle
6) With kitty facing away from you, holding the needle rest your dominant hand on your kitty's back with the needle facing toward his head
7) Lift and make a tent with the skin between kitty's shoulders using your non-dominant hand
8) Exhale and firmly pull that skin tent over the needle
9) Open the IV line wheel and administer the volume of fluids as directed by your doctor
10) Once the needle is in place, because the fluids are warmed, kitty should be comfortable. Giving treats and praise doesn't hurt either!
11) Once you've given half of the fluid volume, back the needle out partially (but remain under the skin), so you can redirect it over the other shoulder and insert it fully again. This helps with weight distribution
12) Close the IV line, remove and discard the needle safely recapping the line with the sterile cap
13) Pinch the skin together with your non dominant hand when you remove the needle

Congratulations! You've Done It!

Notes:

1) While you are getting used to this procedure, it may help to have the fur shaved over two places at the back of the neck. That way you can be sure the needle is getting under the skin. The fur will grow back.
2) Your kitty will look like she/he is wearing shoulder pads. The fluids will drop to one side down a leg, even to the paw. These will be absorbed over 12–24 hours. If the fluids have NOT been absorbed, a smaller volume is needed. Contact your veterinarian.
3) If some of the fluids or even a bit of blood leak from the injection site, there is no need to worry.

References

1 Volk JO, Thomas JG, Colleran EJ, Siren CW. Executive summary of phase 3 of the Bayer veterinary care usage study. *J Am Vet Med Assoc.* 2014;244(7):799–802.
2 Overall K. Facing fear head on: Tips for veterinarians to create a more behavior-centered practice dvm360.com, September 30, 2013 (accessed June 30, 2020).
3 Bradshaw J. Normal feline behaviour:... and why problem behaviours develop. *J Feline Med Surg.* 2018;20(5):411–421.
4 Bayer HealthCare. Bayer Veterinary Care Usage Study III: Feline Findings. 2012.
5 Heath S. Understanding feline emotions:... and their role in problem behaviours. *J Feline Med Surg.* 2018;20(5):437–444.
6 Mellor DJ. Updating animal welfare thinking: Moving beyond the "five freedoms" towards "a life worth living". *Animals.* 2016;6:21. doi:10.3390/ani6030021.
7 Overall K. Fear factor: Is routine veterinary care contributing to lifelong patient anxiety? dvm360.com, August 31, 2013 (accessed June 15, 2020).
8 McMillan FD. A world of hurts – is pain special? *J Am Vet Med Assoc.* 2003;223(2):183–186.

9 Hargrave C. Anxiety, fear, frustration and stress in cats and dogs – Implications for the welfare of companion animals and practice finances. *Companion Anim*. 2015a;20(3):136–141.

10 Hargrave C. In-practice management of stress in cats and dogs – Improving the welfare of companion animals and practice finances. *Companion Anim*. 2015b;20(5):292–299.

11 Mariti C, Bowen JE, Campa S, Grebe G, Sighieri C, Gazzano A. Guardians' perceptions of cats' welfare and behavior regarding visiting veterinary clinics. *J Appl Anim Welf Sci*. 2016;19(4):375–384.

12 Habacher G, Gruffydd-Jones T, Murray J. Use of a web-based questionnaire to explore cat owners' attitudes towards vaccination in cats. *Vet Rec*. 2010;167(4):122–127.

13 Johnson JT, Williamson JA. Faculty development with integration of low stress pet handling techniques into a veterinary school curriculum. *MedEdPublish*. 2018;7.

14 Jeyaretnam J, Jones H. Physical, chemical and biological hazards in veterinary practice. *Australian Vet J*. 2000;78(11):751–758.

15 Levine AD. Feline fear and anxiety. *Vet Clin Small Anim*. 2008;38:1065–1079.

16 Quimby JM, Smith ML, Lunn KF. Evaluation of the effects of hospital visit stress on physiological parameters in the cat. *J Feline Med Surg*. 2011;13:733–737.

17 Lauler DP. Stress hypokalemia. *Conn Med*. 1985;49(4):209–213.

18 Rand JS, Kinnaird E, Baglioni A et al. Acute stress hyperglycemia in cats is associated with struggling and increased concentrations of lactate and norepinephrine. *J Vet Intern Med*. 2002;16:123–132.

19 European Society of Veterinary Medicine. Project Alive. https://www.esve.org/alive/search.aspx (accessed May 30, 2020).

20 Cauvin AL, Witt AL, Groves E et al. The urinary corticoid: Creatinine ratio (UCCR) in healthy cats undergoing hospitalisation. *J Feline Med Surg*. 2003;5:329–333.

21 Carlstead K, Brown JL, Strawn W. Behavioral and physiological correlates of stress in laboratory cats. *Appl Anim Behav Sci*. 1993;38:143–158.

22 Buffington CT. External and internal influences on disease risk in cats. *J Am Vet Med Assoc*. 2002;220(7):994–1002.

23 Westropp JL, Kass PH, Buffington CA. Evaluation of the effects of stress in cats with idiopathic cystitis. *Am J Vet Res*. 2006;67(4):731–736.

24 McMillan FD Emotional pain: Why it matters more to animals than physical pain and what the animals want us to do about it. VMX Proceedings 2018:314–317.

25 Stella J, Croney C, Buffington T. Effects of stressors on the behavior and physiology of domestic cats. *Appl Anim Behav Sci*. 2013;143:157–163.

26 Zeiler GE, Fosgate GT, Van Vollenhoven E, Rioja E. Assessment of behavioural changes in domestic cats during short-term hospitalisation. *J Feline Med Surg*. 2014;16(6):499–503.

27 Gourkow Nadine. Emotions, mucosal immunity and respiratory disease in shelter cats. PhD thesis, Univ Queensland 2012. https://espace.library.uq.edu.au/data/UQ_284698/s41334931_phd_ finalthesis.pdf?dsi_version=c1b69c9518c3b7e9b2eac3aae0b333d6&Expires=1644204798& Key-Pair-Id=APKAJKNBJ4MJBJNC6NLQ&Signature=gEMiEuCTq3jT2kcS8Ajg-1~zN7tGB1-njN MbKv0fNTZfoFSQ61zTBdvcEGix6Q0YaNqVmL8FD7bzSWqUn46ZxeC29OGg4iWBw2ndLmzzbZ npYOjqYxUjyAw0ofIqlP5xpthSn~4LWOApsOCNkKMkWgk34Ouf36wN79iOk2nMIuNnZnkNpkD bYFrAVx63oPrCaJusT4yu6Se5XSaxn624YXUsGcW55MEwxd-k58iGSAOb9FrHtmWIdExiG6Lxm8 PHvJZmhQPxzK79SHbVung2RF-T0npTE53NOceaqig4eBOpXjrF9ib64A2FV0jITKAYVNENTJY5S KXSDrxzJIQOoA__ (accessed February 6, 2022).

28 Belew AM, Barlett T, Brown SA. Evaluation of the white-coat effect in cats. *J Vet Intern Med*. 1999;13(2):134–142.

29 Nibblett BM, Ketzid JK, Grigg EK. Comparison of stress exhibited by cats examined in a clinic versus a home setting. *Appl Anim Behav Sci*. 2015;175:68–75.

30 Herron ME, Shreyer T. The pet-friendly veterinary practice: A guide for practitioners. *Vet Clin North Am Small Anim Pract.* 2014;44:451–481.

31 Rollin BE. Integrating science and well-being. *Vet Clin N Am Sm Anim.* 2020;50(4):899–904.

32 Lloyd JFK. Minimising stress for patients in the veterinary hospital: Why it is important and what can be done about it. *Vet Sci.* 2017;4:1–19.

33 Heath S. Environment and feline health: At home and in the clinic. *Vet Clin Small Anim.* 2020;50(4):663–693.

34 Rochlitz I. A review of the housing requirements of domestic cats (*Felis silvestris catus*) kept in the home. *Appl Anim Behav Sci.* 2005;93:97–109.

35 Hewson C. Evidence-based approaches to reducing in-patient stress – Part 2: Synthetic pheromone preparations. *Vet Nurs J.* 2014;29(6):204–206.

36 Pereira JS, Fragoso S, Beck A, Lavigne S, Varejão AS, da Graça Pereira G. Improving the feline veterinary consultation: The usefulness of Feliway spray in reducing cats' stress. *J Feline Med Surg.* 2016;18(12):959–964.

37 Ellis SL, Thompson H, Guijarro C, Zulch HE. The influence of body region, handler familiarity and order of region handled on the domestic cat's response to being stroked. *Appl Anim Behav Sci.* 2015;173:60–67.

38 Griffin F, Mandese W, Reynolds P et al. Evaluation of clinical exam location on stress in cats: A randomized crossover trial in review. *J Feline Med Surg.* 2020. doi:10.1177/1098612X20959046

39 Mayes ER, Wilkinson A, Pike TW, Mills DS. Individual differences in visual and olfactory cue preference and use by cats (Felis catus). *Appl Anim Behav Sci.* 2015;173:52–59.

40 Bradshaw JW, Casey RA, Brown SL. *The behaviour of the domestic cat.* Oxfordshire: Cabi; 2012.

41 Vitale Shreve KR, Udell MA. Stress, security, and scent: The influence of chemical signals on the social lives of domestic cats and implications for applied settings. *Appl Anim Behav Sci.* 2017;187:69–76.

42 Bol S, Caspers J, Buckingham L, Anderson-Shelton GD, Ridgway C, Buffington CT, Schulz S, Bunnik EM. Responsiveness of cats (Felidae) to silver vine (Actinidia polygama), Tatarian honeysuckle (Lonicera tatarica), valerian (Valeriana officinalis) and catnip (Nepeta cataria). *BMC Vet Res.* 2017;13(1):70.

43 Clark DL, Clark RA. Neutral point testing of color vision in the domestic cat. *Experimental Eye Res.* 2016;153:23–26.

44 Lewis HE. https://www.dvm360.com/view/fear-free-what-you-see-not-what-cat-or-dog-gets (accessed February 6, 2022).

45 Bradshaw J. 2014 How Do Cats Use Their Whiskers? Slow-Motion | Cats Uncovered | BBC Earth https://www.bbc.co.uk/programmes/p027rmq3 (accessed February 6, 2022).

46 Heffner RS, Heffner HE. Hearing range of the domestic cat. *Hear Res.* 1985;19(1):85–88.

47 Mira F, Costa A, Mendes E, Azevedo P, Carreira LM. A pilot study exploring the effects of musical genres on the depth of general anaesthesia assessed by haemodynamic responses. *J Feline Med Surg.* 2016;18(8):673–678.

48 Snowdon CT, Teie D, Savage M. Cats prefer species-appropriate music. *Appl Anim Behav Sci.* 2015;166:106–111. doi:10.1016/j.applanim.2015.02.012.

49 Hampton A, Ford A, Cox III RE, Liu CC, Koh R. Effects of music on behavior and physiological stress response of domestic cats in a veterinary clinic. *J Feline Med Surg.* 2020;22(2):122–128.

50 Paz JE, da Costa FV, Nunes LN, Monteiro ER, Jung J. Evaluation of music therapy to reduce stress in hospitalized cats. *J Feline Med Surg.* 2021;20:1098612X211066484.

51 Soennichsen S, Chamove AS. Responses of cats to petting by humans. *Anthrozoös.* 2002;15(3):258–265.

52 Moody CM, Picketts VA, Mason GJ, Dewey CE, Niel L. Can you handle it? Validating negative responses to restraint in cats. *Appl Anim Behav Sci.* 2018;204:94–100.

53 Rodan I, Sundahl E, Carney H, Gagnon AC, Heath S, Landsberg G, Seksel K, Yin S. AAFP and ISFM feline-friendly handling guidelines. *J Feline Med Surg*. 2011;13(5):364–375.

54 Horwitz DF, Rodan I. Behavioral awareness in the feline consultation: Understanding physical and emotional health. *J Feline Med Surg*. 2018;20:423–426.

55 Bartoshuk LM, Harned MA, Parks LH. Taste of water in the cat: Effects on sucrose preference. *Science*. 1971;171(3972):699–701.

56 Bradshaw JW. The evolutionary basis for the feeding behavior of domestic dogs (Canis familiaris) and cats (Felis catus). *J Nutr*. 2006;136(7):1927S–1931S.

57 Stevens BJ, Frantz EM, Orlando JM, Griffith E, Harden LB, Gruen ME, Sherman BL. Efficacy of a single dose of trazodone hydrochloride given to cats prior to veterinary visits to reduce signs of transport-and examination-related anxiety. *J Am Vet Med Assoc*. 2016;249(2):202–207.

58 Orlando JM, Case BC, Thomson AE, Griffith E, Sherman BL. Use of oral trazodone for sedation in cats: A pilot study. *J Feline Med Surg*. 2016;18(6):476–482.

59 Yin S. Handling the challenging cat. In: Rodan I, Heath S, eds. *Feline behavioral health and welfare*. St. Louis: Elsevier; 2016:306–318.

60 Sundahl E, Rodan I, Heath S. Providing feline-friendly consultations. In: Rodan I, Heath S, eds. *Feline behavioral health and welfare*. St. Louis: Elsevier; 2016:269–286.

61 Whittemore JC, Nystrom MR, Mawby DI. Effects of various factors on Doppler ultrasonographic measurements of radial and coccygeal arterial blood pressure in privately owned, conscious cats. *J Am Vet Med Assoc*. 2017;250(7):763–769.

62 Slingerland LI, Robben JH, Schaafsma I, Kooistra HS. Response of cats to familiar and unfamiliar human contact using continuous direct arterial blood pressure measurement. *Res Vet Sci*. 2008;85(3):575–582.

63 Ellis SL, Rodan I, Carney HC, Heath S, Rochlitz I, Shearburn LD, Sundahl E, Westropp JL. AAFP and ISFM feline environmental needs guidelines. *J Feline Med Surg*. 2013;15(3):219–230.

Appendix 1

Feline Psychopharmacology

Elizabeth Stelow

The purpose of this appendix is to provide useful and accurate basic information regarding the use of psychotropic medications in cats in a quick-reference style. For the clinician in search of greater understanding of the key neurotransmitters targeted, the chemical structure of the medications presented here, or subtle differences in mechanisms of action among medication in the same class, the references presented below are a wonderful place to continue that exploration.

Abbreviations

For this Appendix, the following abbreviations will be very useful:

BZD = Benzodiazepine
CYP450 = Cytochrome P450
SARI = Serotonin Antagonist and Reuptake Inhibitor
SSRI = Selective Serotonin Reuptake Inhibitor
TCA = Tricyclic Antidepressant
MAOI = Monoamine Oxidase Inhibitor

Introduction and Considerations

Studies have shown that the introduction of an appropriate psychotropic medication into a treatment plan for a behavior problem can lead to a more rapid and more satisfactory resolution.[1,2]

How, then, does a clinician recognize the need for medication, select a best-fit starting point, and monitor the results? Much like all other areas of medicine, it's important to start with a thorough understanding of the problem based on diagnostic assessments, an accurate diagnosis, and a comprehensive treatment plan. If the clinician and the client agree that the treatment plan may not be successful given the current level of arousal or reactivity of the patient, there is a good indication that medications may be useful. The client must be counseled that medications may improve the cat's response to the plan but will not be a substitute for the work of implementing the necessary elements.[1]

There are a few limitations to prescribing psychotropic medications to cats:

1) Limited Research. Ideally, a clinician will pair their clinical expertise with a critical appraisal of available medications based on high-quality data from well-designed clinical trials. Together, these form the evidence-based decision making that leads to best outcomes.[3]

   Unfortunately, there is a lack of research supporting the use of psychotropic medications in cats. What limited research there is has focused on a few medications in a few drug classes treating a few behavior problems. Most research to date has been testing selective serotonin reuptake inhibitors (SSRIs, primarily fluoxetine), tricyclic antidepressants (TCAs), benzodiazepines (limited testing), buspirone (in the azapirone class), and trazodone (a serotonin antagonist and reuptake inhibitor, or SARI). The indications researched have been mainly urine marking and stress during veterinary visits. Still, clinicians use these medications and see results. In the discussion below, the current understanding about indications for these medications and side effects and contraindications are presented.

2) Owner Attitudes. Clients' beliefs about and understanding of psychotropic medications will influence their willingness to agree to begin these medications, their willingness to give the medication consistently, and their view of the positive and negative effects they see. Some owners will be clear during the appointment that they are not comfortable with psychotropic medications in general, often due to the person having made negative associations based on what they have heard or read about their use in human psychiatry. Some will be concerned that the side effects they predict (or actually see) will be harmful to the pet. Still others will be interested in trying the medications in the treatment plan but not be prepared for the sometimes lengthy time to effect of some of the newer, more targeted medications.[4]

3) There are no psychopharmaceuticals approved for use in cats.

Despite these limitations, psychopharmaceuticals are often a crucial aspect of a comprehensive treatment plan for problem behaviors is cats.

Determining the Need for a Psychotropic Medication

There are four steps to determining the need for a psychoactive medication:

- Make an accurate diagnosis based on history and physical exam.
- Develop a complete treatment plan to address that diagnosis, taking into consideration the details of the presenting problems and owner lifestyle.
- Assess whether the patient is likely to be successful in completing the treatment plan in a timely manner without the aid of medication. Indications for the need for medications include a combination of excessive arousal, unavoidable triggers, moderate to severe anxiety in some or all circumstances, limited impulse control, compulsive behaviors, and the infrequent presentation of substantial triggers like fireworks or veterinary visits.
- Verify that a medication exists that supports the diagnosis *as it manifests in this patient*. Not all cases of urine marking require medication. Not all diagnoses of play-related aggression require medication.

While it may be tempting to try to diagnose through the response to medication, this is usually not an effective path.[4]

It is crucial that the clinicians remember that medications are one aspect of a treatment plan and cannot replace careful management and the efforts of behavior modification in achieving a satisfactory resolution.[1,4]

Selecting a Medication

There are a few things to consider when selecting a medication.

- The most obvious consideration is the list of medications that have historically been efficacious in treating the diagnosis.
- Another is whether there are restrictions on how the medication must be delivered; for instance, some owners struggle to pill their cats while others can't get their cats to take liquids. Occasionally, these limitations can be overcome with client and patient training or desensitization and counter-conditioning. But, it's important to take note of them.
- Finally, it is crucial that the clinicians know whether the ideal medication must be fast-acting (Is the problem episodic or based on an event, like vet visits? Is the owner's impatience with the problem a threat to the cat's life?) or whether delayed onset medications (like the SSRIs and TCAs) can be considered.

This appendix provides two ways for the clinician to select a medication based on diagnosis. First, the descriptions of the drug classes below each list the indications for which that class is most commonly used.

Second, the dose chart included at the end of this appendix includes current information on the forms and doses currently available for the medications listed. The sections on each drug class includes likely time to effects, since that is something that varies between classes but very little within them.

Patient Workup

All of the medications discussed in this book are metabolized by the liver and/or kidneys. Some affect cardiac function and others alter the tested levels of circulating thyroid analytes. It is, therefore, crucial for the clinician to assess the appropriateness of a patient for a given medication. This starts with a minimum database (complete blood count, serum biochemistry panel) and any other test indicated based on the contraindications of the medication or its class.[2]

Owner Education

Owner compliance is predicated on their good understanding of the plan. This is especially true of medications, and, in particular, those that are meant to be given for a lifetime or that may cause unwanted effects. For each psychotropic medication to be dispensed, the owner must fully understand:

- The goal of prescribing the medication. How will this medication aid in the treatment of the problems presented during the appointment?
- The possible positive and negative effects. When will they likely be seen? Which undesirable effects are "deal-breakers" and which should be tolerated for a day or two to see if they resolve? Most will be mild and transient.[2] Which effects would require immediate or near-term veterinary attention?
- When the medication is likely to begin to work. It is very important that owners are not looking for improvement too early; their disappointment may undermine their confidence in the plan, which may alter compliance.

- How to know if the medication is meeting expectations. Shifts in behavioral responses due to the addition of medication can be subtle. It's important to remind the client that the medication is not the entire plan, but typically only lays the groundwork for behavior modification. Many clients will assert that the medication isn't working because the pet is still doing "the thing" they brought it in for; closer questioning often uncovers some interesting improvements in the extent, duration, or scope of the problem. So, it's best to set the stage for the owners to look for even the subtlest improvements as a sign that the medications "is working."
- When and how often the clinician would like an update.

The better educated the owner is about the medication and what to expect, the better they will be at monitoring and using the medication as directed.[2]

Patient Monitoring

Clinicians have an obligation to monitor patients taking medications they prescribe. Current recommendations include:

Annual lab work and physical exam. This should be even more frequent in older pets whose liver may not remain as competent to metabolizing medications.

Any special tests needed based on contraindications for the medication.

Serotonin Syndrome

"Serotonin Syndrome" is an uncommon response to a significant (10–50 times above baseline) increase in levels of serotonin due to the use of one or more serotonin-enhancing medications. The clinical signs of Serotonin Syndrome may include disorientation, restlessness, tremoring, ataxia, myoclonus, diarrhea, and hyperthermia.[2] These signs typically occur shortly after the start of a medication or an increase in its dose; therefore, owners should watch for any of these signs when starting or increasing a serotonin-enhancing medication in their cat.

Serotonin syndrome is a diagnosis of exclusion.

If diagnosed, supportive care should be instituted based on specific clinical presentation. A serotonin antagonist like cyproheptadine (1.1 mg/kg PO) may be useful in reversing effects.[2]

Anesthesia

Patients taking psychopharmaceuticals should not be tapered off of them prior to an anesthesia event. Doing so could exacerbate the reason for anesthesia and result in an unapproachable patient. Instead, the anesthesia should be tailored to the medications they are taking:

- If the patient is already taking a benzodiazepine, avoid using one in the pre-anesthesia cocktail.
- If the patient is taking a TCA or SARI that affects cardiovascular tone, avoid any anesthesia agents that might do the same.
- If the patient is taking an SSRI or TCA, it is possible that they will require less propofol due to CYP3A4 inhibition. Clinicians should verify which SSRIs and TCAs can cause this effect before using propofol in these cats.

Constant respiratory rate and ECG monitoring is recommended during all anesthesia events with cats taking psychoactive medications.[2]

Polypharmacy

If a cat does not respond as desired to the first psychopharmaceutical prescribed, the clinician can do one of three things:

1) Increase the dose of the first medication to the highest recommended dose in hopes of seeing the desired response
2) Taper the first medication and trying a different one of the same or different drug class
3) Add a second medication to the first to amplify the desired effects.

Although very little research has been done on combinations of these medications in animals, research in humans has shown some helpful combinations:

- SSRI/TCA + BZD when the person is anxious overall but also experiences fear in certain predictable situations
- Fast acting medication (gabapentin, BZD, or trazodone) started at the same time as an SSRI or TCA, so that the person can experience relief while the slower-acting medication takes effect
- SSRI + memantine (not discussed in detail in this appendix) for compulsive behaviors that do not respond to an SSRI alone.

Other possible combinations exist.

As one might guess, combining medications increases the likelihood of increased side effects. Sometimes these are additive (the side effects of a BZD + those of an SSRI); other times, we see worsened side effects if the two medications happen to share a metabolic enzyme, like a specific CYP450 isoform. A very serious side effect when combining two serotonin-enhancing medications, like and SSRI/TCA and SARI, is serotonin syndrome.[5]

Tapering to Change Medications

There is little evidence about how to gradually discontinue one medication to begin an incompatible one. It is wise, then, to proceed cautiously. If a long-acting medication like SSRI or TCA has been used for several weeks, tapering should take a few weeks.[5] If no new medication will be started, tapering can be slowed to take months. In the discussion of each medication, any recommended "washout" before starting a new medication is given. These washouts are necessary between serotonin-enhancing medications.

Specific Drug Classes and Medications

Following is a brief summary of the pertinent facts about the most commonly used classes of psychotropic medications in the cat. For additional information, please refer to one of the books listed in the reference section. The classes included are:

- Anticonvulsants
- Azapirones
- Benzodiazepines
- Monoamine Oxidase-B Inhibitors
- Serotonin Antagonist and Reuptake Inhibitors

- Selective Serotonin Reuptake Inhibitors
- Tricyclic Antidepressants

This is by no means a complete list of psychoactive medications that can be used in cats; it is merely a list of the most-commonly-used medications. Resources listed may include others.

   Note: Dosing listed below is oral, unless otherwise specified; any IV or IM dosing is meant for in-hospital use only.

Class: Anticonvulsants

Medications in Class
This class includes gabapentin, which is the only medication in this class commonly used for behavior diagnoses in cats. Gabapentin, while structurally similar to γ-aminobutyric acid (GABA), is not active at GABA receptors. Instead, its effects appear to be due to a reduction of glutamate release in the amygdala. Since glutamate is, in part, responsible for fear response, that response is lessened.[6]

Indications
Gabapentin is commonly used to treat neuropathic pain. In addition, it is effective in treating anxiety and other "behavior" conditions, like panic, stereotypic behaviors, and compulsive behaviors. It is a good choice as a pre-visit medication for veterinary visits.

Mechanism of Action and Time to Effect
Gabapentin takes effect within 90–120 minutes when given on an as-needed basis. It can also be given every 8–24 hours, depending on the diagnosis and treatment plan.

Cat Dose Range
The starting daily dose for gabapentin in cats is 3–5 mg/kg every 12–24 hours,[2] with a total daily dose range being 3–10 mg/kg every 8–24 hours.[7,8] For as-needed dosing, 5–20 mg/kg and 50–100 mg/cat given 90–120 minutes before the target event have both been reported.[7,9]

Common Side Effects
Relatively few side effects have been reported for gabapentin in cats. A dose-dependent sedation and ataxia appear to be most common. If withdrawn rapidly, there appears to be concerns about triggering seizures.[10]

Contraindications and Drug Interactions
Do not give gabapentin to cats with severe renal or hepatic disease.

Supporting Research and Additional Discussions Affecting Use
In her 2017 research, Dr. van Haaften found that gabapentin given to cats before a routine veterinary visit scored lower on stress scales and were more compliant for physical exams.[9]

   In 2018, Dr. Katherine Pankratz found that gabapentin calmed the fear responses in the treatment groups of 53 community cats that were trapped for desexing surgery. There was limited sedation and the only reported side effect was hypersalivation.[11]

Class: Azapirones

This class includes buspirone, a partial serotonin agonist, and the only medication in this class commonly used in cats. Azapirones are relievers of anxiety with less decrease in cognitive function or memory impairment than is seen in some other drug classes, particularly the benzodiazepines.[2,12]

Medications in Class
The one commonly used medication in this class is buspirone.

Indications
This medication is used to treat urine marking, toileting problems, overgrooming, and inter-cat aggression. In the latter diagnosis, it is used to treat the less confident (typically more nervous) "victim" cat so that it will stand up for itself to that cat that is harassing it.[2,13]

Mechanism of Action and Time to Effect
The effects of buspirone can be seen after approximately one week.[12]

Cat Dose Range
0.5–1 mg/kg PO q8–24 h[7]

Common Side Effects
Buspirone can result in bradycardia or tachycardia, nervousness, GI disturbances, stereotypic behaviors in cats.[12]

Contraindications and Drug Interactions
Use with caution with MAOIs. In humans, this medication is used with caution with erythromycin and itraconazole, as both increase the circulating concentration of buspirone.

Supporting Research and Additional Discussions Affecting Use
In 1993, Hart found that, when given to 62 urine marking cats, buspirone resulted a greater than 75% reduction in marking in 55% of the cats in the study. Moreover, many of these cats did not return to urine marking when the buspirone was discontinued two months later.[13]

Class: Benzodiazepines

Medications in Class
This class includes alprazolam, clonazepam, clorazepate, diazepam, lorazepam, midazolam, oxazepam. Each has a subtly different set of effects, side effects, and contraindications.

Indications
This class of drug is among the strongest for profound relief of episodic anxiety and panic. These medications are also useful in treating urine marking and overgrooming.[12]

Mechanism of Action and Time to Effect
These medications potentiate the effect of GABA at GABA receptors by increasing that receptor's affinity for the GABA molecule.[2]

These medications are rapid onset (~60 minutes) and are, therefore, good for as-needed use.[14] Due to a number of factors, such as physiologic tolerance and difficulty in forming new memories, they are not ideal for long-term chronic use.

According to at least one resource,[2] these medications have the following dose-dependent benefits:

Low dose: calms and tempers excitement
Moderate dose: reduces anxiety to facilitate social interactions
High dose: hypnotic

Cat Dose Range[2,7]
Alprazolam: 0.125–0.25 mg q 8 hours
Clonazepam: 0.05–0.2 mg/kg q 12–24
Clorazepate: 0.2–0.4 mg/kg q 12–24 hours; 0.5–2.2 mg/kg PRN for profound distress.
Diazepam: 0.2–0.5 mg/kg q 12–24 hours
Lorazepam: 0.03–0.08 mg/kg q 12–24 hours; up to 0.125–0.25 mg/cat/dose
Midazolam: 0.05–0.3 mg/kg IV, IM, or SC
Oxazepam: 0.2–0.5 mg/kg q 12–24 hours; 3 mg/kg for appetite stimulation

Common Side Effects
The primary side effects of medications of this class in cats are dose-related sedation and ataxia. They have been noted to cause disinhibition of undesirable behaviors, like aggression. Use of these medications may not be compatible with learning new skills due to reported amnestic properties. Paradoxical excitation is a frustrating side effect for clients.

Contraindications and Drug Interactions
Use with care in cats with hepatic or renal deficiencies. Clonazepam, lorazepam, and oxazepam have no intermediate metabolites – so they may be better for patients with hepatic insufficiency.[12]

    There is history of hepatic necrosis in some cats after oral administration of these medications.

Supporting Research and Additional Discussions Affecting Use
Frequent daily dosing of benzodiazepines requires gradual withdrawal at the end of treatment.[7]

    Physiologic tolerance can occur with these medications; this requires dose increases over time.[2]

    Clinicians are cautioned to be aware that medications in this class are all subject to potential human abuse.[2] Before prescribing, the clinician must feel comfortable that the entirety of the medication will be given to the cat.

Class: Monoamine Oxidase B Inhibitors (MAOI-Bs)

Medications in Class
This class includes selegiline, an irreversible inhibitor of MAO-B and the only medication in this class commonly used in cats.

Indications
This medication is most commonly used for cats with cognitive dysfunction. It is licensed for dogs with that diagnosis – not so for cats.

Mechanism of Action and Time to Effect
The roles of monoamine oxidases in general include breaking down serotonin, norepinephrine, and dopamine; altering their receptors; and increasing their release from pre-synaptic neurons. Due to its structure as an inhibitor of MAO-B, selegiline affects mainly dopamine. Additionally, MAOIs may reduce free radicals in brain tissue.[15]

Cat Dose Range
0.25-1.0 mg/kg q 24 hours[7] Can be split q 12 hours.[2]

Common Side Effects
Selegiline can cause restlessness, agitation, vomiting, diarrhea, disorientation, and hearing loss.[15]

Contraindications and Drug Interactions
MAOIs should not be used in conjunction with any other serotonin-enhancing medication, including SSRIs and TCAs. Combining these medications can lead to life-threatening health problem like serotonin syndrome. If selegiline is to be given following treatment with fluoxetine, allow 5 weeks of washout between the medications; this can be reduced to 2 weeks for the other SSRIs.[15]
  Avoid combining with metronidazole, prednisolone, and sulfamethoxazole-trimethoprim.

Supporting Research and Additional Discussions Affecting Use
A small amount of selegiline metabolizes to amphetamine-like metabolites. This may be a problem for animals not diagnosed with cognitive dysfunction.[2]
  In one study, Landsberg et al. found that older cats had a reduction in clinical signs of cognitive decline while taking Selegiline.[16]

Class: Serotonin Antagonist and Reuptake Inhibitors (SARIS)

Medications in Class
This class includes trazodone HCl, which is the only medication in the class commonly used in cats.

Indications
Anxiety, post-operative sedation, pre-veterinary visit anxiolysis.

Mechanism of Action and Time to Effect
Trazodone blocks serotonin 2_A and 2_C receptors and reduces the reuptake of serotonin into presynaptic neurons. On an empty stomach, trazodone takes 60 minutes to initial effect; this latency to effect is twice as long when given with food.

Cat Dose Range
For as-needed dosing, give 50–100 mg/cat or 10.6–33.3 mg/kg prior to an event.[17] If given daily, the recommended cat dose is 1–2 mg/kg every 12 hours.[7]

Common Side Effects
Sedation is the most common side effect seen in clinical trial with trazodone in cats.[17–19]

Contraindications and Drug Interactions
Avoid giving with MAOIs and with caution with SSRIs or TCAs to avoid serotonin syndrome.
  Use with caution in cats with renal disease, hepatic disease, cardiac disease, or glaucoma.
  Do not use with azole antifungals, macrolide antibiotics, or phenothiazides, as they inhibit CYP450(3A4), which is used in trazodone metabolism.[17]

Supporting Research and Additional Discussions Affecting Use

There are two studies of the effects of single-use trazodone in cats. In one study (Orlando 2015), cats were given 50–100 mg trazodone; they were seen to reduce their activity but did not show a difference in response to physical exam.[18]

In a second study (Stevens 2016), cats were given either 50 mg trazodone or a placebo before being placed in a carrier and transported to a physical exam; a crossover was completed three weeks after the initial test. Trazodone resulted in a decrease in anxiety during transport and increased ease of handling. The primary side effect seen was sedation.[19]

Class: Selective Serotonin Reuptake Inhibitors (SSRIs)

Medications in Class

This class includes fluoxetine, fluvoxamine, paroxetine, and sertraline.

Indications

SSRIs are most often used in cats to treat anxiety, aggression, compulsive behaviors, and urine marking.[2,20]

Mechanism of Action and Time to Effect

Early in the course of daily treatment, SSRIs reduce the reuptake of serotonin into the presynaptic neuron. Over time, they also downregulate serotonin 1_A receptors in the postsynaptic neuron. This delayed effect has more therapeutic benefit than the reuptake inhibition; therefore, efficacy should not be assessed until at least 4 weeks after the start of daily treatment.[20]

Cat Dose Ranges[2,7,20]

SSRIs are typically give every 24 hours[2], but can be split into 12 hours doses to minimize side effects, where necessary.[2]

Fluoxetine: 0.5–1.0 mg/kg q24 hours or 0.5–1.5 mg/kg q 24 hours[7]

Fluvoxamine: 0.25–0.5 mg/kg q 24 hours

Paroxetine: 0.5 mg/kg q 24 × 6–8 wk then 1.0 mg/kg q 24[2] or 0.5–1.0 mg/kg q 24 hours[7] or 0.5–1.5 mg/kg q 24 hours[20]

Sertraline: 0.5–1.5 mg/kg q 24 hours[7] or 0.5 mg/kg q 24 × 6-8 wk then 1.0 mg/kg q 24 hours[2]

Common Side Effects

The most common side effects of SSRI use in cats include appetite suppression, constipation (esp paroxetine), urinary incontinence/retention, tremors, nausea, anxiety, agitation, and aggression.

Contraindications and Drug Interactions

Do not combine any SSRI with any MAOI, including Amitraz products, due to the likelihood of serotonin syndrome.

Do not give fluoxetine or fluvoxamine with Cisapride.

Fluoxetine uses the same Cytochrome enzymes as benzodiazepines and tricyclic antidepressants; so, when combining these medications, plan to keep the doses of each in the low-to-mid range.

Paroxetine has less liver enzyme inhibition than the others. Paroxetine should not be used in animals with glaucoma.

Supporting Research and Additional Discussions Affecting Use

The bulk of the research on SSRIs in cats has been done on the first one to become available as a generic: fluoxetine. There are no studies on the use of sertraline in cats.

Transdermal formulations of these medications have proved to be ineffective.[21]

Class: Tricyclic Antidepressants (TCAs)

Medications in Class

This class includes amitriptyline, clomipramine, doxepin, imipramine, and nortriptyline.

Indications

Anxiety, compulsive behaviors, aggression, excessive vocalization, overgrooming.

Mechanism of Action and Time to Effect

TCAs inhibit the reuptake of serotonin and norepinephrine, with variations in percentages among individual medications. They are also variably antihistaminic, anticholinergic, and α-1 antagonistic. They take 3–8 weeks to achieve full effect and should not be assessed for efficacy before 8 weeks.

Cat Dose Ranges[2,7,22]

Amitriptyline: 0.5–2.0 mg/kg q 12–24 hours

Clomipramine: 0.25–1.3 mg/kg q 24 hours[22] or 0.25–0.5 mg/kg q 24 hours[2] or 0.25–1.0 mg/kg q 24 hours[7]

Doxepin: 0.5–1.0 mg/kg q 12–24 hours

Imipramine: 0.5–1.0 mg/kg q 12–24 hours

Nortriptyline: 0.5–2.0 mg/kg q 12–24 hours

Common Side Effects

The most common side effects of TCA use in cats include sedation, reduced appetite, ataxia, constipation, diarrhea, urinary retention, and tachycardia.

Contraindications and Drug Interactions

Do not combine and TCA with any MAOI, including Amitraz products, due to the likelihood of serotonin syndrome.

TCAs can interfere with the measurement of circulating T4; they, therefore, should not be given to cats who require frequent, accurate T4 readings.[2]

Avoid using amitriptyline in cats with seizures or cardiac arrhythmias.[7]

Supporting Research and Additional Discussions Affecting Use

In one study of urine marking cats, clomipramine was found to be as effective at reducing marking incidents as fluoxetine.[23] A similar study found a decrease urine marking in over 80% of the 25 subjects, with 25% of cats to be calmer and more affectionate on clomipramine.[24] Finally, a prospective randomized clinical trial with 67 cats found that clomipramine ranging in dose from 0.125–1.0 mg/kg daily was associated with reduction in urine marking; sedation was noted as the most common side effect, occurring in half the cats.[25]

Drug Dose Chart[2,7–10,14,17,20,22]

Class	Drug name	Cat dose	Contraindications	Side effects
Anticonvulsants Behavioral dx: anxiety	Gabapentin	Daily: 3–5 mg/kg every 12–24 h to start. 3–10 mg/kg q 8–24 h. PRN: 5–20 mg/kg and 50–100 mg/cat given 90–120 minutes before.	Rapid withdrawal may lead to seizure activity. Avoid use with severe renal disease.	Sedation, ataxia
Azapirones Behavioral dx: anxiety, urine marking, over-grooming, intercat aggression.	Buspirone	0.5–1 mg/kg PO q 8–24 h		Changes in heart rate, nervousness, GI disturbances, stereotypic behaviors.
Benzodiazepines (BZDs) Behavioral dx: anxiety, panic, urine marking, overgrooming	Alprazolam	0.125–0.25 mg q 8 h	Duration: 24 hours	Sedation and ataxia, paradoxical excitation, polyphagia, possible disinhibition of aggression.
	Clonazepam	0.05–0.2 mg/kg q 12–24 h	Duration: 24–48 hours	
	Clorazepate	0.2-0.4 mg/kg q 12–24 h; 0.5–2.2 mg/kg PRN for profound distress.	Duration:	
	Diazepam	0.2–0.5 mg/kg q 12–24 h	Duration: 24–48 hours	has caused hepatic necrosis when given orally.
	Lorazepam	0.03–0.08 mg/kg q 12–24 h; up to 0.125–0.25 mg/cat	Duration:	
	Midazolam	0.05–0.3 mg/kg IV, IM, or SC	Hospital use only	
	Oxazepam	0.2–0.5 mg/kg q 12–24 h; 3 mg/kg for appetite stimulation	Duration: 12–18 hours	
Monoamine Oxidase-B Inhibitors Behavioral dx: cognitive dysfunction	Selegiline (L-deprenyl)	0.25–0.5 mg/kg q 12–24 h; up to 1 mg/kg PO q 24h; start low	Avoid using with SSRIs or TCAs.	Restlessness, agitation, vomiting, diarrhea, disorientation, and hearing loss

(Continued)

(Continued)

Class	Drug name	Cat dose	Contraindications	Side effects
Serotonin Antagonist and Reuptake Inhibitors Behavioral dx: anxiety, post-operative sedation, pre-veterinary visit fear	Trazodone	50–100 mg/cat or 10.6–33.3 mg/k PRN for events. 1–2 mg/kg q 12 hs if given daily	Do not use with macrolide antibiotics, azole antifungals, phenothiazides. Use in caution with renal and hepatic disease, cardiac disease, and glaucoma.	Sedation
Selective Serotonin Reuptake Inhibitors Behavioral dx: anxiety, panic, urine marking, overgrooming	Fluoxetine	0.5–1.0 mg/kg q 24 h or 0.5–1.5 mg/kg q 24 h	Avoid use with MAOIs, Cisapride. Use with care with TCAs, trazodone, tramadol, and BZDs.	Appetite suppression, constipation (esp paroxetine), urinary incontinence/ retention, tremors, nausea, anxiety, agitation, and aggression.
	Fluvoxamine	0.25–0.5 mg/kg q 24 h	Avoid use with MAOIs, Cisapride. Use with care with TCAs, trazodone, tramadol.	
	Paroxetine	0.5 mg/kg q 24 h x 6–8 wk then 1.0 mg/kg q 24 h or 0.5–1.0 mg/ kg q 24 h or 0.5–1.5 mg/kg q 24 h	Avoid use with MAOIs. Use with care with TCAs, trazodone, tramadol. Avoid with glaucoma.	
	Sertraline	0.5–1.5 mg/kg q24 or 0.5 mg/ kg q 24 × 6–8 wk then 1.0 mg/kg q 24 h	Avoid use with MAOIs. Use with care with TCAs, trazodone, tramadol.	
Tricyclic Antidepressants Behavior dx: anxiety, compulsive behaviors, aggression, excessive vocalization, overgrooming	Amitriptyline	0.5–2.0 mg/kg q 12–24 h	Avoid use with MAOIs. Use with care with SSRIs, trazodone, tramadol.	Sedation, reduced appetite, ataxia, constipation, diarrhea, urinary retention, and tachycardia.
	Clomipramine	0.25–1.3 mg/kg q 24 h or 0.25–0.5 mg/kg q 24 h or 0.25–1.0 mg/kg q 24 h	Avoid use with MAOIs. Use with care with SSRIs, trazodone, tramadol.	

(Continued)

(Continued)

Class	Drug name	Cat dose	Contraindications	Side effects
	Doxepin	0.5–1.0 mg/kg q 12–24 h	Avoid use with MAOIs. Use with care with SSRIs, trazodone, tramadol.	
	Imipramine	0.5–1.0 mg/kg q 12–24 h	Avoid with seizures. Avoid use with MAOIs. Use with care with SSRIs, trazodone, tramadol.	
	Nortriptyline	0.5–2.0 mg/kg q 12–24 h	Avoid use with MAOIs. Use with care with SSRIs, trazodone, tramadol.	

References

1 King JN, Simpson BS, Overall KL, et al. Treatment of separation anxiety in dogs with clomipramine: Results from a prospective, randomized, double-blind, placebo controlled, parallel-group, multicenter clinical trial. *J Appl Anim Behav Sci*. 2000;67:255–275.

2 Overall K. Pharmacological Approaches to changing behavior and neurochemistry: Roles for diet, supplements, nutraceuticals, and medication. In: *Manual of clinical behavioral medicine for dogs and cats*. St Louis (MO): Elsevier; 2013:458–512.

3 Kochevar DT, Fajt V. Evidence-based decision making in small animal therapeutics. *Vet Clin North Am Small Anim Pract*. 2006;36:943–959.

4 Overall KL. Pharmacological treatment in behavioral medicine: The importance of neurochemistry, molecular biology, and mechanistic hypotheses. *Vet J*. 2001;162:9–21.

5 de Souza Dantas L. Mattos, Crowell-Davis SL, Ogata N. Combinations. In: Crowell-Davis SL, Murray TF, de Souza Dantas LM, eds. *Veterinary psychopharmacology*, 2nd ed. Hoboken, NJ: John Wiley & Sons Inc.; 2019:281–290.

6 Stahl SM. *Stahl's essential psychopharmacology: Neuroscientific basis and practical applications*, 4th ed. Cambridge: Cambridge University Press; 2013.

7 Perrin C, Seksel K, Landsberg GM. Appendix: Drug dosage chart. *Vet Clin North Am Small Anim Pract*. 2014;44(3):629–632.

8 Crowell-Davis SL, Irimajiri M, de Souza Dantas L. Mattos. Anticonvulsants and mood stabilizers. In: *Veterinary psychopharmacology*, 2nd ed. Hoboken, NJ: John Wiley & Sons Inc.; 2019:147–156.

9 van Haaften KA, Eichstadt LR, Stelow EA, et al. Effects of a single preappointment dose of gabapentin on signs of stress in cats during transportation and veterinary examination. *J Am Vet Med Assoc*. 2017;251(10):1175–1181.

10 KuKanich B. Outpatient oral analgesics in dogs and cats beyond nonsteroidal antiinflammatory drugs. *An Evidence-based Approach. Vet Clin North Am Small Anim Pract*. 2013;43(5):1109–1125.

11 Pankratz KE, Ferris KK, Griffith EH, et al. Use of single-dose oral gabapentin to attenuate fear responses in cage-trap confined community cats: A double-blind, placebo-controlled field trial. *J Feline Med Surg*. 2017;20(6).

12 Seksel K, Landsberg G, Ley JM. Behavioral therapeutics. In: Little S, ed. *The cat: Clinical medicine and management*. St. Louis (MO): Elsevier Saunders; 2012:227–234.

13 Hart BL, Eckstein RA, Powell KL, Dodman NH. Effectiveness of buspirone on urine spraying and inappropriate urination in cats. *J Am Vet Med Assoc*. 1993;203:254–258.

14 de Souza Dantas L. Mattos, Crowell-Davis SL. Benzodiazepines. In: Crowell-Davis SL, Murray TF, de Souza Dantas LM, eds. *Veterinary psychopharmacology*, 2nd ed. Hoboken, NJ: John Wiley & Sons Inc.; 2019:67–102.

15 de Souza Dantas L. Mattos, Crowell-Davis SL. Monoamine oxidase inhibitors. In: Crowell-Davis SL, Murray TF, de Souza Dantas LM, eds. *Veterinary psychopharmacology*, 2nd ed. Hoboken, NJ: John Wiley & Sons Inc.; 2019:185–199.

16 Landsberg G. Feline housesoiling: Marking and inappropriate elimination. *Proceedings of the Atlantic Veterinary Conference*. Atlantic City, NJ: 1999.

17 de Souza Dantas L. Mattos, Crowell-Davis SL. Miscellaneous serotonergic agents. In: Crowell-Davis SL, Murray TF, de Souza Dantas LM, eds. *Veterinary psychopharmacology*, 2nd ed. Hoboken, NJ: John Wiley & Sons Inc.; 2019:129–146. *[Azapirones, SARIs]*.

18 Orlando JM, Case BC, Thomson AE, et al. Use of oral trazodone for sedation in cats: A pilot study. *J Feline Med Surg*. 2016;18(6):476–482.

19 Stevens B, Frantz ES, Orlando JM, et al. Efficacy of a single dose of trazodone hydrochloride given to cats prior to veterinary visits to reduce signs of transport- and examination-related anxiety. *J Am Vet Med Assoc*. 2016;249(2):202–207.

20 Ogata N, de Souza Dantas L. Mattos, Crowell-Davis SL. Selective serotonin reuptake inhibitors. In: Crowell-Davis SL, Murray TF, de Souza Dantas LM, eds. *Veterinary psychopharmacology*, 2nd ed. Hoboken, NJ: John Wiley & Sons Inc.; 2019:103–128.

21 Ciribassi J, Luescher A, Pasloske KS, et al. Comparative bioavailability of fluoxetine after transdermal and oral administration to healthy cats. *Am J Vet Res*. 2003;64(8):994–998.

22 Crowell-Davis SL. Tricyclic Antidepressants. In: Crowell-Davis SL, Murray TF, de Souza Dantas LM, eds. *Veterinary psychopharmacology*, 2nd ed. Hoboken, NJ: John Wiley & Sons Inc.; 2019:231–256.

23 Hart BL, Cliff KD, Tues V, et al. Control of urine marking by use of long-term treatment with fluoxetine or clomipramine in cats. *J Am Vet Med Assoc*. 2005;226(3):378–382.

24 Landsberg GM, Wilson AL. Effects of clomipramine on cats presented for urine marking. *J Am Anim Hosp Assoc*. 2005;41:3–11.

25 King J, Steffan J, Heath S, et al. Determination of the dosage of clomipramine for the treatment of urine spraying in cats. *J Am Vet Med Assoc*. 2004;225:881.

Appendix 2

Medications for Pain Management in Cats

Elizabeth Stelow

Pain can be difficult to identify in cats. With proper guidance, clients can learn to detect changes in their cat's normal mobility and behavior patterns indicative of pain.
— Ray/AAFP Senior Care Guidelines[1]

Introduction

Failure to identify and treat pain in cats can reduce their quality of life, and lead to more adverse outcomes like central sensitization and chronic pain.[2] In fact, the AAFP, in its Senior Care Guidelines, states, "The Task Force proposes that pain be thought of as a disease itself that can greatly influence quality of life." Chapter 7 of this volume considers the causes and presentations of both acute and chronic pain in cats, as well as accepted approaches to treatment. Most pain prevention or control strategies currently involve medications (meds), which are the subject of this Appendix. In addition, a comprehensive update on pain management guidelines for dogs and cats recently (2022) was published.[3]

The recent development and validation of a number of pain-scoring systems for cats, newer analgesic drugs, innovative pain-relief techniques, and increasing understanding of feline-specific pharmacokinetics and pharmacodynamics of pain meds have greatly enhanced feline pain prevention and treatment.[4]

Historically, selecting and administering pain meds to cats has been challenging. This is due, in part to the fact that feline drug metabolism sometimes differs from that in most other species. For instance, cats metabolize drugs that rely on conjugation (glucuronidation, etc.), such as carprofen and morphine, more slowly than many other species, whereas they metabolize analgesics, like piroxicam and buprenorphine, which undergo oxidation, more rapidly. Finally, cats excrete drugs that are passed unchanged in the urine or bile (like gabapentin) at rates similar to other species.[2] This variation has resulted in misunderstandings – and so requires a thorough awareness of the effects of each drug used on cats.

Overall Strategy for Managing Pain in Cats

As discussed in Chapter 7, pain may be acute, like traumatic injury or surgical wounds, or chronic, like osteoarthritis, FIC, or cancer. Acute pain, when it is foreseeable, requires a combination of pre-emptive as well as multimodal relief.[5] Unforeseen acute and chronic pain management must rely on relief after the fact; each management approach has its own strategy based on the duration and intensity of the pain. Strategies are best presented based on the source and predictability of the pain:

Perioperative Pain

Start pain meds at the time of surgery to reduce post-operative pain.[2] Multimodal pain management. Includes two or more meds or other treatments with different mechanisms of action; e.g., Opioid + NSAID or Opioid + cooling therapy may act synergistically. Remember also to consider anxiolytics (gabapentin/trazodone) and antiemetics (maropitant/ondansetron).

Acute Pain (non-perioperative):[2]

- Orofacial: NSAIDs, Opioids, Locoregional anesthesia
- Neuropathic: NSAIDs, Opioids, NMDA receptor antagonists, Alpha-agonists, Locoregional anesthesia. Gabapentinoids[6,a]
- Visceral: ± NSAIDs, Opioids, Alpha-2 agonists, locoregional anesthesia
- Oncologic: NSAIDs, Opioids, NMDA receptor antagonists, Alpha-agonists, Locoregional anesthesia.
- Somatic: NSAIDs, Opioids, NMDA receptor antagonists, Locoregional anesthesia.

Chronic Pain

Particularly in senior cats, chronic pain may come from the following:[1]

- Osteoarthritis (OA) and spondylosis are the two most common degenerative joint disease (DJD) causes of pain and the behavioral changes associated with it. These conditions currently are incurable, and require ongoing treatment to maintain comfort, mobility, and good welfare. Drugs with published efficacy include nonsteroidal anti-inflammatory drugs (NSAIDs), gabapentin, and tramadol.
- Other causes: Constipation (and the posturing associated with it), dental disease, myofascial pain, dermatitis, otitis, corneal ulcers, glaucoma, inflammatory bowel disease (IBD), pancreatitis, megacolon, constipation, FIC, neoplasia, post-op pain.

Non-Pharmaceutical Therapies

Environmental enrichment, regular (voluntary ± coaxed) activity, massage, acupuncture, extracorporeal shock wave therapy, cold therapy, and electrical nerve stimulation are adjunctive treatments for acute and chronic pain.[1,3,7]

Additionally, the emerging treatment of feline-specific monoclonal anti-nerve growth factor antibodies has been reported to address the neuropathic component of OA and relieve the pressure of daily medication administration with subcutaneous injections once every four to six weeks in pilot studies.[8,9]

---

a Gabapentin is particularly helpful in cases of neuropathic pain, as it can be used long-term to good effect.

Specific Drug Classes and Medications

The most common analgesics used in cats fall into the following drug classes: anticonvulsants, nonsteroidal anti-inflammatory drugs (NSAIDS), N-methyl-D-aspartate (NMDA) receptor antagonists, opioids, and tricyclic antidepressants. Each class has different indications, durations of effect, and contraindications.

Medications and Doses

Class: Anticonvulsants

Medications in Class

Gabapentin is the only medication in this class commonly used for behavior or pain therapy in cats. Gabapentin is structurally similar to γ-aminobutyric acid (GABA), but is not active at GABA receptors. Instead, it appears to reduce glutamate release in the amygdala. Since glutamate is, in part, responsible for fear responses, these are lessened.[10]

Indications

Gabapentin is commonly used to treat neuropathic pain. In addition, it is effective in treating anxiety and other problematic "behavior" conditions, like panic, stereotypical behaviors, and compulsive behaviors. It is a good choice as a pre-visit medication for veterinary visits.

Common Side Effects

Relatively few side effects have been reported for gabapentin in cats. A dose-dependent sedation and ataxia appear to be most common.[7] Abrupt discontinuation after chronic administration reportedly may result in withdrawal and seizures.[11]

Contraindications and Drug Interactions

Do not give gabapentin to cats with severe renal or hepatic disease.

Supporting Research and Additional Discussions Affecting Use

In her 2017 research, Dr. Karen van Haaften found that cats given gabapentin given before a routine veterinary visits scored lower on stress scales and were more compliant for physical exams.[12]

In 2018, Dr. Katherine Pankratz reported that gabapentin calmed the fear responses in the treatment groups of 53 community cats that were trapped for desexing surgery. Limited sedation was observed, and the only reported side effect was hypersalivation.[13]

Class: Nonsteroidal Anti-inflammatory Drugs (NSAIDS)

NSAIDS inhibit cyclo-oxygenase (COX) enzymes, which facilitate the synthesis of prostanoids that participate in some forms of pain and inflammation. Thus, inhibiting either or both of the COX-1 and COX-2 enzymes should result in reduced pain and inflammation. NSAIDs are best used for the treatment of mild-to-moderate pain.

NSAIDs have been considered to be a challenging drug class to use in cats. "Adverse effects include gastrointestinal irritation, protein-losing enteropathy, and renal damage. However, NSAID-induced acute kidney injury in healthy cats receiving NSAIDs is a myth."[4]

According to Monteiro,[7] "They are widely used in the treatment of chronic pain in cats, and enough data exist to support long-term use in cats with OA. Particularly, meloxicam and robenacoxib have been shown to be safe when administered to cats with concomitant OA and stable chronic kidney disease."[7]

They do, however, have a lower safety margin than opioids, and are not reversible.[14]

Contraindications: Do not use in cats with gastrointestinal ulceration or bleeding, platelet dysfunction, or severe renal dysfunction, and avoid concurrent corticosteroid use.[14]

Medications in Class

Please note that, as of this writing, no NSAID medication is approved for long-term use in cats in the United States. Both meloxicam and Robenacoxib are approved for long-term use for musculoskeletal pain in cats in the United Kingdom and other European countries, as well as elsewhere in the world.[3]

Meloxicam. This is a COX-2 (preferential) NSAID. The injectable form is licensed in the United States for use in cats. The oral form is used frequently in cats with osteoarthritis, particularly in the United Kingdom,[15] but is not yet approved for cats in the United States.

Robenacoxib. This COX-2 (specific) NSAID is licensed for a 6-day course for acute pain in cats in the United Kingdom and a 3-day course in the United States. Chronic oral use is permitted in the European Union, per the European Medicines Agency.[16]

Carprofen. This NSAID is licensed in the United Kingdom. It is given as a single dose subcutaneously; repeat doses are not recommended.

Ketoprofen. This COX-1 inhibitor has been used for up to five days in cats to treat musculoskeletal pain.[14] Its use perioperatively is not recommended due to possible interference with platelet function.[14]

Indications

NSAIDs are useful for mild-to-moderate musculoskeletal pain, including osteoarthritis, and perioperative pain and inflammation from soft-tissue surgeries.[2,14] The method of administration and national permitting dictates which medications may be used to treat chronic pain.

Neuropathic pain is not responsive to NSAIDs.[17]

Common Side Effects

Possible side effects include loss of appetite, nausea, vomiting, lethargy or depression, diarrhea and/or hematochezia, icterus. These can be signs of toxicity, so advise clients not to take them lightly.[2]

Supporting Research and Additional Discussions Affecting Use[1]

Approximately 68% of cats with degenerative joint disease have some degree of chronic kidney disease, making the use of NSAIDs in this population controversial. Retrospective studies found no adverse effects on renal function (sequential serum creatinine concentration and USG) or longevity in cats with stable CKD (IRIS stages 1–3) receiving meloxicam at a median daily dose 0.02 mg/kg,[18] and no adverse effects were reported in cats with CKD (IRIS stages 1–2) given robenacoxib 1.0–2.4 mg/kg q24h for 28 days in a prospective study.[19] In contrast, a recent prospective study (meloxicam 0.02 mg/kg q24h for 6 months or placebo) in cats with CKD reported a higher urinary protein-creatinine ratio at 6 months in meloxicam-treated cats.[20]

Medications in Class
Ketamine, and to a lesser extent amantadine (the oral counterpart to ketamine), are the most commonly used NMDA receptor antagonists in feline pain management.

Indications
Ketamine blocks the effects of glutamate, therefore reducing central sensitization.[5] It has been used perioperatively at subanesthetic doses in combination with opioids to reduce postoperative pain.[5,14]

Amantadine exerts a pain modifying effect through blockade of spinal postsynaptic NMDA receptors,[21] which are involved in the process of central and peripheral sensitization and visceral pain.[22]

Common Side Effects
Little has been reported about the side effects of amantadine in cats. Ketamine is delivered typically as a CRI perioperatively; to our knowledge side effects have not been reported for this use.

Supporting Research and Additional Discussions Affecting Use
Mainly anecdotal reports of amantadine use, as well as concern that clinical assessment of the pain control provided by ketamine may be difficult.[14]

We found few toxicity, safety, efficacy, or dose titration studies for amantadine in cats.[3]

Medications in Class
Opioid drugs bind to receptors in both the central and peripheral nervous system. They decrease the release of excitatory neurotransmitters, activate inhibitory pathways, and alter the postsynaptic cell membrane resulting in analgesia.

The most commonly used opioid medications for acute pain management in cats include morphine, hydromorphone, methadone, fentanyl, and buprenorphine. Long-term use of oral opioids is not recommended for chronic pain control.[3]

Indications
The full μ-agonist opioids are suitable for the management of moderate-to-severe pain associated with surgeries and visceral pain due to inflammatory conditions (such as pancreatitis). Partial μ-agonist opioids are best for mild-to-moderate pain, such as that associated with osteoarthritis, castration or ovariohysterectomy, and invasive imaging. Mixed μ-agonist/antagonist opioids are best for mild pain or the facilitation of venipuncture, cystocentesis, and the collection of other laboratory samples and examinations.[2]

Common Side Effects
Morphine, hydromorphone: Nausea and vomiting are the most common side effects.

"Tricyclic Antidepressants (TCAs) are a complex drug class, with serotoninergic, noradrenergic, antihistamine, anticholinergic, antimuscarinic, NMDA receptor antagonistic, and sodium channel blocking actions."[17]

Medications in Class
While there are other medications in this class, amitriptyline is the tricyclic antidepressant most commonly used for pain management in cats.

Indications
In humans, amitriptyline (and, occasionally other tricyclic antidepressants) is used in the treatment of neuropathic pain.

Mechanism of Action
Per Epstein 2020, "clinical improvement is attributed to antisensitization and pain modification."[17]

Common Side Effects
Sedation and weight gain are the most commonly observed side effects.[7,23]

Supporting Research and Additional Discussions Affecting Use
A 1998 study investigated amitriptyline treatment for severe recurrent idiopathic cystitis in cats.[23] Each cat received 10 mg of amitriptyline, PO, every 24 hours in the evening for 12 months, or until lower urinary tract signs recurred. During the first 6 months of treatment, 11 of the 15 cats had no owner-observed lower urinary tract signs, and during the next 6 months, 9 of 15 cats remained free of signs. Unfortunately, no placebo or usual care control was included in this study, and subsequent studies have demonstrated that the placebo effect in cats with FIC can be large.[24,25]

Drug Dose Chart Adapted from[4,5,7,12,15,26,27]

Class	Drug	Dose/Route	Important information
Anticonvulsants	Gabapentin	5–10 mg/kg PRN or q8–12 hours	Also shown to reduce fear and anxiety.
Non-steroidal anti-inflammatory drug	Meloxicam, 5 mg/ml injectable	0.3 mg/kg SC ONCE	Approved dose in the United States.
	Meloxicam, 2 mg/ml injectable	0.2 mg/kg SC once, then 0.05 mg/kg PO q 24 h x 4 days	
	Meloxicam, 0.5 mg/ml oral	0.1 mg/kg PO once then 0.05 mg/kg PO q 24 h thereafter	Titrate to lowest effective dose if used chronically. Avoid higher dose in cats with renal disease. Approved in the European Union but not the United States.
	Carprofen	1–4 mg/kg SC ONCE	
	Robenacoxib, 20 mg/ml	2 mg/kg SC q 24 h up to 3 days	
	Robenacoxib, 6 mg tablets	1 mg/kg PO q 24 h up to 6 days	Best for acute pain.
	Ketoprofen, 10 mg/ml	2 mg/kg SC q 24 h up to 3 days	
	Ketoprofen, 5 mg tablets	1 mg/kg PO q 24 h up to 5 days	Best for acute musculoskeletal pain.

(Continued)

(Continued)

Class	Drug	Dose/Route	Important information
NMDA receptor antagonists	Amantadine	3–5 mg/kg PO q 12–24 h	Best in combination with other analgesics
Tricyclic antidepressants	Amitriptyline	1–2 mg/kg PO q 12–24 h	
Full μ-agonist opioids	Fentanyl	5 μg/kg bolus with 3–20 μg/kg/h IV. Available in a patch	Duration: duration of the infusion
	Hydromorphone	0.025–0.1 mg/kg IV/IM	Duration: 2–6 hours. May induce nausea/vomiting. Higher doses may induce hyperthermia.
	Methadone	0.2–0.6 mg/kg IV/IM/oral (transmucosal)	Duration: 6 hours. Give lower doses IV and higher transmucosally. Less likely to induce nausea.
	Morphine	0.05–0.2 mg/kg IV/IM/epidural	Duration: 3–6 h IV/IM, 24 h epidural. Give slowly IV. May induce nausea/vomiting.
Partial μ-Agonist Opioids	Buprenorphine (0.3 mg/ml concentration)	0.01–0.04 mg/kg IV/IM/Oral (transmucosal)	Duration: 8 hours. Do not give SC.
	Buprenorphine (1.8 mg/ml concentration)	0.24 mg SC	Duration: up to 24 hours. Simbadol brand licensed for use in cats in the US
Mixed μ-receptor agonist/ antagonist	Butorphanol	0.2–0.4 mg/kg IV/IM/SC	Duration 1–2 hours.

Nerve blocks are not covered in this appendix.

References

1 Ray M, Carney HC, Boynton B, et al. AAFP feline senior care guidelines. *JFMS*. 2021;23:613–638.
2 Steagall PV, Robertson S, Simon B, et al. ISFM consensus guidelines on the management of acute pain in cats. *JFMS*. 2022;24:4–30.
3 Gruen ME, Lascelles BDX, Colleran E, et al. AAHA pain management guidelines for dogs and cats. *J Am Anim Hosp Assoc*. 2022;58:55–76.
4 Steagall PV. Analgesia: What makes cats different/challenging and what is critical for cats? *Vet Clin: Small Anim Pract*. 2020;50:749–767.
5 Lamont LA. Feline perioperative pain management. *Vet Clin: Small Anim Pract*. 2002;32:747–763.
6 Lorenz ND, Comerford EJ, Iff I. Long-term use of gabapentin for musculoskeletal disease and trauma in three cats. *JFMS*. 2013;15:507–512.
7 Monteiro BP. Feline chronic pain and osteoarthritis. *The Vet\Clin North Am Small Anim Pract*. 2020;50(4):769–788.
8 Gruen ME, Myers JA, Lascelles BDX. Efficacy and safety of an anti-nerve growth factor antibody (frunevetmab) for the treatment of degenerative joint disease-associated chronic pain in cats: A multisite pilot field study. *Front Vet Sci*. 2021;8:610028.

9 Gruen M, Thomson A, Griffith E, et al. A feline-specific anti-nerve growth factor antibody improves mobility in cats with degenerative joint disease–associated pain: A pilot proof of concept study. *JVIM*. 2016;30:1138–1148.

10 Stahl SM. *Stahl's essential psychopharmacology: Neuroscientific basis and practical applications,* 4th ed. New York: Cambridge University Press; 2013.

11 KuKanich B. Outpatient oral analgesics in dogs and cats beyond nonsteroidal anti-inflammatory drugs: An evidence-based approach. *Vet Clin: Small Anim Pract*. 2013;43:1109–1125.

12 Van Haaften KA, Forsythe LRE, Stelow EA, et al. Effects of a single preappointment dose of gabapentin on signs of stress in cats during transportation and veterinary examination. *J Am Vet Med Assoc*. 2017;251:1175–1181.

13 Pankratz KE, Ferris KK, Griffith EH, et al. Use of single-dose oral gabapentin to attenuate fear responses in cage-trap confined community cats: A double-blind, placebo-controlled field trial. *JFMS*. 2018;20:535–543.

14 Robertson SA. Managing pain in feline patients. *Vet Clin North Am Small Anim Pract*. 2008;38:1267–1290, vi.

15 Bennett D, Zainal Ariffin SMb, Johnston P. Osteoarthritis in the cat: 2. How should it be managed and treated. *JFMS*. 2012;14:76–84.

16 Onsior (robenacoxib). In: European Medicines Agency; 2021.

17 Epstein ME. Feline neuropathic pain. *The Vet Clin North Am Small Anim Pract*. 2020;50(4):789–809.

18 Gowan RA, Baral RM, Lingard AE, et al. A retrospective analysis of the effects of meloxicam on the longevity of aged cats with and without overt chronic kidney disease. *JFMS*. 2012;14:876–881.

19 King JN, King S, Budsberg SC, et al. Clinical safety of robenacoxib in feline osteoarthritis: Results of a randomized, blinded, placebo-controlled clinical trial. *JFMS*. 2016;18:632–642.

20 KuKanich K, George C, Roush JK, et al. Effects of low-dose meloxicam in cats with chronic kidney disease. *JFMS*. 2021;23:138–148.

21 Banpied T, Clarke R, Johnson J. Amantadine. *J Neurosci*. 2005;25:3312–3322.

22 Petrenko AB, Yamakura T, Baba H, et al. The role of N-methyl-D-aspartate (NMDA) receptors in pain: A review. *Anesth & Analg*. 2003;97:1108–1116.

23 Chew D, Buffington C, Kendall M, et al. Amitriptyline treatment for severe recurrent idiopathic cystitis in cats. *J Am Vet Med Assoc*. 1998;213:1282–1286.

24 Chew DJ, Bartges JW, Adams LG, et al. Randomized, placebo-controlled clinical trial of pentosan polysulfate sodium for treatment of feline interstitial (idiopathic) cystitis In: 2009 ACVIM Forum. Montreal, Quebec: JVIM; 2009:674.

25 Delille M, Fröhlich L, Müller RS, et al. Efficacy of intravesical pentosan polysulfate sodium in cats with obstructive feline idiopathic cystitis. *JFMS*. 2016;18:492–500.

26 Crowell-Davis SL, Irimajiri M, de Souza Dantas LM. Anticonvulsants and mood stabilizers. In: Crowell-Davis SL, Murray TF and de Souza Dantas LM, eds. *Veterinary psychopharmacology*, 2nd ed. Hoboken, NJ: John Wiley & Sons; 2019:147–156.

27 Perrin C, Seksel K, Landsberg GM. Appendix: Drug dosage chart. *Vet Clin North Am Small Anim Pract*. 2014;44(3):629–632.

Index

Clinical Handbook of Feline Behavior Medicine, First Edition. Elizabeth Stelow.
© 2023 John Wiley & Sons, Inc. Published 2023 by John Wiley & Sons, Inc.
Companion Website: www.wiley.com/go/stelow/behavior

Multicat households   16, 17, 22, 24, 31, 33, 34, 40, 51,
 55, 59–60, 67, 71, 90, 91, 98, 174, 178, 188, 202
Multimodal environmental modification (MEMO)   50,
 119–121
Musculoskeletal pain   112–114, 292, 294